CORPUS LINGUISTICS FOR HEALTH COMMUNICATION

Corpus Linguistics for Health Communication provides an accessible and practical introduction to the use of corpus linguistics methods to analyse health-related language use across various contexts and genres. Offering a critical review of the field, discussion of extended case studies, and practical exercises based on spoken, written, and digital language data, this book:

- introduces the fields of health communication and corpus linguistics and critically reviews cutting-edge studies in the burgeoning area of corpus-based health communication;
- describes the processes involved in planning a corpus linguistics study of health communication, including designing and building a corpus, selecting tools, and implementing techniques of analysis;
- demonstrates how corpus linguistics methods can – and have – been applied to the study of spoken, written, and digital health communication, offering critical reflections and suggesting areas for future development.

Corpus Linguistics for Health Communication is essential reading for those working at the interface of corpus linguistics and health communication. Both those with a little or a lot of experience in either field will find value in its pages.

Gavin Brookes is a Reader in Linguistics at Lancaster University, UK.

Luke Curtis Collins is a Senior Research Associate at Lancaster University, UK.

ROUTLEDGE CORPUS LINGUISTICS GUIDES

Series Editor: Anne O'Keeffe

Anne O'Keeffe is Professor in Applied Linguistics and Director of the Inter-Varietal Applied Corpus Studies (IVACS) Research Centre at Mary Immaculate College, University of Limerick, Ireland. She is co-editor of *The Routledge Handbook of Corpus Linguistics* and co-editor of the Routledge Applied Corpus Linguistics series.

Series Editor: Niall Curry

Niall Curry is Senior Lecturer in TESOL and Applied Linguistics at Manchester Metropolitan University, UK, at the Manchester Centre for Research in Linguistics and the Department of Languages, Information and Communications. He is co-editor of the Routledge Applied Corpus Linguistics series.

Series Co-Founder: Ronald Carter

Ronald Carter (1947–2018) was Research Professor of Modern English Language in the School of English at the University of Nottingham, UK. He was also the co-editor of the Routledge Applied Corpus Linguistics series, Routledge Introductions to Applied Linguistics series and Routledge English Language Introductions series.

Routledge Corpus Linguistics Guides provide accessible and practical introductions to using corpus linguistic methods in key sub-fields within linguistics. Corpus linguistics is one of the most dynamic and rapidly developing areas in the field of language studies, and use of corpora is an important part of modern linguistic research. Books in this series provide the ideal guide for students and researchers using corpus data for research and study in a variety of subject areas.

Other Titles in this Series

Corpus Linguistics for World Englishes
Claudia Lange and Sven Leuckert

Corpus Linguistics for Education
Pascual Pérez-Paredes

Corpus Linguistics for English for Academic Purposes
Vander Viana and Aisling O'Boyle

Corpus Linguistics for Writing Development
Philip Durrant

Corpus Linguistics for Health Communication
Gavin Brookes and Luke Curtis Collins

More information about this series can be found at www.routledge.com/series/RCLG

CORPUS LINGUISTICS FOR HEALTH COMMUNICATION

A Guide for Research

Gavin Brookes and Luke Curtis Collins

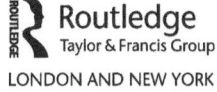
Routledge
Taylor & Francis Group

LONDON AND NEW YORK

First published 2024
by Routledge
4 Park Square, Milton Park, Abingdon, Oxon OX14 4RN

and by Routledge
605 Third Avenue, New York, NY 10158

Routledge is an imprint of the Taylor & Francis Group, an informa business

© 2024 Gavin Brookes and Luke Curtis Collins

British Library Cataloguing-in-Publication Data
A catalogue record for this book is available from the British Library

ISBN: 9780367568450 (hbk)
ISBN: 9780367568436 (pbk)
ISBN: 9781003099659 (ebk)

DOI: 10.4324/9781003099659

Typeset in Galliard
by Deanta Global Publishing Services, Chennai, India

CONTENTS

TABLES

ABBREVIATIONS

BNC1994	British National Corpus (1990s version)
BNC2014	British National Corpus (2010s version)
CA	Conversation analysis
CDA	Critical discourse analysis
EEBO	Early English Books Online
IEN	Internationally educated nurse
KD	Ketogenic diet
LIWC	Linguistic Inquiry Word Count
LMEMT	Corpus of Late Modern English Medical Texts
MIP	Metaphor identification procedure
NHS	National Health Service (UK)
NLP	Natural language processing
OSCE	Objective structured clinical examination
PrEP	Pre-exposure prophylaxis
SARS	Severe acute respiratory syndrome
THF	Teenage Health Freak
USAS	UCREL Semantic Analysis System
USN	United States nurse
WHO	World Health Organization

ACKNOWLEDGEMENTS

We would like to thank the series editors, Anne O'Keeffe and Niall Curry, for their supportive and insightful feedback on drafts of this book. We would also like to thank the former series editor, Mike McCarthy, for his enthusiasm and support during the proposal stage and the book's initial design.

The research underpinning Chapter 3 was carried out as part of the UK Research and Innovation (UKRI) funded project, 'Public Discourses of Dementia: Challenging Stigma and Promoting Personhood' (grant reference: MR/V022954/1).

1

INTRODUCING HEALTH COMMUNICATION AND CORPUS LINGUISTICS

1.1. Introduction

It is difficult to imagine an aspect of health and illness that does not involve language use. We use language to communicate our beliefs and experiences relating to our health, our bodies, and the illnesses that befall us. We are advised on how to maintain our health and how we can avert illness through language deployed in public health campaigns, which also implore us to monitor our health risks through language-based mediums such as fitness apps and DNA testing kits. If we become ill, we are likely to use language to communicate our pain and distress, initially to our relatives and friends, and then, in most cases, to a healthcare professional. That professional will, in turn, diagnose and (hopefully) treat our ailments using any number of tools or therapies which are likely to involve at least some element of language use and communication.

Linguists working within the field of health communication are interested in studying the language used in precisely these types of contexts, and plenty more besides, in order to better understand how such language use contributes to the creation, representation, and negotiation of health-related beliefs, practices, and experiences. Researchers interested in health communication, thus, have available to them infinitely vast amounts of language data for study. On the one hand, the wide availability of potential health-related language data can be viewed as a positive – opening up ever-widening possibilities for research and, with that, opportunities to continually extend and enrich our understanding of the relationship between language, health, and illness. Yet, on the other hand, we may also be daunted by the prospect of collecting and storing such large volumes of language data, let alone doing justice to it in our analysis.

DOI: 10.4324/9781003099659-1

In this book, we explore how methods from corpus linguistics can support the linguistic analysis of large volumes of health-related language data. Corpus linguistics is a field of linguistics research which offers a set of methods for analysing (typically) very large amounts of naturally occurring language use (McEnery and Wilson 2001; McEnery and Hardie 2012; Brookes and McEnery 2020). The word *corpus* is Latin for 'body'. A corpus is, therefore, a metaphorical 'body' of texts or language use that is designed to represent, at scale, how language is used in particular contexts. One of the main appeals of using large collections of data is that it allows the researcher to account for a wide range of variation in the type of language or texts being studied and, therefore, produce more generalisable findings based on more substantial and representative textual evidence. Corpora are, as noted, typically very large in size. Indeed, many of the corpora we will encounter throughout this book consist of many thousands of texts and amount to millions of words. For example, the 2014 update of the British National Corpus (BNC2014), which represents general British English language use, contains more than 100 million words of speech and writing collected in the United Kingdom (UK) between 2012 and 2016 (Love et al. 2017; Brezina et al. 2021).

The storage and analysis of large corpora such as the BNC2014 is made easier by advances in technology and data management. In modern corpus linguistics research, corpora are stored electronically and analysed using specialist software or, increasingly, computer programming (introduced in Chapter 3). With computational assistance, corpus linguistics methods allow information about the frequency and patterning of language in vast corpora to be obtained quickly and reliably. Such approaches can tell us, for example, how frequent particular words or chains of words are in a corpus, which words tend to co-occur together in a corpus with marked frequency, and which words occur with a markedly high frequency in one corpus when compared against another. These procedures, and many more, can be carried out with greater speed and accuracy than would be possible using a purely manual approach to linguistic analysis. Moreover, the relationships between linguistic phenomena can be subjected to complex statistical measurement.

Because, at this point, we risk presenting corpus linguistics as a solely quantitative analytical pursuit, it is important to point out that research in corpus linguistics routinely involves combining quantitative and qualitative perspectives on the language in a corpus. Indeed, as well as counting and quantifying, corpus analytical software tools provide, as we will see, relatively unique ways of visualising language data to bring new perspectives to qualitative analyses. Therefore, in addition to bringing practical benefit in terms of enabling rapid and reliable analysis of vast datasets of health-related language, corpus linguistics methods can also bring significant benefit to the analysis of such datasets, by enabling novel quantitative and qualitative perspectives on them.

Over the past 40 or so years, corpus linguistics approaches have risen to prominence in an ever-widening range of disciplines and professions which involve some element of linguistic or textual analysis. In this book, we will explore some of the ways in which corpus linguistics methods can support research in the field of health communication. This book sets out to demonstrate how the novel perspectives provided by corpus linguistics, hinted at above, can enhance existing approaches to health-related language. The aim of this book, therefore, is to demonstrate how corpus linguistics methods can contribute to – and, indeed, enhance – the study of health communication. This will be achieved through a series of thematically organised chapters that report on a mixture of existing and original studies in which researchers have applied corpus linguistics methods in the study of language taking place in a diverse range of health(care) contexts and in relation to an ever wider range of contemporary health and illness concerns. Over the course of the next six chapters, we will consider how to select or build a corpus, become familiar with the analytical techniques that we can use to subject corpora to quantitative and qualitative linguistic analyses, and then explore how such techniques can and have been applied to examine language in a wide range of spoken, written, and digital contexts of health communication.

The present chapter will lay the theoretical foundations for those to come. Following the brief introduction given above, Section 1.2 provides a more detailed introduction to the field of health communication. Section 1.3 then elaborates on the field of corpus linguistics, before Section 1.4 reviews the main benefits (and some limitations) of applying corpus linguistics methods to the study of health communication. Section 1.5 then concludes this opening chapter by providing a brief overview of the subsequent chapters in this book.

1.2 What is health communication?

As introduced briefly above, the term *health communication* broadly refers to all aspects and modes of communication that take place within medical contexts or which relate, in some way, to issues surrounding health and illness. The concept of health communication is, therefore, all-embracing, as it accounts for a vast and diverse range of communicative activities. This ranges from language taking place in so-called 'everyday' contexts, such as in conversations about health and illness over the dinner table or in online support groups and adverts for health products, to those which take place in more institutionalised domains, such as consultations with medical professionals and health policy documents. The study of health communication is a broad and often interdisciplinary field of enquiry that spans a variety of disciplines, including linguistics, anthropology, communication studies, ethics, psychology, sociology, medicine, and many more besides. In this book, we focus on health communication research which examines naturally occurring linguistic routines, in contrast with more theoretical approaches and research which seeks to describe what constitutes 'effective' health communication (see, for example, Berry 2006).

The concept of *discourse* has emerged as a central concern in the types of linguistic studies of health communication described above and, as such, is drawn upon across much of the research we present and discuss over the course of the coming chapters. *Discourse* is a rather nebulous term, and it can be difficult to define, as it is used in a variety of (often inconsistent) ways within and across disciplines. Over the past 50 or so years, the concept of discourse has been appropriated within a diverse range of disciplines all concerned with analysing language or text in some way. This, of course, includes linguistics but also disciplines such as cultural studies, history, literature, media studies, philosophy, and psychology, to give just a few examples (see Mills (1997) and Baker (2023) for an overview of conceptualisations of discourse). Gwyn (2002) helpfully identifies two broad and interrelated senses in which *discourse* has been utilised within studies of health communication: a micro sense and a macro sense. The micro sense refers to the lexico-grammatical choices that speakers or writers make in order to create meaning – that is, 'the particular means by which individuals express themselves in language' (ibid., p. 31). Meanwhile, the macro sense refers to more generic styles of representation – 'constrained ways of thinking and talking within a given sociocultural orbit' (ibid.; see also: Candlin et al. 1999; Gee 2010, p. 34). While the micro definition is likely to be most familiar to linguists, the macro definition orients broadly to poststructuralist approaches and might be more familiar to those working within disciplines such as cultural studies.

The distinction between micro and macro definitions of discourse was blurry when Gwyn provided his account and has become blurrier since. Many researching health communication, including Gwyn himself, and many of the studies introduced across the coming chapters, combine micro and macro approaches together in order to 'capture both the linguistic routines that constitute the discourse of particular healthcare contexts, as well as how such discourses both draw upon and reproduce societal understandings of, and attitudes toward, health, illness and the body' (Brookes et al. 2023, p. 553).

From a broadly poststructuralist perspective, then, discourse is viewed not as just *reflecting* but actively constructing 'entities and relations in social life' (Candlin et al. 1999, p. 323). Importantly, this includes entities and social relations surrounding health and illness. As Fox (1993), in an oft-cited passage, puts it,

> [I]llness cannot be just illness, for the simple reason that human culture is constituted in language [...] and that health and illness, being things which fundamentally concern humans, and hence need to be 'explained', enter

into language and are constituted in language, regardless of whether or not they have some independent reality in nature.

(Fox 1993, p. 6)

Lupton (2013) also articulates this point – perhaps in a way that makes the connection between health, illness, and discourse even clearer – by drawing on the example of how the discourses around mothers and foetuses can shape understandings, beliefs, and even experiences relating to pregnancy and childbirth.

[A]n integral and intertwined relationship exists between discourses – the way we speak or visually represent phenomena – and practices – the actions and activities surrounding these phenomena. For example, the ways in which the maternal body and the foetus are described, visually represented, and treated in western societies tend to make an explicit separation between woman and foetus which is not evident in some other cultures. Debates over abortion in popular and legal settings, accusations made against women for smoking or drinking alcohol while pregnant, the training of medical students in obstetrics and gynaecology, the use of ultrasound that represents the foetus as an image separate from the maternal body, colour photographs in books and popular science magazines that show the foetus in the womb, seemingly floating in space, the way that people speak of the foetus as having a potential gender and name before birth, all serve to reinforce this division between mother and foetus. Practices constitute and reinforce existing discourses, and vice versa.

(Lupton 2013, p. 14)

Gwyn (2002) also makes this argument and, in so doing, provides a glimpse at the kinds of contexts in which we are likely to encounter health discourses which we may then recycle in our own health-related interactions:

Illness is constructed, reproduced and perpetuated through language. We get to know about our own illnesses through the language of doctors and nurses, friends and relatives, and we often recycle the words picked up from our consultations in the doctor's surgery into conversation, sprinkling our stories of sickness with epithets that give the impression of a grander knowledge of medical science. When we open the newspapers or switch on the television or radio, we encounter an increasing variety of articles and programmes offering information, advice and warnings about every conceivable dimension of health and care of the body.

(Gwyn 2002, p. 13)

Discourse, including language use but also practices involving other modes of communication, can, therefore, be regarded as a central activity within healthcare that plays 'a significant role in constituting practices that take place within a range of medical settings' (Brookes et al. 2023, pp. 553–554). By way of demonstrating the centrality of discourse to health and illness, earlier in this chapter we considered some common discursive activities through which people's understandings and experiences of health and illness are constructed, mediated, and negotiated, including, *inter alia*, conversations over the dinner table, interactions within online support groups, and consultations with health professionals.

Indeed, the very nature of healthcare itself unavoidably involves communication between various participants. Sarangi (2004, p. 1) observes how the relationship between health professionals and patients is a primarily 'communicative' one. This is because, as Harvey and Adolphs (2012, p. 471) elaborate, '[c]ommunication is a central aspect of health and healthcare provision, especially, as Sarangi points out, in terms of how discourse produces a cause and effect, given that the professional causes the patient to adopt or modify certain behaviours'. Yet, over time, the discourses around health have become more complex, as they not only permeate an ever-expanding range of domains of social and institutional life, but they also reflect the ever more complex and technologised means through which our bodies and health are mediated. If we consider the various ways in which our experiences of our bodies are mediated through technology in the form of tests, scans, and medical records, then, as Jones (2015, p. 842) points out, 'the body as an object of medical knowledge has itself become more discursive, a collection of texts that are increasingly separated from the actual physical body of the patient'.

Importantly, from the blended micro and macro view of discourse that characterises much contemporary health communication research, the discourses identified within micro level (healthcare) contexts can be interpreted as being at once constitutive of and constituted by the macro level contexts in which they occur. Thus, the language used in documents and conversational turns that take place in a localised healthcare context is linked to the wider healthcare landscape (and sociocultural context). For example, Brookes and Harvey (2016a) and Chałupnik and Brookes (2021) demonstrate how the ongoing privatisation of UK healthcare services has been both reflected in and constituted by a rhetoric of 'deliverology' in UK healthcare providers' websites. Baker et al. (2019), in a corpus-based study of online patient feedback on UK healthcare services, demonstrated how some patients drew upon discourses of customer satisfaction to frame and legitimate the feedback they gave. In another example, Jones (2013, pp. 4–5) observed a connection between the increased emphasis on preventable diseases within industrial societies and discourses which position illnesses as outcomes of individual behaviours, arguing that 'health has become not just a matter of physical, mental and social well-being, but primarily a discursive exercise of constantly reproducing "health" in our daily lives as part of ongoing identity projects'.

A consequence of this refocusing of emphasis *away* from the eradication of disease and *towards* the maintenance of health is *medicalisation*, which refers to the process by which 'non-medical problems become defined and treated as medical problems, usually in terms of illnesses or disorders' (Conrad 1992, p. 209). Conrad (2007) and others have argued that society has become increasingly medicalised, with more and more aspects of life coming to be viewed as medical phenomena. Evidence for the influence of medicalisation in society is offered by health communication research which demonstrates of its effects both at the macro level, such as in pharmaceutical advertising (Harvey 2013b), and the micro level, for example, in interactions taking place in online support groups (Hunt and Brookes 2020). Analysis of health discourse taking place across different contexts can, therefore, help us to achieve a better understanding of the nature and, indeed, the effects of broad changes to social and health(care) landscapes and how these refract at the micro level, in terms of interactions taking place between individuals.

The discourses that surround health and illness at both the micro and macro level are numerous and variable and can relate to each other in complex ways; they are often contradictory, affording us with different ways to interpret, explain, and act in relation to our health (Gwyn 2002). Any single health topic can be surrounded by a plethora of discourses which can result in that thing being experienced and understood differently by individuals, depending on which discourses they are exposed/have access to and which ones resonate and gain 'traction' with them personally. This point is made by Brookes and Hunt (2021, p. 6), using ongoing anxiety and scepticism regarding vaccinations as an example:

> [W]hile it is the case that some discourses enjoy dominance over others within societies, individuals can engage with these dominant discourses in various ways, including by challenging them and by drawing on alternative ways of thinking and communicating about health.

Indeed, while discourses can produce effects, including those which constitute public health advice, the effects that are produced are not always predictable or, in fact, in the health interests of the populations they target (Koteyko 2014). This represents an important distinction between how discourse is understood by discourse analysts as compared to health educators and medical practitioners, who have

> [T]raditionally viewed the relationship between discourse and action in a rather straightforward way, assuming that discourse leads (or should lead) rather directly and unproblematically to some kind of desired action, and that the 'better' the discourse (in the form of information) the better the health outcomes. Unfortunately, time and time again in the area of health

we are confronted with situations in which the relationship between what is said, written, or otherwise communicated and what people actually do is complicated, indirect, or utterly contrary to what is expected.

(Jones 2015, p. 842)

It is these features of discourse, i.e., that it can shape our health-related knowledge, belief, and behaviours, but also that it can vary depending on the topics, individuals, and contexts involved that make discourse an important object of study for those interested in exploring the social realities of health.

The aim of any discourse analytical account of health communication is, thus, to not only describe the discourses that surround a particular health or illness topic, or which constitute communication and practice taking place within particular healthcare contexts (and increasingly beyond), but, importantly, it is also concerned with identifying the discourses that are brought to bear on health and illness by a range of social actors and institutions and unravelling the complexities and contradictions that these discourses might represent.

Contemporary health communication research can be situated against a backdrop of what has come to be known as the 'communicative turn' in medical practice. As Lupton (2013, p. 13) observes,

All areas of the humanities and social sciences have experienced a heightened interest in language and discourse over the past three decades or so. There has been an increasing preoccupation with recognizing and understanding the role of language in constituting and maintaining social order and notions of reality.

As part of this movement, researchers and healthcare practitioners have focused increasingly on patients' voices and perspectives (or put another way, their discourses) in a shared acknowledgement of the limitations of adopting purely, singularly biomedical perspectives on health and illness which prioritise technical and scientific understandings above what can be learned from patients' articulations of their lived experience of the given health or illness concern under focus. Relatedly, the 'narrative medicine' movement (see Greenhalgh and Hurwitz 1998) in clinical settings advocates approaches that focus on the discourses on which people draw to make sense of their embodied experiences, on the premise that this can lead to a better understanding of patients' subjective experiences of illness and, subsequently, improve treatment.

Research that is informed by the communicative and narrative turns, which 'prioritizes the role of discourse in patients' accounts of health and illness [by] exploring the discursive means by which people articulate and make sense of their condition' (Harvey and Adolphs 2012, p. 471), not only characterises the focus of much contemporary health communication research in general but also, as we will see throughout this book, health communication research taking a corpus-aided approach specifically.

In responding to the pervasiveness of health- and illness-related discourse throughout society, research on health communication engages with a wide and ever-expanding range of genres and modes. As Jones (2015, pp. 841–842) observes,

> Over the past several decades there has been considerable interest among discourse analysts in various aspects of health communication, including physician–patient interaction, the discourse of health promotion texts, the construction of health and risk in the media, and the discursive negotiation of health and risk in everyday life.

(For detailed discussions about the contexts and text types addressed in contemporary health communication research, see Brown et al. (2006), Harvey and Koteyko (2012), Jones (2013), and Demjén (2020).)

TASK 1.1

Take a few minutes to consider where and with whom you communicate about health and illness and encounter others' communication about health and illness. Then, consider the questions below:

- *Where* does this communication take place (i.e., in what kinds of situations and texts)?
- With *whom* does this communication occur (i.e., what individuals and institutions are involved)?
- Think of a particular health-related topic. If you were to plan a study looking at the language used to represent this topic, what kinds of texts might you want to consider in your study? Would you anticipate some kinds of texts being easier to collect than others?

The study of health communication has largely been dominated by investigations of interactions involving doctors and patients (e.g., Mishler 1984; ten Have 1995; Atkinson 1995). The interest in doctor–patient interactions, as the prototypical health exchange, has been maintained to this day. However, by the mid-1990s, the foci in health communication began to diversify, as health communication studies started to account for healthcare interactions involving other allied health professionals, such as nurses (Crawford et al. 1998), pharmacists (Pilnick 1999), and physiotherapists (Parry 2004). Beyond spoken interactions, written texts analysed within health communication research include genres such as medical note taking (Hobbs 2003), patient case notes (Heartfield 1996), patient information leaflets (Fage-Butler 2011), and healthcare provider websites (Brookes and Harvey 2016a). More recently, in response to the influence that digital technologies have had in facilitating and, indeed, shaping health-related discourses (Lupton 2017), researchers have explored the language utilised in online health communication environments, such as email interactions between patients and healthcare providers (Harvey 2012), health- and illness-related support groups (Stommel and Koole 2010), online feedback platforms (Baker et al. 2019), social media sites (Hunt 2015), and health apps (Thomas and Lupton 2016).

Research on health communication draws on a wide range of approaches, with those from within discourse analysis proving to be particularly popular (see Brookes and Hunt 2021). Much of this discourse-oriented health communication research has taken what Harvey and Adolphs (2012, p. 472) broadly describe as 'an applied linguistic perspective'. Applied linguistics is a broad and interdisciplinary field of intellectual inquiry and practice that is concerned with addressing 'real-world problems in which language is a central issue' (Brumfit 1995, p. 27). Demjén (2020, p. 2) argues that the focus of applied linguistics on the role of language in practical issues and decision-making

> makes it ideally suited for the investigation of healthcare contexts where language and communication can, when they work well, improve information-provision, self-esteem, support and even diagnosis and self-management but, when they work poorly, can also be a source of confusion, isolation, anxiety, stigma and even misdiagnosis.

Conversation analytical approaches have proven to be particularly useful for interrogating the linguistic routines that constitute healthcare interactions (see Barnes and van der Scheer 2021), as have approaches from interactional sociolinguistics (see Stubbe et al. 2021). Other established approaches that have proved effective in the study of spoken health communication, particularly healthcare encounters and interviews, include those from discursive psychology (Seymour-Smith 2015; Lamerichs 2021) and narrative analysis (Arribas-Ayllon 2021).

Approaches from within critical discourse analysis have also been used to examine the discourse of healthcare interactions, as exemplified by Fairclough's (1992) analysis of a doctor–patient interaction that was originally studied by Mishler (1984). Broadly, critical discourse analysis is an interdisciplinary field of research which offers approaches for integrating critical perspectives into discourse analysis with the emancipatory aim of identifying and challenging how discourse is used to create and sustain uneven power relations within society (Fairclough 2015). Critical discourse analytical approaches have been applied by researchers attempting to understand and critique power relations relating to health in a wide range of contexts both within and beyond health-care sites, such as public health policy documents (Brookes 2021), media representations of illness (Bilić and Georgaca 2007), and psychiatric nurses' notes (Galasiński and Ziółkowska 2021).

More recently, multimodal approaches to critical discourse analysis have been increasingly used to examine how issues relating to power and inequalities are produced and challenged through multimodal discourse (i.e., involving language but also modes other than language, such as imagery, layout, font, and sound). Multimodal approaches to critical discourse analysis have been used to interrogate representations of a variety of health-related topics across an ever-expanding range of text types, including, for example, health provider websites (Thompson 2012; Brookes and Harvey 2016a), health promotion material (Brookes et al. 2016), and health-related charity texts (Brookes et al. 2021).

In recent years, approaches to studying health communication have become even more diverse, with further approaches to discourse analysis proving popular for interrogating the language within a wider range of texts produced about health and in health(care) and illness contexts. Such emergent approaches include, for example, mediated discourse analysis (Jones 2013, 2015), discursive ethnography (Jones 2016; Ringer and Holen 2021), cognitive linguistic analysis (Knapton et al. 2021; Knapton and Rundblad 2014), and stylistic analysis (Hunt and Carter 2011; Demjén and Semino 2021).

The approach to analysing health communication that is taken is likely to have a strong bearing on the view of discourse that we take. For example, the macro view of discourse identified by Gwyn (2002) described earlier can be associated closely with approaches that are influenced by poststructuralist thinking, such as critical discourse analysis, while the micro view of discourse is more characteristic of approaches which involve focusing more intently on the text than on context, such as conversation analysis. We might opt for a particular analytical approach because it suits the view of discourse that we have, or, alternatively, we might inherit the view of discourse we take from an analytical approach that we find appealing, or which suits the needs of our research and the type of data on which we are focusing (Brookes and Hunt 2021).

While the approaches discussed above have been presented separately, many studies of health communication involve combining different approaches to discourse in their analyses. For example, McHoul and Rapley (2001) note how approaches from conversation analysis and interactional sociolinguistics have been informed by principles from critical discourse analysis in studies in which researchers aim at not just describing but also actually critiquing and changing the practices that constitute healthcare interactions (e.g., Francis and Kramer-Dahl 2004). Similarly, Chałupnik and Atkins (2020) and Atkins and Chałupnik (2021) supplemented a conversation analytical approach with perspectives from pragmatics in order to examine the performance of leadership practices in emergency medicine training in the UK. Along with interdisciplinarity and theoretical eclecticism, much health communication research can, thus, be characterised as bringing together different methodological approaches in order to provide more nuanced and theoretically eclectic accounts of the communicative contexts under study. One area in which this methodological pluralism has been particularly productive is in corpus studies of health communication in which, as we will see over the course of the coming chapters, quantitative corpus linguistics techniques can supplement and, indeed, enhance the perspectives provided by the kinds of qualitative approaches described above.

1.3 What is corpus linguistics?

The definition of corpus linguistics given at the start of this chapter, while useful for understanding the field in broad terms, conceals the fact that the status and very conceptualisation of corpus linguistics continue to be the subject of lively debate within the field. The area of greatest contention perhaps concerns the distinction between 'corpus-driven' and 'corpus-based' linguistics, and whether corpus linguistics should be considered a theory or methodology. The field of corpus linguistics in the 'corpus-driven' sense involves using the corpus in an inductive way in order to form hypotheses about language, typically in reference to existing linguistic frameworks (e.g., Sinclair 2004). Proponents of this approach regard corpus linguistics as a theory with corpus enquiries revealing hitherto unknown features of language use, thus challenging the 'underlying assumptions behind many well-established theoretical positions' (Tognini Bonelli 2001, p. 48). The 'corpus-based' approach, on the other hand, involves using corpora in order to test or refine existing hypotheses about language taken from other sources. From this view, corpus linguistics is regarded less as a theory and more as a methodology for testing and refining existing descriptions of language (e.g., McEnery and Hardie 2012). However, McEnery et al. (2006) argue that the distinction is somewhat 'over-stated' and that these positions should be viewed as extremes. Indeed, most corpus linguists take a less extreme view, including McEnery et al. (2006, p. 8) who, while viewing corpus linguistics as a methodology and not a theory, also acknowledge its status as a 'new philosophical approach to language'. Today, corpus linguistics is generally regarded as a methodology, and 'corpus-based' is often used as an umbrella term for a range of corpus enquiries, including in much of the research we will explore over the course of the coming chapters. Recent years have also witnessed the emergence and increasing popularity of a sub-field known as corpus-assisted discourse studies (Partington et al. 2013). Research within this paradigm seeks to explore non-obvious meaning in corpora and embraces the use of wider sources beyond the corpus (e.g., dictionaries, historical records, and other texts) as a way of contextualising the discourse observed within it.

The object of analysis in corpus linguistics is the corpus (pl. *corpora*). Corpora are not, strictly speaking, randomly compiled collections of language (Leech 1992) but are carefully designed datasets which strive to represent a particular language or language variety. While definitions of a corpus vary somewhat, McEnery et al. (2006, p. 4) point out that there is an increasing consensus that a corpus should:

(1) Be machine-readable (i.e., rendered in a digital format so that it can be stored and analysed using a computer);
(2) Contain authentic language use (i.e., real-life speech and/or writing as opposed to researcher-invited examples);
(3) Be sampled (i.e., contain texts or parts of texts that have been selected according to principled criteria);
(4) Be representative (i.e., it should represent a clearly defined language or language variety).

Based on the above, then, we can consider a corpus to be a *machine-readable* collection of *authentic language use* that has been *sampled* so that it *represents* a language or language variety. We will now expand upon each of these points in more detail.

Storing corpora in an electronic, machine-readable format is important because doing so allows them to be analysed using a computer. Because corpora tend, as we have noted, to be very large, it is usually not possible or, at the very least, practical for researchers to analyse their corpora by hand and eye alone. With the help of computers and specialist analytical software (many of which are free to access and easy to use – see Chapter 3), the human analyst can carry out a range of analytical procedures that they would otherwise be unable to perform manually. These procedures allow us to perform a range of functions to help us to identify linguistic patterns and trends in the corpus. Such procedures, which are introduced in more detail in Chapter 3, include (but are not limited to) searching for every occurrence of a given word or combination of words; generating frequency information about words, chains of words, and grammatical types; performing statistical tests on those frequencies (i.e., to measure the significance or strength of relationships between phenomena); and presenting observed patterns in the corpus in ways that render them more amenable to manual analysis.

Another important feature of a corpus is that the language it contains should be authentic or 'naturally occurring'. In other words, corpora contain real language use – that is, language produced by humans in real-world contexts. The range of domains in which humans produce language is almost incomprehensively vast, and corpora can theoretically represent language produced in almost any mode (e.g., spoken, written, computer-mediated, and gestural communication) or genre (e.g., casual conversations, books, online message boards, television dialogues, etc.). A single corpus can also represent multiple languages, modes, and genres together. Whatever type of language use a corpus contains, a key consideration is its representativeness. At this point, we will address the final two key features of a corpus – that they are sampled and representative – together.

Biber (1993, p. 243) defines representativeness as the 'extent to which a sample includes the full range of variability in a population'. When designing a corpus, variability, as Biber terms it, can be considered both from situational and linguistic perspectives. For a corpus to be deemed representative of a target language or variety, it needs to contain texts or samples of texts which represent (i) the range of text types in that language or variety and (ii) the range of linguistic distributions in that language or variety (Biber 1993). The language or language variety that the corpus is intended to represent will, therefore, influence decisions relating to sampling – that is, what texts we include in our corpus and to what extent each variable of interest will be represented.

At this point, it is useful to consider the difference between general and specialised corpora. A general corpus is one that aims to be representative of an entire language or variety. An example of such a corpus is the aforementioned BNC2014, which contains approximately 100 million words of spoken and written British English (Love et al. 2017; Brezina et al. 2021). Such corpora tend to be extremely large (they are typically millions, and occasionally billions, of words in size) and are usually constructed over a long period of time by entire teams of researchers. General corpora can be used for a wide range of purposes. Specialised corpora, on the other hand, are designed to represent language as it is used in a more specific context. For example, a specialised corpus might represent just a single genre (e.g., just newspaper articles), time (e.g., just texts that were published in 2020), and/or place/language variety (e.g., just texts published in the UK). Specialised corpora tend to be constructed for specific research projects and are designed to help researchers to answer specific research questions. An example of such a resource is Harvey's (2012, 2013a) 1-million-word corpus of health advice-seeking emails sent by adolescents to UK health practitioners. As the studies discussed in the coming chapters demonstrate, both general and specialised corpora can provide insight into the language surrounding particular health-related topics, and, in many cases, specialised and general corpora are, in fact, used in conjunction with one another, with the general corpus acting as a 'benchmark' regarding what might be expected in general language use.

The theoretical and practical considerations attending to corpus design and construction are explored in more detail in Chapter 2 of this book. For now, it is sufficient to note that if a corpus is well-designed so that it offers a strong representation of the target language or language variety, then that corpus offers the distinct advantage that findings based on its contents can be generalised to the entire language or variety under study (Leech 1991).

It is difficult to overstate the impact that corpus linguistics has had on the study of language. It is certainly no exaggeration to state, as Leech (2000, p. 677) does, that the availability of large datasets and the tools with which to analyse them have 'revolutionised' how we can analyse and now even conceptualise language. Corpora have been utilised by researchers working in a wide range of areas of linguistics, including (but not limited to) contrastive linguistics (Johansson 2007; Curry 2023), discourse analysis (Baker 2023; Partington et al. 2013; Marchi and Taylor 2018), critical discourse analysis (Baker et al. 2008; Mautner 2015; Wright and Brookes 2019), language teaching and learning (O'Keeffe et al. 2007; Flowerdew 2012; Curry et al. 2022), semantics (Ensslin and Johnson 2006; Glynn and Robinson 2014; Stubbs 1995), pragmatics (Aijmer and Rühlemann 2014; Rühlemann 2018; Jucker 2022), sociolinguistics (Baker 2010; Friginal and Hardy 2013; Murphy 2010), historical linguistics (Leech et al. 2009; Jenset and McGillivray 2017; McEnery et al. 2022), theoretical linguistics (Xiao and McEnery 2004; Mahlberg 2005; Barlow 2011), literary linguistics (Semino and Short 2004; Mahlberg 2013; Mastropierro 2017), psycholinguistics (Ellis and Simpson-Vlach 2009; Ellis 2019; Gries and Wulff 2021), and translation studies (Baker 2004; Laviosa 2011; Hartwell and Kraif 2022).

In addition to their application within linguistics, corpus linguistics approaches have been applied to research in an ever-expanding range of other disciplines, too. To offer just a handful of examples, corpus linguistics has been applied in areas such as history (McEnery and Baker 2017), geography (Paterson and Gregory 2018), psychiatry (Lustig et al. 2021), and clinical psychology (Collins et al. 2022). Such disciplinary diversity is also evident in interdisciplinary corpus linguistics research, which brings together insights and theories from within linguistics with those from other disciplines (see Ancarno (2018) for a discussion of interdisciplinary corpus linguistics research).

Corpus linguistics has, then, had a profound influence on the study of language and text within the field of linguistics and increasingly beyond it. This book is about a relatively recent but burgeoning application of corpus linguistics: the study of health communication. Mirroring, to some extent, the evolution in the focus of health communication research in a general sense, early corpus studies of health communication were primarily based on spoken interactions involving patients and clinical staff. In one such study, Thomas and Wilson (1996) examined a 1.25-million-word corpus of such exchanges. Their objective was to show how 'computer content analysis' could overcome the 'shortcomings of straight quantitative analysis' and has 'the potential to provide results which are in some respects comparable to manual discourse analysis' (Thomas and Wilson 1996, p. 92). This study, while pioneering in the sense that it applied corpus linguistics techniques to the analysis of health-related communication, was largely quantitative in focus and paid little attention to how the observed linguistic features actually functioned in dialogic contexts.

This kind of focus, however, was adopted by Skelton and colleagues who, in a series of studies, combined quantitative corpus analysis with a more qualitative approach in order to explore a range of linguistic features of primary care consultations involving doctors and patients (Skelton and Hobbs 1999a, 1999b; Skelton et al. 1999, 2002). These researchers assembled a corpus of 373 consultations involving 40 doctors based in practices in the UK. Their studies utilised information about the frequency of words and the co-occurrence of word pairings (known as 'collocation', introduced in Chapter 3) as means of identifying the occurrence of features such as first-person pronouns, medical jargon, and metaphorical expressions, and then considered how these were distributed across the doctors' and the patients' talk in their corpus. Importantly, these researchers complemented such quantitative findings with qualitative explorations of how these features operated in the context of interaction. Another important feature of this collection of studies, as observed by Hunt (2021), is that their research aims were oriented to matters that were not just of linguistic interest but which had clear practical relevance to clinicians and medical educators. As he puts it,

> Rather than simply noting the preponderance of several linguistic features in general practice, Skelton and colleagues focus on the role of pronouns in a discourse of shared decision making, the function of mitigated directives to foster patient adherence, and the practitioners' use of vague expressions and discourse markers to reassure patients.
>
> *(Hunt 2021, p. 137)*

Much like the field of health communication in general, applications of corpus linguistics approaches to the study of health communication have expanded in focus over time. For example, while the interest in analysing corpora of spoken healthcare interactions initiated by the likes of Thomas and Wilson (1996) and Skelton and colleagues has been maintained, corpus studies of spoken health communication have also begun to consider the interactional routines of an ever-expanding range of clinical professionals, such as nurses (Staples 2015) and specialists working to treat hearing impairment (Collins 2015). Moreover, the mediums and genres of spoken health communication represented and analysed in corpora have also expanded to include, for example, telemedicine (Adolphs et al. 2004), focus groups (Hunt 2021), and interviews (Collins et al. 2022), to give just a few examples. We will take a closer look at these and many other corpus studies of spoken health communication in Chapter 4.

The focus of corpus studies of health communication has expanded not only in terms of its focus on spoken health communication but has also been applied to other modes of interaction; namely, written and computer-mediated communication. Again, this is another way in which the expansion of corpus studies of health communication mirrors the expansion of the field of health communication in general. As we will see in Chapter 5, in which we explore corpus studies of written health communication, such studies have contributed particularly to the ongoing widening of the lens of health communication research to capture contexts *away from* medical institutions, incorporating discourses produced by other institutions. For example, news media representation of health and illness has become a popular area of interest (Brookes and Baker 2021; Balfour 2020; Price 2022).

A substantial amount of contemporary corpus linguistics research into health communication addresses health-related language produced in computer-mediated interaction, and this is the focus of Chapter 6. As we will see in that chapter, the range of digital contexts of health-related interaction available for study, while presenting new ethical challenges for corpus linguists, has been particularly beneficial in terms of further widening the scope of (corpus linguistics) health communication research. This has enabled a focus not only on the digital discourse produced by medical institutions, such as in Chałupnik and Brookes's (2021) study of marketising discourse in UK health providers' websites and Baker et al. (2019) and Evans's (2021) studies which explored how healthcare providers respond to patients' feedback on health services, but has importantly facilitated large-scale investigations into the kinds of so-called 'layperson' discourses that ordinary people use to make sense of various health-related matters. Such studies have helped to shed new light on how individuals with first-hand, 'lived' experiences of a given illness discursively construct and negotiate their identities in relation to those illnesses. For example, various studies have noted the influence of medicalising discourses in the way that individuals articulate their experiences of mental illness online (e.g., Brookes 2018, 2020; Hunt and Brookes 2020), while Harvey and colleagues' corpus analyses of online adolescent health inquiries have highlighted some of the folk conceptualisations of health through which this group are liable to filter other (official) health messages (Harvey et al. 2007; Harvey 2012, 2013a; Mullany et al. 2015; Brookes and Harvey 2016b).

TASK 1.2

Thinking about what we have learnt about corpus linguistics so far, consider the following questions:

- What would you consider to be the main strengths of corpus linguistics approaches to language analysis?
- Do any potential limitations of corpus linguistics approaches come to mind, especially compared to more qualitative approaches to language analysis?
- Are any of the strengths of corpus linguistics approaches likely to be particularly appealing for the study of health communication (if so, why)? Likewise, might any of the limitations of these approaches be particularly concerning for health communication research?

Towards the end of this section, we have tried to summarise some of the main trends in corpus studies of health communication. This has been a necessarily brief summary but it is important in laying the groundwork for the rest of the book, as the forthcoming chapters explore in considerably more depth some of the ways in which corpus linguistics approaches can and have been applied to the analysis of health-related language in a range of spoken (Chapter 4), written (Chapter 5), and computer-mediated (Chapter 6) communicative settings. Before exploring these applications, in the next section we consider some of the main reasons why we might want to use a corpus to analyse health communication, before considering some of the limitations of corpus linguistics methods and how we might overcome these.

1.4 Why use a corpus to analyse health communication?

In the previous section, we considered how one of the defining features of a corpus is that it contains authentic language use and that corpus linguistics as a field of research is, thus, committed to analysing, and basing theories on, such real-life language use. In this sense, corpus linguistics is firmly rooted not only within the field of applied linguistics but also within empirical linguistics research more generally (as opposed to forms of analysis that rely on researcher intuition and invented examples). There are, as Baker (2010, p. 94) points out, 'sound theoretical justifications for this approach: humans do not always make accurate introspective judgements regarding language, instead relying on cognitive and social biases'. Furthermore, corpus data can also reveal patterns in language use that might be unexpected or which otherwise run counter to our intuition (Sinclair 2003).

Of course, by this we do not mean to undermine the value of human intuition to (corpus) linguistic analyses. In fact, our intuitions about language can be useful when making sense of the linguistic patterns we observe in a corpus. As Hunston (2002, p. 22) puts it, '[a]lthough an over-reliance on intuition can be criticised, it would be incorrect to argue that intuition is not important. Indeed, it is an essential tool for extrapolating important generalisations from a mass of specific information in a corpus'. While intuitions can, therefore, play a role in corpus analysis, one of the most appealing features of a corpus is that the authentic language use it contains provides evidence with which hypotheses about language use can be generated, tested and, if needs be, confirmed, rejected, or refined. Thus, McEnery et al. (2006, p. 7) argue that '[t]he key to using corpus data is to find the balance between the use of corpus data and the use of one's intuition'.

Some researchers interested in investigating health communication have argued corpus linguistics approaches to be suitably aligned to the principles of evidence-based medicine (Adolphs et al. 2004; Crawford et al. 2014). This refers to the 'conscientious, explicit, judicious and reasonable use of modern, best evidence in making decisions about the care of individual patients. [Evidence-based medicine] integrates clinical experience and patient values with the best available research information' (Masic et al. 2008, p. 219; see also: Brown et al. 2006). This is because empirical corpus linguistics methods are able to support researchers working in the domain of health(care) by providing 'data driven' approaches to naturally occurring language use. It has also been argued that such corpus approaches may be able to contribute to professional healthcare practice. For example, in their corpus study of UK telephone healthcare consultations, Adolphs et al. (2004, p. 23) describe the power of corpus linguistics approaches to reveal 'recurrent features of healthcare communication over and above what we can find in models of good consultation practice which have been developed *a priori*'.

As well as the fact that they contain authentic language use, one of the main appeals of using corpora is that, if they are assembled in a careful way, they can offer greater representativeness of a language or variety of interest than, say, a single or handful of texts. As we have noted already, the benefit of analysing representative corpora is that they usually allow analysts to claim that their findings are more generalisable with respect to the type of language that is under investigation. Relatedly, large and representative corpora can also provide analysts with the means for identifying what is often referred to as the "incremental effect" of discourse – that is, the propensity for discourses to be subtly established through linguistic patterns that might feature sparingly in one or two texts but become significant when considered as part of a broader discourse type or collection of texts (see also: Baker 2023; Stubbs 1994).

Like the other advantages of corpus linguistics discussed in this section, the benefits associated with being able to look at vast and more representative amounts of language data, of course, apply to all areas of linguistics in which corpus linguistics approaches have been put to use. For the study of health communication, though, these benefits are particularly clear (if, as yet, somewhat under-utilised). As we discussed earlier in this chapter, health-related communication can take place not only in the clinic but in an almost incomprehensibly wide and diverse range of non-clinical settings too (see Jones 2013). This produces, as Hunt (2021, p. 133) points out, 'an incalculably huge volume of data for discourse analysts'. Yet, perhaps as a result of the previously discussed predominance of studies focusing on spoken healthcare encounters within the field of health communication research, studies in the area have tended to employ relatively small datasets and purely qualitative approaches to analyse these. Another reason for the strong preference for qualitative approaches among linguistic studies of health communication might be that researchers more accustomed to working within this qualitative paradigm might not know where to start in terms of beginning to sample some of this language use at any scale, and, if they do, they might be understandably daunted by the prospect of analysing a dataset comprising thousands of texts and millions of words (ibid.).

While the relatively small datasets that are commonplace in health communication research have enabled rich and detailed insights into the linguistic dynamics of health(care) communication across a range of contexts, the use of such limited data has been criticised for not providing findings that can be generalised to wider communication taking place within the particular domains under study. In response to this criticism, since the late 1990s an increasing number of researchers working in the area of health communication have advocated using, and, indeed, have themselves used, corpus linguistics approaches in order to study more widely representative datasets and obtain more generalisable findings about health-related language use in a variety of clinical and non-clinical contexts (e.g., Skelton et al. 1999a, 1999b; Adolphs et al. 2004; Crawford et al. 2014; Brookes et al. 2022; Hunt 2021).

As well as facilitating the analysis of vast bodies of language data, the computational assistance on which modern corpus linguistics rests can also bring other advantages to the analytical process. Some of these advantages are practical. For example, the analytical software underpinning corpus studies offers the practical advantage that they can perform frequency counts and complex statistical calculations considerably faster and more reliably than the human mind alone (McEnery et al. 2006). Indeed, with computational assistance, corpus linguists are able to quantify linguistic patterns which can help to understand the prevalence of particular linguistic features in a corpus, including what is frequent or infrequent or characteristic or uncharacteristic. For example, if we took a claim such as 'doctors ask more questions than patients in medical encounters', a corpus analysis can help us to confirm or reject such a hypothesis. Furthermore, we could explore, proportionally, how often doctors ask questions in their talk relative to patients, the types of questions they ask, and what similarities and differences can be observed with respect to the types or functions of questions in medical encounters as compared to other contexts of interaction. In addition to what is frequent or characteristic, large corpora also allow researchers to determine and find evidence for linguistic phenomena that might be rare or atypical in a particular context of language use.

The power to quantify and assess statistically the frequency of and relationships between linguistic phenomena in a corpus has been argued to be particularly advantageous to researchers working on health communication, who might find themselves working with or presenting their findings to others working within medicine and related disciplines (Brown et al. 2006). For example, Crawford and colleagues (2014, pp. 75–76) argue that

Dominated by a positivist, biomedical ambit, modern healthcare organizations and cultures of research and clinical practice have been largely closed to purely interpretive investigations. Funding agencies and review boards have tended to favour investigations planned in the manner of an experimental trial.

They contend that corpus linguistics approaches, in permitting statistical analyses of linguistic patterns across vast and representative language datasets, might offer something of a 'Trojan horse' to this mentality, enabling linguistics research that has clear implications for clinical and healthcare practice, as well as unlocking funding (hitherto largely inaccessible to linguists) in order to support such work.

Being guided by more objective criteria, such as frequency and statistical significance, analyses carried out using corpus linguistics approaches also bring the considerable advantage that they can help to reduce the influence of researcher bias on the analysis (Baker 2023). The increased objectivity afforded by corpus linguistics approaches is supported by an underlying commitment to methodological transparency, which is underpinned by two guiding principles: (i) no systematic bias in the selection of texts included in the corpus (i.e., do not exclude a text because it does not fit a pre-existing argument or theory) and (ii) total accountability (all data gathered must be accounted for) (McEnery and Hardie 2012). Abiding by these principles, users of corpus linguistics approaches can make their methodological choices and procedures more transparent, in the process helping them to overcome the accusation, often directed at discourse analysts – particularly those working in a critical way – that their analyses are based on convenient texts or examples that they have cherry-picked in order to support their own argument or theory (see, for example, Widdowson 2004). Again, the methodological transparency of corpus linguistics approaches has been viewed as being particularly attractive to those working in health communication. This is because, as Carter (2013, p. xiv) argues, as a series of approaches predicated on examining large amounts of authentic language data, corpus linguistics methods are able to provide the kind of substantial quantitative evidence that is accepted by the scientific, evidence-based world of medicine.

However, and importantly, it should be acknowledged that it is not possible for the influence of human bias to be removed from the corpus linguistics research process completely. Human researchers are, as we will see over the next two chapters in particular, required to make a number of important decisions over the course of any corpus linguistics study. These include, not least, those involved in selecting or designing a corpus as well as choosing which analytical techniques to use and what parameters will be employed. These are all decisions which will shape the findings produced in any corpus linguistics study. Moreover, the frequency and statistical output that corpus linguistics techniques provide are not ends in themselves. The computer can help us to identify and find evidence for patterns in a corpus, but it cannot explain why those patterns exist nor what their wider significance might be for the type of language use or context being examined. The human analyst must arrive at these explanations themselves.

When interpreting and explaining the quantitatively observed patterns in a corpus, it can be useful to supplement the aforementioned quantitative approaches with more qualitative analysis of linguistic features of interest in their original contexts of use (Baker 2023). In fact, such mixed-methods approaches, which combine (particularly quantitative) techniques within corpus linguistics with more qualitative approaches to linguistic – and particularly discourse – analysis are becoming increasingly standard in corpus research, not least in health communication research (Crawford et al. 2014). Typically, such studies begin by quantitatively surveying the patterns and trends in a corpus before following that up with qualitative interrogation of those patterns within their wider textual (and sometimes institutional and sociocultural) contexts of use, though many studies also employ a cyclical approach which involves oscillating between quantitative and qualitative perspectives on the corpus data (discussed in Chapter 3).

This productive synthesis of corpus linguistics with other forms of analysis demonstrates another strength of corpus linguistics approaches; namely, their versatility. Indeed, Hardie and McEnery (2010) observe the flexibility of corpus linguistics approaches when they point out that 'different theoretical frameworks may be used in explaining corpus observations, with whatever theory seems most appropriate to the task at hand' (2010, pp. 386–387). Hunt (2021, p. 139) argues that there are 'few limitations on the type of qualitative analysis that may be undertaken' as part of a corpus study and, furthermore, that an upshot of this flexibility is that corpus linguistics approaches to discourse are 'inherently interdisciplinary, with corpus methods working in conjunction with other discourse analytic approaches' (ibid.). These facets of corpus linguistics – that it is open to methodological pluralism, theoretically diverse, and interdisciplinary – are all, as we have seen, features that it shares in common with discourse-based approaches to health communication (ibid.). Crawford et al. (2014, p. 76) argue that in this way, corpus linguistics approaches are

> proving a subversion point to traditional, anti-intellectual hierarchies of knowledge formation which are strongly marked in health care, where randomized control trials have been seen as the 'gold standard' (Timmermans and Berg 2003) and more highly valued than qualitative or interpretive investigations.

They point out that, while qualitative approaches in medico-scientific research are often framed merely as 'laying the groundwork' for subsequent quantitative analysis, the use of corpus linguistics approaches in health communication research 'promotes a different frame – with quantitative research (computational analysis) acting as a diagnostic for richer qualitative investigation' (Crawford et al. 2014, p. 76; see also: Hunt and Brookes 2020).

1.5 What are the limitations of using corpus linguistics approaches to analyse health communication?

Our foregoing discussion does not mean to suggest that corpus linguistics approaches necessarily trump all other approaches to linguistic analysis. Indeed, like any methodology, corpus linguistics is not free of limitations, and it is important to acknowledge these and bear them in mind before embarking on a corpus study (and, indeed, throughout it). First, on a practical note, constructing corpora can be a time-consuming and resource-intensive process, as we will discuss in the next chapter. It also requires a number of careful decisions to be made, particularly during the design stage, and mistakes can be costly both in terms of time and resources. For these reasons, major corpus projects are typically carried out by large teams of researchers and with financial support from institutions or research grants. Of course, smaller, specialised corpora are generally much less costly to construct and, as such, do not require the efforts of entire teams; specialised corpora are often designed, assembled, and then analysed all by a small team or even a single researcher working alone.

Another limitation of corpora, and one that is more theoretical in nature, concerns what they have the power to represent. The conversion of collection of texts into a corpus is a transformative process, and the product of this process (i.e., the corpus) bears important differences from the original texts. Because corpora tend to contain written material or transcripts of spoken language, modes such as gesture (for example, in face-to-face communication), visuals (for example, images in newspaper texts), and sound (for example, in television or film texts) are more difficult to analyse using corpus linguistics approaches. As we will see in Chapter 2, representing such features of communication in a corpus is not impossible, though, at present, designing such corpora does present additional challenges to the relatively more straightforward compilation of corpora comprising spoken or written communication.

Another limitation related to the process of rendering texts into a corpus is that this process involves divorcing those texts from the social contexts in which they originally took place (see Widdowson 2000). This point is articulated particularly well by Hunt (2021) in relation to corpora representing health(care) communication specifically, when he writes,

The grouping of texts into a corpus can obfuscate important contextual factors from the original discourse. [...] [S]imply examining a concordance line containing a mitigated directive [(see Skelton and Hobbs 1999a,b)] obscures factors such as the patients' condition, the length and quality of their relationship with the doctor and the placement of that directive in a longer interactional sequence, all of which may help to elucidate the occurrence and function of the mitigation.

(Hunt 2021, p. 138)

Hunt (2021) also points out that the challenges posed by this detachment of the texts in a corpus from their original contexts are likely to be rendered more acute when dealing with a corpus that is compiled from hundreds or even thousands of individual texts, in which 'identifying salient aspects of their original contexts becomes prohibitively difficult' (p. 138).

Additional work is therefore required by the corpus compiler if they wish to retain contextual elements in their corpus design, for example by recording relevant contextual features at the time of data collection and representing these in the corpus through the use of annotation (discussed in Chapter 2). Through this process, some contextual metadata can be retained in a corpus which can aid the interpretation of observed linguistic patterns. For example, if we want to compile a corpus of clinical encounters between general practitioners (GPs) and their patients, as well as recording and transcribing interactions to put in our corpus, we may want to annotate or 'tag' those texts for information such as the identity variables of the interactants (e.g., age, sex, nationality, ethnicity, and so on) as well as information that might be relevant to the clinical context specifically (e.g., the reason for the patient's visit, the GP's years in service, and so on). As we will see in the next chapter, whether we annotate a corpus – and what kinds of information we include if we do – will depend on our specific research questions and what uses we intend or envisage for our corpus. Yet even if we carry out extensive annotation based on careful observation and recording made at the point of data collection, it is not possible to capture everything, and some aspects of the context will inevitably be lost from our corpus, not least those which might not be observable or accessible to us as researchers in the first place.

In addition to using annotation, corpus analysts can also integrate context into their analyses by drawing on extra-corpus theories and resources which can provide clues about the historical and sociopolitical contexts in which the texts in the corpus were originally situated. For example, in their study of historical representations of nationality-driven names for venereal disease in seventeenth-century England, McEnery and Baker (2022) coupled corpus data with theories and supporting data from beyond linguistics to gain a deeper insight into how the naming practices for the disease came about in that historical and sociocultural context. This allowed them to move from merely describing to interpreting and *explaining* such naming practices.

As well as the corpus itself, some of the limitations of corpus linguistics concern the analytical process. First, and perhaps foremost, people are often put off using corpus linguistics approaches in their research because they do not feel that they are sufficiently computer literate to operate the analytical software and/or sufficiently statistically literate to carry out and interpret statistical tests in their analyses. Although corpus linguistics approaches are often perceived as quantitative in nature, as we noted earlier in this chapter, input of the human analyst is essential and is required in every stage of a corpus project – from designing and collecting the data, to analysing that data and interpreting and reporting results. While it is the case that modern corpus linguistics relies on computer software as a way of storing and analysing the kinds of vast datasets that are now commonplace in the field, it is important to stress that many of the software tools currently available are relatively easy to learn how to use, through accompanying instructional documentation and videos that are designed for beginners. Furthermore, these tools can carry out statistical tests for users, sparing human analysts the task of performing complex equations. Nevertheless, it is important for human users to understand what the statistical tests measure and which ones they should use for their analyses. We will explore some of these considerations in Chapter 3 and advise on accessible resources which can help in understanding statistical measures and deciding on which ones to use.

A further limitation of analytical techniques in corpus linguistics is that they are best suited to identifying certain types of patterns but are less effective at identifying other phenomena. For example, words and chains of words can be identified and counted relatively unproblematically. This is also the case for identifying words and word combinations belonging to particular grammatical classes, and even semantic domains, provided that our corpus is annotated for this information. Yet other, more complex phenomena, such as pragmatic meaning (i.e., implied meaning) and metaphor, are difficult to identify automatically and will necessitate some qualitative, manual analysis by the researcher. Furthermore, in a more general sense, corpora and the techniques used to analyse them are also much better at telling us what linguistic features are present in the data than they are at telling us what is absent. Indeed, corpus users should be cognisant that most established analytical techniques in corpus linguistics will direct our focus to what is present in the corpus and that identifying absences will require additional work. In recent years, advances have been made in developing approaches to identifying these and other complex phenomena in corpora, including pragmatic features (Rühlemann 2018), metaphor (Demmen et al. 2015), and absence (Duguid and Partington 2018). While such advancements open up possibilities for some automated assistance, identifying such phenomena will inevitably require that considerable manual work be undertaken by the analyst.

Finally, while computers can be useful for identifying frequent and statistically interesting linguistic patterns in a vast corpus of texts, computers cannot interpret those patterns or tell us why they are significant or otherwise noteworthy. Therefore, it is up to the human analyst to dig deeper (and often wider – drawing on corpus-external sources) to make sense of and explain the significance of the linguistic patterns in their corpus. At this stage in the analysis, Harvey and Koteyko (2013) recommend supplementing quantitative analysis of health communication data with qualitative analysis of the texts in the corpus. They write,

> Identifying the occurrence rates of linguistic features is an effective means of revealing the properties of a text [...], but quantitative inquiries alone, which deprive linguistic data of context, are unlikely to be sufficient for providing an understanding of communication. Conducting qualitative analysis (that is, scrutinising linguistic features in their original context of use) in conjunction with quantitative analysis is able to provide robust and sensitive insights into communication.
>
> *(Harvey and Koteyko 2013, p. 197)*

As we have noted already, and will see in more depth over the course of the coming chapters, the majority of corpus studies of health communication effectively integrate qualitative and quantitative perspectives on their data, typically beginning with more quantitative techniques which are used to 'take the pulse' (Adolphs et al. 2004) of the corpus data before drilling down to interrogate frequent and statistically salient patterns with more qualitative, theoretically diverse approaches (Hunt 2021; Brookes et al. 2023).

The criticisms discussed in this section should not discourage the use of corpus linguistics approaches. All methodological approaches have shortcomings, and it is important that users of those approaches are aware of such limitations. With this in mind, then, it is important for users of corpus linguistics approaches to be cognisant of what corpus linguistics can and cannot do – where its strengths lie but also where its weaknesses are. Having this awareness is important for critically evaluating our own corpus research as well as that of others, and can provide the starting point for beginning to think about how such shortcomings might be at least mitigated or even overcome altogether when planning a project using corpus linguistics methods. In this spirit, we have, in this section, focused not only on raising awareness of the limitations of corpus linguistics approaches but also suggested some ways that these might be addressed. It is our view that the strengths of corpus linguistics certainly outweigh its weaknesses, and that many of these weaknesses can be overcome through the 'triangulation' of corpora with other sources of data and of corpus linguistics approaches with other forms of analysis. This is something that we will witness more in the coming chapters as we explore how corpus linguistics approaches can and have been used to inter-rogate health-related discourse across a range of contexts.

1.6 Chapter summary

In this chapter, we have introduced the core concepts and themes that are explored in this book; namely, health communication and corpus linguis-tics. The starting point for the broadly applied linguistic approach to health communication we have set out in this chapter, and which guides the case studies described in this book (as well as the majority of the wider research discussed across its pages), is the view that language is relevant to under-standing not only the ways in which we make sense of the social experience of health, but it is also of clear practical importance to health(care) profes-sionals who must communicate medical ideas on a regular basis. The field of health communication is thus characterised by research which examines the linguistic and discursive routines that constitute health and illness in a wide range of contexts, both within and beyond the clinic. The range of contexts in which health-related communication takes place is, as we have discussed, very broad indeed. This gives rise to an almost insurmountable amount of health language data being available to health communication researchers (Crawford et al. 2014).

In the second half of this chapter, we introduced corpus linguistics as a field of research which offers a set of methods for analysing large amounts of naturally occurring language data. We discussed its main strengths and limitations and suggested ways in which the latter might be mitigated or overcome. Most importantly, we argued that corpus linguistics can offer a useful methodology for exploring vast collections of health-related texts (i.e., corpora) which, if designed well, can provide a better representation of the broad range of contexts in which health-related communication takes place and, with that, the otherwise 'insurmountable' amounts of language data that such communicative contexts produce. This means that findings are more generalisable to the particular healthcare context or clinical group under study. We also considered arguments that, by affording the opportu-nity to examine large volumes of authentic language data, corpus linguistics approaches can also be said to go some way towards appeasing the commit-ment to more objective and empirical approaches to large datasets now com-monplace in the domain of evidence-based health communication research. This is an argument to which we will return in the concluding chapter of this book.

The central aim of this book is to develop the appeal for the use of corpus linguistics methods in the study of health communication in more detail, through demonstration of, and critical engagement with, the myr-iad ways in which corpus linguistics approaches can and have been applied in the study of health communication. With this central aim in mind, we will learn more about corpus linguistics approaches over the course of the coming chapters and, in particular, the next two chapters of this book. In Chapter 2, we consider the principles and practices underpinning corpus design and construction, and in Chapter 3 we familiarise ourselves with staple corpus techniques. We will then see these techniques in action in corpus studies of health communication research across Chapters 4 to 6, in which we both discuss existing research and report on more extensive case studies.

In line with the applied linguistic perspective set out earlier in this chapter, this book is concerned with research that analyses naturally occurring discourse that relates in some way to health and occurs across a range of clinical and non-clinical contexts. As noted, the book does not engage directly with research belonging to the more theoretical tradition of health communication research which seeks, for example, to establish what counts as effective communicative practice in healthcare settings. That said, much of the research described in this book belongs to the applied linguistics tradition as defined above and, as such, has an 'applied' agenda in terms of producing insights which are of practical relevance to those working within healthcare in some way or who otherwise seek to improve the effectiveness of their health-related communicative practices. Nevertheless, we envisage this book to be of primary benefit to those who either approach health communication from an applied linguistics per-spective, wishing to enrich their research by incorporating corpus linguis-tics methods into their analyses or, conversely, those who employ corpus linguistics methods routinely in their research who might be interested in extending their current applications to explore discourses around health and illness. As we hope is clear by this point, we have tried to write this book without assuming any prior knowledge of either corpus linguistics or health communication on the part of the reader. However, naturally, those with a background in either, or in applied linguistics and discourse analysis in a more general sense, may find it easier to navigate the pages of this book than those who are newcomers in the truest sense. We have pro-vided a series of reflective tasks and recommended further reading at the end of each chapter which we hope will help beginners to get to grips with the approaches and concepts introduced. At the same time, some of these tasks and suggested further reading will provide opportunities for more advanced readers to develop a more detailed understanding. Whatever your disciplinary background, we hope that you find the approaches, con-cepts, and studies introduced in this book as interesting as we do, and that in these you find the inspiration to carry out your own corpus linguistic explorations of health communication.

Further reading

- Harvey, K. & Koteyko, N. (2013). *Exploring health communication: Language in action*. Routledge. https://doi.org/10.4324/9780203096437

This book provides an accessible introduction to the field of health communication, written from an applied linguistic perspective. It also presents case studies applying corpus linguistics approaches to health communication data.

- Baker, P. (2023). *Using corpora in discourse analysis* (2nd edition). Bloomsbury.

This book, now in its second edition, provides an accessible demonstration of how corpus linguistics approaches can be used to analyse discourse occurring across a range of contexts. We particularly recommend Chapter 1 as a general introduction to the area.

- McEnery, T. & Hardie, A. (2012). *Corpus linguistics: Method, theory and practice*. Cambridge University Press. https://doi.org/10.1017/CBO9780511981395

This book provides a comprehensive introduction to corpus linguistics. It is written with more advanced readers in mind, so it is perhaps best suited for those wanting to learn more about critical debates in corpus linguistics. It is best read *following* the first chapter of Baker (2023).

References

Adolphs, S., Brown, B., Carter, R., Crawford, P. & Sahota, O. (2004). Applying corpus linguistics in a health care context. *Journal of Applied Linguistics, 1*(1), 9–28. http://dx.doi.org/10.1558/japl.1.9.55871

Aijmer, K. & Rühlemann, C. (Eds.). (2014). *Corpus pragmatics: A handbook*. Cambridge University Press. https://doi.org/10.1017/CBO9781139057493

Ancarno, C. (2018). Interdisciplinary approaches in corpus linguistics and CADS. In C. Taylor & A. Marchi (Eds.), *Corpus approaches to discourse: A critical review* (pp. 130–156). Routledge. https://doi.org/10.4324/9781315179346

Arribas-Ayllon, M. (2021). Narrative analysis: DNA testing and collaborative knowledge-building in a CFS/ME forum. In G. Brookes & D. Hunt (Eds.), *Analysing health communication: Discourse approaches* (pp. 81–110). Palgrave Macmillan. https://doi.org/10.1007/978-3-030-68184-5_4

Atkins, S. & Chałupnik, M. (2021). Pragmatics: Leadership and team communication in emergency medicine training. In G. Brookes & D. Hunt (Eds.), *Analysing health communication: Discourse approaches* (pp. 271–299). Palgrave Macmillan. https://doi.org/10.1007/978-3-030-68184-5

Atkinson, P. (1995). *Medical talk and medical work: The liturgy of the clinic*. Sage.

Baker, M. (2004). A corpus-based view of similarity and difference in translation. *International Journal of Corpus Linguistics*, *9*(2), 167–193. https://doi.org /10.1075/ijcl.9.2.02bak

Baker, P. (2010). Corpus methods in linguistics. In L. Litosseliti (Ed.), *Research methods in linguistics* (pp. 92–113). Continuum.

Baker, P. (2023). *Using corpora in discourse analysis* (second edition). Continuum.

Baker, P., Brookes, G. & Evans, C. (2019). *The language of patient feedback: A corpus linguistic study of online health communication*. Routledge. https://doi.org /10.4324/9780429259265

Baker, P., Gabrielatos, C., KhosraviNik, M., Krzyżanowski, M., McEnery, T. & Wodak, R. (2008). A useful methodological synergy? Combining critical discourse analysis and corpus linguistics to examine discourses of refugees and asylum seekers in the UK press. *Discourse & Society*, *19*(3), 273–306. https://doi.org/10.1177 /0957926508088962

Balfour, J. (2020). Representation of people with schizophrenia in the British press. In E. Friginal & J.A. Hardy (Eds.), *The Routledge handbook of corpus approaches to discourse analysis*. (pp. 537–553). Routledge. https://doi.org/10.4324/9780429259982-31

Barlow, M. (2011). Corpus linguistics and theoretical linguistics. *International Journal of Corpus Linguistics*, *16*(1), 3–44. https://doi.org/10.1075/ijcl.16.1.02bar

Barnes, R.K. & Van der Scheer, I.Z. (2021). Conversation Analysis: Questioning patients about prior self-treatment. In G. Brookes & D. Hunt (Eds.), *Analysing health communication: Discourse approaches* (pp. 19–48). Palgrave MacMillan. https://doi.org/10.1007/978-3-030-68184-5_2

Berry, D. (2006). *Health communication: Theory and practice*. Open University Press.

Biber, D. (1993). Representativeness in corpus design. *Literary and Linguistic Computing*, *8*(4), 243–257. https://doi.org/10.1093/llc/8.4.243

Bilić, B. & Georgaca, E. (2007). Representations of 'mental illness' in Serbian newspapers: A critical discourse analysis. *Qualitative Research in Psychology*, *4*(1–2), 167–186. https://doi.org/10.1080/14780880701473573

Brezina, V., Hawtin, A. & McEnery, T. (2021). The written British National Corpus 2014 – Design and comparability. *Text & Talk*, *41*(5–6), 595–615. https://doi.org /10.1515/text-2020-0052

Brookes, G. (2018). Insulin restriction, medicalisation and the Internet: A corpus-assisted study of diabulimia discourse in online support groups. *Communication & Medicine*, *15*(1), 14–27. https://doi.org/10.1558/cam.33067

Brookes, G. (2021). Empowering people to make healthier choices: A critical discourse analysis of the Tackling Obesity policy. *Qualitative Health Research*, *31*(12), 2211–2229. https://doi.org/10.1177/10497323211027536

Brookes, G., Atkins, S. & Harvey, K. (2022). Corpus linguistics and health communication: Using corpora to examine the representation of health and illness. In A. O'Keeffe & M. McCarthy (Eds.), *The Routledge handbook of corpus linguistics* (second edition, pp. 615–628). Routledge. https://doi.org/10.4324 /9780367076399-43

Brookes, G. & Baker, P. (2021). *Obesity in the news: Language and representation in the press*. Cambridge University Press. https://doi.org/10.1017/9781108864732.012

Brookes, G. & Harvey, K. (2016a). Opening up the NHS to market: Using multimodal critical discourse analysis to examine the ongoing corporatisation of health care communication. *Journal of Language and Politics*, *15*(3), 288–302. https://doi. org/10.1075/jlp.15.3.04bro

Brookes, G. & Harvey, K. (2016b). Examining the discourse of mental illness in a corpus of online advice-seeking messages. In L. Pickering, E. Friginal & S. Staples (Eds.), *Talking at work: Corpus-based explorations of workplace discourse* (pp. 209–234). Palgrave Macmillan. https://doi.org/10.1057/978-1-137-49616-4_9

Brookes, G., Harvey, K. & Adolphs, S. (2023). Discourse and health(care). In M. Handford & J.P. Gee (Eds.), *The Routledge handbook of discourse analysis* (second edition, pp. 553–567). Routledge. https://doi.org/10.4324/9781003035244-46

Brookes, G., Harvey, K. & Mullany, L. (2016). 'Off to the best start'? A multimodal critique of breast and formula feeding health promotional discourse. *Gender and Language*, *10*(3), 340–363. https://doi.org/10.1558/genl.v10i3.32035

Brookes, G. & Hunt, D. (2021). Discourse and health communication. In G. Brookes & D. Hunt (Eds.), *Analysing health communication: Discourse approaches* (pp. 1–17). Palgrave Macmillan. https://doi.org/10.1007/978-3-030-68184-5_1

Brookes, G. & McEnery, T. (2020). Corpus linguistics. In S. Adolphs & D. Knight (Eds.), *The Routledge handbook of English language and digital humanities* (pp. 378–404). Routledge. https://doi.org/10.4324/9781003031758

Brookes, G., Putland, E. & Harvey, K. (2021). Multimodality: Examining visual representations of dementia in public health discourse. In G. Brookes & D. Hunt (Eds.), *Analysing health communication: Discourse approaches* (pp. 241–269). Palgrave Macmillan. https://doi.org/10.1007/978-3-030-68184-5_10

Brown, B., Crawford, P. & Carter, R. (2006). *Evidence based health communication*. Open University Press.

Brumfit, C.J. (1995). Teacher professionalism and research. In G. Cook & B. Seidlhofer (Eds.), *Principle and practice in applied linguistics* (pp. 27–42). Oxford University Press.

Candlin, C., Maley, Y. & Sutch, H. (1999). Industrial instability and the discourse of enterprise bargaining. In S. Sarangi & C. Roberts (Eds.), *Talk, work and institutional order: Discourse in medical, mediation and management settings* (pp. 323–349). Mouton De Gruyter.

Carter, R. (2013). Foreword. In K. Harvey, *Investigating adolescent health communication: A corpus linguistics approach*. Bloomsbury. http://dx.doi.org/10.5040/9781472541970.ch-003

Chałupnik, M. & Atkins, S. (2020). 'Everyone happy with what their role is?': A pragmalinguistic evaluation of leadership practices in emergency medicine training. *Journal of Pragmatics*, *160*, 80–96. https://doi.org/10.1016/j.pragma.2020.02.014

Chałupnik, M. & Brookes, G. (2021). 'You said, we did': A corpus-based analysis of marketising discourse in healthcare websites. *Text & Talk*, *41*(5–6), 643–666. https://doi.org/10.1515/text-2020-0038

Charteris-Black, J. & Seale, C. (2010). *Gender and the language of illness*. Palgrave Macmillan. https://doi.org/10.1057/9780230281660

Collins, L.C. (2015). *Language, Corpus and Empowerment: Applications to deaf education, healthcare and online discourses*. Routledge.

Collins, L.C., Brezina, V., Demjén, Z. Semino, E. & Woods, A. (2022). Corpus linguistics and clinical psychology: Investigating personification in first-person accounts of voice-hearing. *International Journal of Corpus Linguistics*, *28*(1), 28–59. https://doi.org/10.1075/ijcl.21019.col

Conrad, P. (1992). Medicalization and social control. *Annual Review of Sociology*, *18*, 209–232. http://www.jstor.org/stable/2083452

Conrad, P. (2007). *The medicalization of society: On the transformation of health Conditions into treatable disorders.* The Johns Hopkins University Press.

Crawford, P., Brown, B. & Harvey, K. (2014). Corpus linguistics and evidence-based health communication. In H.E. Hamilton & W.S. Chou (Eds.), *The Routledge handbook of language and health communication* (pp. 75–90). Routledge. https://doi.org/10.4324/9781315856971

Crawford, P., Brown, B. & Nolan, P. (1998). *Communicating care: The language of nursing.* Stanley Thornes.

Curry, N. (2023). Question illocutionary force indicating devices in academic writing: A corpus-pragmatic and contrastive approach to identifying and analysing direct and indirect questions in English, French, and Spanish. *International Journal of Corpus Linguistics, 28*(1), 91–119. https://doi.org/10.1075/ijcl.20065.cur

Curry, N., Love, R. & Goodman, O. (2022). Adverbs on the move: Investigating publisher application of corpus research on recent language change to ELT. *Corpora, 17*(1), 1–38. https://dx.doi.org/10.3366/cor.2022.0233

Demjén, Z. (Ed.). (2020). *Applying linguistics in illness and healthcare contexts.* Bloomsbury. http://dx.doi.org/10.5040/9781350057685

Demjén, Z. & Semino, E. (2021). Stylistics: Mind style in an autobiographical account of schizophrenia. In G. Brookes & D. Hunt (Eds.), *Analysing health communication: Discourse approaches* (pp. 333–356). Palgrave Macmillan. https://doi.org/10.1007/978-3-030-68184-5_13

Demmen, J., Semino, E., Demjén, Z., Koller, V., Hardie, A., Rayson, P. & Payne, S. (2015). A computer-assisted study of the use of Violence metaphors for cancer and end of life by patients, family carers and health professionals. *International Journal of Corpus Linguistics, 20*(2), 205–231. https://doi.org/10.1075/ijcl.20.2.03dem

Duguid, A. & Partington, A. (2018). ABSENCE: You don't know what you're missing. Or do you? In A. Marchi & C. Taylor (Eds.), *Corpus approaches to discourse: A critical review* (pp. 38–59). Routledge. https://doi.org/10.4324/9781315179346

Ellis, N.C. (2019). Usage-based theories of Construction Grammar: Triangulating corpus linguistics and psycholinguistics. In J. Egbert & P. Baker (Eds.), *Using corpus methods to triangulate linguistic analysis* (pp. 239–267). Routledge. https://doi.org/10.4324/9781315112466

Ellis, N.C. & Simpson-Vlach, R. (2009). Formulaic language in native speakers: Triangulating psycholinguistics, corpus linguistics, and education. *Corpus Linguistics and Linguistic Theory, 5*(1), 61–78. https://doi.org/10.1515/CLLT.2009.003

Ensslin, A. & Johnson, S. (2006). Language in the news: Investigating representations of 'Englishness' using WordSmith Tools. *Corpora, 1*(2), 153–185. https://doi.org/10.3366/cor.2006.1.2.153

Evans, C. (2021). A corpus-assisted discourse analysis of NHS responses to online patient feedback. Doctoral Thesis. Lancaster University. https://doi.org/10.17635/lancaster/thesis/1276.

Fage-Butler, A.M. (2011). The discursive construction of risk and trust in patient information Leaflets. *HERMES - Journal of Language and Communication in Business, 24*(46), 61–73. https://doi.org/10.7146/hjlcb.v24i46.97368

Fairclough, N. (1992). *Discourse and social change.* Cambridge: Polity Press.

Fairclough, N. (2015). *Language and power* (third edition). Routledge.

Flowerdew, L. (2012). *Corpora and language education.* Palgrave Macmillan.

Fox, N. (1993). *Postmodernism, sociology and health.* Open University Press.

Francis, G. & Kramer-Dahl, A. (2004). Grammar in the construction of medical case histories. In C. Coffin, A. Hewings & K. O'Halloran (Eds.), *Applying English grammar: Functional and corpus approaches* (pp. 172–196). Arnold. https://doi.org/10.4324/9780203783801

Friginal, E., & Hardy, J. (Eds.). (2013). *Corpus-based sociolinguistics: A guide for students*. Routledge. https://doi.org/10.4324/9780203114827

Galasiński, D., & Ziółkowska, J. (2021). Critical discourse studies: Mad, bad or nuisance? Discursive constructions of detained patients in Polish nursing notes. In G. Brookes & D. Hunt (Eds.), *Analysing health communication: Discourse approaches* (pp. 215–239). Palgrave Macmillan. https://doi.org/10.1007/978-3-030-68184-5

Gee, J.P. (2010). *An introduction to discourse analysis: Theory and method* (third edition). Routledge. https://doi.org/10.4324/9780203847886

Glynn, D. & Robinson, J.A. (Eds.). (2014). *Corpus methods for semantics: Quantitative studies in polysemy and synonymy*. John Benjamins. https://doi.org/10.1075/hcp.43

Greenhalgh, T., & Hurwitz, B. (Eds.). (1998). *Narrative based medicine: Dialogue and discourse in clinical practice*. BMJ Books.

Gries, S. & Wulff, S. (2021). Examining individual variation in learner production data: A few programmatic pointers for corpus-based analyses using the example of adverbial clause ordering. *Applied Psycholinguistics, 42*(2), 279–299. https://doi.org/10.1017/S014271642000048X

Gwyn, R. (2002). *Communicating health and illness*. Sage. https://doi.org/10.4135/9781446219553

Hardie, A., & McEnery, T. (2010). On two traditions in corpus linguistics, and what they have in common. *International Journal of Corpus Linguistics, 15*(3), 384–394. https://doi.org/10.1075/ijcl.15.3.09har

Hartwell, L.M. & Kraif, O. (2022). Parallel corpora in English language teaching. In R. Jablonkai & E. Csomay (Eds.), *The Routledge handbook of corpora and English language teaching and learning* (pp. 578–594). Routledge. https://doi.org/10.4324/9781003002901

Harvey, K. (2012). Disclosures of depression: Using corpus linguistic methods to examine young people's online health concerns. *International Journal of Corpus Linguistics, 17*(3), 349–379. https://doi.org/10.1075/ijcl.17.3.03har

Harvey, K. (2013a). *Investigating adolescent health communication: A corpus linguistics approach*. Bloomsbury. http://dx.doi.org/10.5040/9781472541970.ch-003

Harvey, K. (2013b). Medicalisation, pharmaceutical promotion and the internet: A critical multimodal discourse analysis of hair loss websites. *Social Semiotics, 23*(5), 691–714. https://doi.org/10.1080/10350330.2013.777596

Harvey, K. & Adolphs, S. (2012). Discourse and healthcare. In M. Handford & J. P. Gee (Eds.), *The Routledge handbook of discourse analysis* (pp. 470–481). Routledge. https://doi.org/10.4324/9780203809068

Harvey, K. Brown, B., Crawford, P., Macfarlane, A. & McPherson, A. (2007). 'Am I normal?' Teenagers, sexual health and the internet. *Social Science & Medicine, 65*, 771–781. https://doi.org/10.1016/j.socscimed.2007.04.005

Harvey, K. & Koteyko, N. (2012). *Exploring health communication: Language in action*. https://doi.org/10.4324/9780203096437

Heartfield, M. (1996). Nursing documentation and nursing practice: A discourse analysis. *Journal of Advanced Nursing, 24*(1), 98–103. https://doi.org/10.1046/j.1365-2648.1996.15113.x

Hobbs, P. (2003). The use of evidentiality in physicians' progress notes. *Discourse Studies, 5*(4), 451–478. https://doi.org/10.1177/14614456030054001

Hunston, S. (2002). *Corpora in applied linguistics.* Cambridge University Press.

Hunt, D. (2015). The many faces of diabetes: A critical multimodal analysis of diabetes pages on Facebook. *Language & Communication, 43,* 72–86. https://doi.org/10.1016/j.langcom.2015.05.003

Hunt, D. (2021). Corpus linguistics: Examining tensions in general practitioners' views about diagnosing and treating depression. In G. Brookes & D. Hunt (Eds.), *Analysing health communication: Discourse approaches* (pp. 133–160). Palgrave Macmillan. https://doi.org/10.1007/978-3-030-68184-5_6

Hunt, D. & Brookes, G. (2020). *Corpus, discourse and mental health.* Bloomsbury.

Hunt, D. & Carter, R. (2011). Seeing through The Bell Jar: Investigating linguistic patterns of psychological disorder. *Journal of Medical Humanities, 33*(1), 27–39. https://doi.org/10.1007/s10912-011-9163-3

Jenset, G., & McGillivray, B. (2017). *Quantitative historical linguistics: A corpus framework.* Oxford University Press.

Johansson, S. (2007). *Seeing through multilingual corpora. On the use of corpora in contrastive studies.* John Benjamins. https://doi.org/10.1075/scl.26

Jones, L. (2016). Policy as discursive practice: An ethnographic study of hospital planning in England. PhD thesis. London School of Hygiene & Tropical Medicine. https://doi.org/10.17037/PUBS.02997234

Jones, R.H. (2013). *Health and risk communication: An applied linguistic perspective.* Routledge. https://doi.org/10.4324/9780203521410

Jones, R.H. (2015). Discourse, cybernetics, and the entextualization of the self. In R. Jones, A. Chik & C. Hafner (Eds.), *Discourse and digital practices: Doing discourse analysis in the digital age* (pp. 28–47). Routledge. https://doi.org/10.4324/9781315726465

Jucker, A.H. (2022). Corpus pragmatics. In J. Verschueren & J.-O. Östman (Eds.), *Handbook of Pragmatics: Manual* (second edition, pp. 1516–1527). John Benjamins. https://doi.org/10.1075/hop.m

Knapton, O., Power, A. & Rundblad, G. (2021). Cognitive approaches to discourse analysis: Applying conceptual blending theory to understandings of disease transmission. In G. Brookes & D. Hunt (Eds.), *Analysing health communication: Discourse approaches* (pp. 301–331). Palgrave Macmillan. https://doi.org/10.1007/978-3-030-68184-5_12

Knapton, O. & Rundblad, G. (2014). Public health in the UK media: Cognitive Discourse Analysis and its application to a drinking water emergency. In C. Hart & P. Cap (Eds.), *Contemporary Critical Discourse Studies* (pp. 559–582). Bloomsbury. http://dx.doi.org/10.5040/9781472593634.ch-024

Koteyko, N. (2014). *Language and politics in post-soviet Russia: A corpus assisted approach.* Palgrave Macmillan. https://doi.org/10.1057/9781137314093

Lamerichs, J.M.W.J. (2021). Discursive psychology: A discursive approach to identity work in online illness talk. In G. Brookes & D. Hunt (Eds.), *Analysing health communication: Discourse approaches* (pp. 111–132). Palgrave Macmillan. https://doi.org/10.1007/978-3-030-68184-5_5

Laviosa, S. (2011). Corpus linguistics and translation studies. In V. Viana, S. Zyngier & G. Barnbrook (Eds.), *Perspectives on corpus linguistics* (pp. 131–153). John Benjamins. https://doi.org/10.1075/scl.48.09lav

Leech, G. (1991). The state of the art in corpus linguistics. In K. Aijmer & B. Altenberg (Eds.), *English corpus linguistics: Studies in honour of Jan Svartvik* (pp. 8–29). Longman. https://doi.org/10.4324/9781315845890

Leech, G. (1992). Corpora and theories of linguistic performance. In J. Svartvik (Ed.), *Directions in corpus linguistics* (pp. 105–22). Mouton de Gruyter. https://doi.org/10.1515/9783110867275

Leech, G. (2000). Grammars of spoken English: New outcomes of corpus-oriented research. *Language Learning*, 50(4), 675–724. https://doi.org/10.1111/0023-8333.00143

Leech, G., Hundt, M., Mair, C. & Smith, N. (2009). *Change in contemporary English: A grammatical study*. Cambridge University Press. https://doi.org/10.1017/CBO9780511642210

Love, R., Dembry, C., Hardie, A., Brezina, V. & McEnery, T. (2017). The Spoken BNC2014: Designing and building a spoken corpus of everyday conversations. *International Journal of Corpus Linguistics*, 22(3), 319–344. https://doi.org/10.1075/ijcl.22.3.02lov

Lupton, D. (2013). Quantifying the body: Monitoring and measuring health in the age of mHealth technologies. *Critical Public Health*, 23(4), 393–403. http://dx.doi.org/10.1080/09581596.2013.794931

Lupton, D. (2017). Editorial: Towards sensory studies of digital health. *Digital Health*, 3, 1–6. https://doi.org/10.1177/2055207617740090

Lustig, A., Brookes, G. & Hunt, D. (2021). Linguistic analysis of online communication about a novel persecutory belief system (Gangstalking): Mixed methods study. *Journal of Medical Internet Research*, 23(3), e25722. https://doi.org/10.2196/25722

Mahlberg, M. (2005). *English general nouns: A corpus theoretical approach*. John Benjamins. https://doi.org/10.1075/scl.20

Mahlberg, M. (2013). *Corpus stylistics and Dickens's fiction*. Routledge. https://doi.org/10.4324/9780203076088

Marchi, A. & Taylor, C. (2018). *Corpus approaches to discourse: A critical review*. Routledge. https://doi.org/10.4324/9781315179346

Masic, I., Miokovic, M. & Muhamedagic, B. (2008). Evidence based medicine - New approaches and challenges. *Acta Informatica Medica*, 16(4), 219–225. https://doi.org/10.5455/aim.2008.16.219-225

Mastropierro, L. (2017). *Corpus stylistics in heart of darkness and its Italian translations*. Bloomsbury. https://doi.org/10.5040/9781350013575

Mautner, G. (2015). Checks and balances: How corpus linguistics can contribute to CDA. In R. Wodak & M. Meyer (Eds.), *Methods of critical discourse analysis* (pp. 154–179). Sage.

McEnery, A. & Baker, H. (2017). *Corpus linguistics and 17th-century prostitution: Computational linguistics and history*. Bloomsbury. https://doi.org/10.5040/9781474295062

McEnery, T. & Baker, H. (2022). 'A geography of names': A genre analysis of nationality-driven names for venereal disease in seventeenth-century England. In T. Hiltunen & I. Taavitsainen (Eds.), *Corpus pragmatic studies on the history of medical discourse* (pp. 23–48). John Benjamins. https://doi.org/10.1075/pbns.330.02mce

McEnery, T., Brookes, G. & Clarke, I. (2022). Corpus studies of language through time: Introduction to the special issue. *International Journal of Corpus Linguistics*, *27*(4), 393–398. https://doi.org/10.1075/ijcl.00050.edi

McEnery, T. & Hardie, A. (2012). *Corpus linguistics: Method, theory and practice*. Cambridge University Press.

McEnery, T. & Wilson, A. (2001). *Corpus linguistics: An introduction* (second edition). Edinburgh University Press.

McEnery, T., Xiao, R. & Tono, Y. (2006). *Corpus-based language studies: An advanced resource book*. Routledge.

McHoul, A. & Rapley, M. (2001). Ghost: Do not forget; this visitation / is but to whet thy almost blunted purpose: Culture, psychology and 'being human'. *Culture & Psychology*, *7*(4), 433–451. https://doi.org/10.1177/1354067X0174002

Mills, S. (1997). *Discourse*. Routledge. https://doi.org/10.4324/9780203131725

Mishler, E. (1984). *The discourse of medicine dialectics in medical interviews*. Ablex.

Mullany, L., Smith, C., Harvey, K. & Adolphs, S. (2015). 'Am I anorexic?' Weight, eating and discourses of the body in online adolescent health communication. *Communication and Medicine*, *12*(2–3), 211–223. https://doi.org/10.1558/cam.16692.

Murphy, B. (2010). *Corpus and sociolinguistics: Investigating age and gender in female talk*. John Benjamins. https://doi.org/10.1075/scl.38

O'Keeffe, A., McCarthy, M. & Carter, R. (2007). *From corpus to classroom: Language use and language teaching*. Cambridge University Press. https://doi.org/10.1017/CBO9780511497650

Parry, R.H. (2004). Communication during goal-setting in physiotherapy treatment sessions. *Clinical Rehabilitation*, *18*(6), 668–682. https://doi.org/10.1191/0269215504cr745oa

Partington, A., Duguid, A. & Taylor, C. (2013). *Patterns and meanings in discourse: Theory and practice in corpus-assisted discourse studies*. Routledge. https://doi.org/10.1075/scl.55

Paterson, L.L. & Gregory, I.N. (2018). *Representations of poverty and place: Using geographical text analysis to understand discourse*. Palgrave. https://doi.org/10.1007/978-3-319-93503-4

Pilnick, A. (1999). "Patient counselling" by pharmacists: Advice, information, or instruction? *Sociological Quarterly*, *40*(4), 613–622. https://doi.org/10.1111/j.1533-8525.1999.tb00570.x

Price, H. (2022). *The language of mental illness: Corpus linguistics and the construction of mental illness in the press*. Cambridge University Press. https://doi.org/10.1017/9781108991278

Ringer, A. & Holen, M. (2021). Discursive ethnography: Understanding psychiatric discourses and patient positions through fieldwork. In G. Brookes & D. Hunt (Eds.), *Analysing health communication: Discourse approaches* (pp. 189–213). Palgrave Macmillan. https://doi.org/10.1007/978-3-030-68184-5_8

Rühlemann, C. (2018). *Corpus linguistics for pragmatics: A guide for research*. Routledge. https://doi.org/10.4324/9780429451072

Sarangi, S. (2004). Editorial: Towards a communicative mentality in medical and healthcare practice. *Communication and Medicine*, *1*(1), 1–11. https://doi.org/10.1515/come.2004.002

Semino, E., & Short, M. (2004). *Corpus stylistics: Speech, Writing and thought presentation in a corpus of English writing*. Routledge.

Seymour-Smith, S. (2015). Applying discursive approaches to health psychology. *Health Psychology*, *34*(4), 371–380. https://doi.org/10.1037/hea0000165

Sinclair, J. (2003). *Reading concordances*. Longman.

Sinclair, J. (2004). *Trust the text: Language, corpus, and discourse*. Routledge. https://doi.org/10.4324/9780203594070

Skelton, J.R. & Hobbs, F.D.R. (1999a). Descriptive study of cooperative language in primary care consultations by male and female doctors. *BMJ*, *318*(7183), 576–579. https://doi.org/10.1136%2Fbmj.318.7183.576

Skelton, J.R. & Hobbs, F.D.R. (1999b). Concordancing: Exploring the uses of language-based research in medical education. *Lancet*, *353*(9147), 108–111. https://doi.org/10.1016/S0140-6736(98)02469-6

Skelton, J.R., Murray, J. & Hobbs, F. (1999). Imprecision in medical communication: Study of a doctor talking to patients with serious illness. *Journal of the Royal Society of Medicine*, *92*, 620–625. https://doi.org/10.1177%2F014107689909201204

Skelton, J.R., Wearn, A.M. & Hobbs, F.D.R. (2002). 'I' and 'we': A concordancing analysis of how doctors and patients use first person pronouns in primary care consultations. *Family Practice*, *19*(5), 484–488. https://doi.org/10.1093/fampra/19.5.484

Staples, S. (2015). *The discourse of nurse- patient interactions: Contrasting the communicative styles of U.S. and international nurses*. John Benjamins. https://doi.org/10.1075/scl.72

Stommel, W. & Koole, T. (2010). The online support group as a community: A micro-analysis of the interaction with a new member. *Discourse Studies*, *12*(3), 357–378. https://doi.org/10.1177/1461445609358518

Stubbe, M., Dew, K., Macdonald, L. & Dowell, A. (2021). Interactional Sociolinguistics: Tracking patient-initiated questions across an episode of care. In G. Brookes & D. Hunt (Eds.), *Analysing health communication: Discourse approaches* (pp. 49–80). Palgrave Macmillan. https://doi.org/10.1007/978-3-030-68184-5_3

Stubbs, M. (1994). Grammar, text, and ideology: Computer-assisted methods in the linguistics of representation. *Applied Linguistics*, *15*(2), 201–223. https://doi.org/10.1093/applin/15.2.201

Stubbs, M. (1995). Collocations and semantic profiles: On the cause of the trouble with quantitative methods. *Function of Language*, *2*(1), 1–33. https://doi.org/10.1075/fol.2.1.03stu

Thomas, G.M. & Lupton, D. (2016). Threats and thrills: Pregnancy apps, risk and consumption. *Health, Risk & Society*, *17*(7–8), 495–509. http://dx.doi.org/10.1080/13698575.2015.1127333

Thomas, J. & Wilson, A. (1996). Methodologies for studying a corpus of doctor–patient interaction. In J. Thomas and M. Short (Eds.), *Using corpora for language research* (pp. 92–109). Longman.

Thompson, R. (2012). Looking healthy: Visualizing disorder & wellness online. *Visual Communication*, *11*(4), 395–420. https://doi.org/10.1177/1470357212453978

Timmermans, S. & Berg, M. (2003). The practice of medical technology. *Sociology of Health & Illness*, *25*(3), 97–114. https://doi.org/10.1111/1467-9566.00342

Tognini-Bonelli, E. (2001). *Corpus linguistics at work*. John Benjamins. https://doi.org/10.1075/scl.6

Widdowson, H.G. (2000). On the limitations of linguistics applied. *Applied Linguistics*, 21(1), 3–25. https://doi.org/10.1093/applin/21.1.3

Widdowson, H.G. (2004). *Text, context, pretext: Critical issues in discourse analysis*. Blackwell. https://doi.org/10.1002/9780470758427

Wright, D. & Brookes, G. (2019). 'This is England, speak English!': A corpus-assisted critical study of language ideologies in the right-leaning British press. *Critical Discourse Studies*, 16(1), 56–83. https://doi.org/10.1080/17405904.2018.1511439

Xiao, R. & McEnery, T. (2004). *Aspect in Mandarin Chinese: A corpus-based study*. John Benjamins. https://doi.org/10.1075/slcs.73

2

DESIGNING AND BUILDING A CORPUS

2.1 Introduction

In the previous chapter, we became acquainted with what corpus linguistics is and we also considered some of the key affordances and applications of the methodology, focusing specifically on why we might want to use corpus linguistics approaches to analyse health communication. We learned that the first step in any corpus study will involve deciding on the topic of the study and on the research questions that will guide it. We will then likely undertake some reading to review relevant literature to inform our understanding of that topic and any previous research that has been done around it to refine our research questions.

Following this step, and perhaps even alongside it, we will have to decide what corpus or corpora we want to analyse in our research. As its name suggests, the concept of the corpus is at the centre of corpus linguistics, as it is the data on which research in corpus linguistics bases its analyses. For certain research projects, suitable publicly available corpora may already exist. The types of general language corpora introduced in Chapter 1, for instance, can be useful for investigating the representations or discourses around a particular health- or illness-related phenomenon in more general contexts of language use. For example, Hamilton et al. (2007) analysed uses of the word 'risk', as a noun and as a verb, across three general corpora containing more than one hundred million words of contemporary English usage. From this, they determined that 'risk' was commonly used in the context of health and that it more consistently carried a negative semantic prosody compared with its more neutral meaning in other contexts (i.e., discussing finance, government, and business).

DOI: 10.4324/9781003099659-2

In most cases, though, studies of health communication are focused on topics and/or communicative contexts that are unlikely to be represented in publicly available corpora. For this reason, most corpus studies of health communication are based on specialised corpora, purpose-built for the study at-hand. As well as being one of the earliest decisions we, as researchers, have to make when embarking on a corpus linguistics project, the selection and design of a corpus is arguably one of the most important decisions we will make, as the design of our corpus will influence our findings and the claims we can make.

In this chapter, we explore the main considerations that underpin the design and construction of specialised corpora. We begin by exploring the considerations that go into the process of designing a corpus. We then move onto more practical matters by exploring ways of collecting texts for a corpus, before considering the processes involved in cleaning and annotating a corpus. Finally, we discuss some of the ethical considerations that are likely to be involved in corpus design and construction. Generally speaking, the ordering of the sections of this chapter reflects the order in which many corpus builders will likely have to approach each of the issues or 'steps' discussed therein. However, this order is certainly not hard and fast; indeed, corpus construction is often an iterative process which involves countering issues as we go, and then returning to a previous step in the process to modify our design in a way that helps to ensure that our corpus optimally represents the kind of language use that we want to investigate. The final topic we consider in this chapter, ethics, pervades all aspects of corpus design and construction and should be considered from the outset. More generally, corpus design and construction are often iterative, involving lots of false starts and lessons that are learnt later in the process – through 'doing' – which then require us to return to our corpus and modify its design. It is to corpus design that we turn first.

2.2 Designing a corpus

A core tenet of corpus linguistics and corpus design is the notion that, as researchers, we seek to engage with and study authentic language use, recognising that language used in real-world contexts tells us something valuable about the users of that language and the social contexts in which the language being studied is used. The notion of *authenticity*, as understood in corpus linguistics research, refers to the quality of a given instance of language use being 'naturally occurring' or existing in 'real life' (McEnery and Wilson 2001). Following McEnery and Hardie (2012), the language use included in a corpus should involve minimal disruption from the corpus builder or researcher, and anything beyond this constitutes a reason to declare that a corpus is 'special' in the sense that it operates with a relatively loose interpretation of the criterion of authenticity. Such special corpora might represent language use that is in some way semi-elicited by researchers, for example, through the use of surveys or questionnaires or language use that has been produced in experimental conditions. This looser operationalisation of the concept of authenticity could be of value for research on health-related contexts which, for ethical or other reasons, might otherwise be difficult or even impossible for researchers to access. In most cases, though, when designing a corpus, we usually want to include in it texts that can be judged as being as authentic as possible in the sense that it involves minimal interference from the researcher. We begin, then, by exploring the considerations that might attend to this issue of authenticity when designing corpora of health communication specifically.

2.2.1 Authenticity in corpus design

One of the principal challenges with collecting authentic, spoken health communication stems from the relative inaccessibility of clinical encounters for researchers. While there are examples of language-based studies that have collected authentic hospital interactions in context (Iedema et al. 2009; Slade et al. 2015), these require substantial resources and time as well as careful measures for minimising the interruption to care. One approach to accessing authentic healthcare interactions with health professionals is to simulate the role of patient or advice-seeker, though this can only be advised in very particular circumstances so as to avoid denying those in real need of care from the services they require. To investigate the language of interactions that take place through the NHS Direct telephone advice-giving service, Adolphs et al. (2004) explain that they were approved by the service providers to make and record calls to its operatives, presenting with a range of different health complaints that had been scripted beforehand. The responding health professionals were not made aware of when these invented cases were presented and, thus, Adolphs et al. (2004) maintain that they were able to elicit data that was authentic to how the service is delivered. While there may be criticisms of researchers occupying services and health practitioners' time when they might otherwise be attending to genuine cases, there is a balance to be struck in securing the type of data that subsequently informs practice. Adolphs et al. (2004, p. 23) stress that data-driven approaches like this, that refer to 'real examples', can 'alert practitioners, educators and researchers to features of accomplished professional practice which were not hitherto obvious' and that once these are rendered visible, they can be critically examined in terms of whether they are desirable, according to intended outcomes for the service.

We can also look to healthcare practices for demonstrations of procedures that facilitate the development of communication skills without interfering with the delivery of care to patients in need. It is an established practice in the training of clinical staff to employ simulated patients in the enactment of role-play exercises, and researchers have arranged to observe the sessions that take place as a routine part of training (see Atkins 2019) or otherwise recruited health professionals to participate in simulations they have engineered themselves. French and Lapointe (2016) describe the compilation of the Multilingual Health Corpora for Training Purposes (MHCTP), which used role-playing with nurses and simulated patients based in Quebec to generate language data in French and English that can be directly compared. In addition to facilitating more directly comparable data, French and Lapointe (2016, p. 260) explain that the scripted scenarios created the type of encounter – and, consequently, language – 'that would normally take years to collect from authentic health communication situations'. They were particularly interested in supporting professionals in emotionally charged moments that they may encounter in their work, and which require particular language skills to navigate. Through documenting the responses that their participant nurses contributed in these role-plays, French and Lapointe (2016), thus, provide evidence-based examples of the language used by practising nurses to communicate empathy.

While representing something of a criterion in corpus design, it is important not to use a concept such as authenticity uncritically. Indeed, some have expressed doubt about the capacity of corpora to represent authentic language use at all. For example, Widdowson (2000) has questioned the extent to which corpora can represent context, while Mishan (2004, p. 219) similarly argues that the process of transposing texts into corpora 'forfeit[s] a crucial criterion for authenticity, namely context'. To an extent, this is a fair criticism; In the pursuit of scale, quantitatively oriented methods almost inevitably involve some element of decontextualisation (it is not possible, or at least not practical, to engage with contexts of text production and consumption when analysing a large corpus to the same extent as it is when analysing a single text or a handful of texts). Furthermore, while there have been advancements in multimodal corpus development in recent years, it is also true that most corpora are monomodal, representing language at the expense of other modes (e.g., imagery and font in written texts, sound and gesture in spoken texts). Such multimodal elements are, as noted, increasingly being incorporated into corpus design, and while such advancements are further along regarding spoken texts (Adolphs and Carter 2013), researchers are increasingly capturing the non-linguistic elements of written texts in corpora through the use of annotation (see Section 2.5).

2.2.2 Text choice in corpus design

Adopting this notion of authenticity as a key criterion in corpus construction, the first decision to make when attempting to design and build a corpus that reflects authentic language use pertains to the selection of the type of texts or language use that we want to include within it. When compared to the design of general language corpora, the decision regarding what texts we include in a specialised corpus can be relatively straightforward and will be driven by the topic of our research and our research questions. For certain types of texts, known as 'closed' or 'finite' texts, this task is even easier, as there is a clearly defined limit to the texts we can include in our corpus, and so we can include everything that is available. An example of such a dataset is Mahlberg's (2013) corpus of the known, published works of Charles Dickens. Because Dickens was deceased at the point at which Mahlberg compiled her corpus, it was possible for her to collect all of the novelist's known, published works in her corpus. However, in most cases it will not be possible to include all relevant texts in a corpus. This is because we, as researchers and corpus builders, tend not to have access to – or even complete knowledge of – the full extent of the texts that could be deemed relevant for our research purposes, even if these purposes are very clearly defined. For this reason, most corpora constitute a mere sample of all the possible texts 'out there' that could have been included.

Designing a corpus, therefore, essentially involves developing a sampling frame to help us to decide which texts will be included in the corpus as well as deciding whether we will include these texts in their entirety or sample material from them. Developing a sampling frame for building a corpus means making decisions surrounding 'the kind of texts included, the number of texts, the selection of particular texts, the selection of text samples from within texts, and the length of text samples' (Biber 2004, p. 174). As such, when designing a sampling frame to address these considerations, the related issue of representativeness comes to the fore.

When deciding which texts to include in the corpus, as well as being as authentic as possible, we can draw on the concept of representativeness as an iterative guide for corpus construction. As discussed in the previous chapter, Biber (1993, p. 244) defines *representativeness* as 'the extent to which a sample includes the full range of variability in a population'. Here, the term 'population' refers not necessarily to a group of people, but more conceptually to the 'notional space within which language is being sampled' (McEnery and Hardie 2012, p. 8). The more representative of the target variety or context of use (i.e., the population) our corpus is, the more confident we can be as analysts that our findings can be generalised to that population. The process of determining representativeness ought to be seen as iterative, whereby researchers develop sampling frames based on representativeness, build corpora, interrogate them, and, if the data appear skewed or unrepresentative, researchers should update the sampling frame, redevelop the corpus, and redo their analyses. For example, if we wanted to study language produced in clinical encounters in England, we would want to assemble a corpus that represents such encounters, in all their variability, as widely as possible. For this purpose, we would want to include in our corpus interactions taking place in different types of provision, involving different types of practitioners from different parts of the country and involving patients from different backgrounds, presenting with a range of health concerns. Upon doing so, we would need to critically reflect on the data, determine what they truly represent, and consider the need to add data to better represent the language we wish to study.

Some types of language use are particularly difficult to represent adequately in a corpus, and much of this is to do with access to texts. For example, texts representing the use of minority or under-resourced languages can be difficult for corpus compilers to access. Of more direct relevance to the study of health communication, certain contexts of health communication and the interactions and texts produced therein can be difficult for researchers to access, foremost due to ethical requirements (discussed later in the chapter). Due in part to such challenges, many corpus studies of health communication have examined the discourse surrounding particular health-related topics in the context of (relatively anonymous) online communication, including on social media platforms but also within online support groups (e.g., Brookes 2019; Hunt and Brookes 2020; Collins and Baker 2023). The anonymous nature of such mediums means that researchers seldom have access to the kinds of demographic metadata about the users that would be required to measure and assess the representativeness of such corpora, at least in terms of demographic characteristics (although, for an example of an exception, see Collins and Baker 2023). In cases such as these, the issue of corpus representativeness is less pressing, and we might want to employ a more opportunistic approach to data collection and gather as many texts as we can.

The above points notwithstanding, representativeness is a central consideration in the compilation of most corpora, and if it is possible to measure representativeness in the target variety, or 'population', and we have access to the contexts and texts required to make our corpus representative, then it is good practice to design a corpus to be as representative as possible. At the very least, it is important to be aware and mindful of the concept of representativeness when designing and using a corpus so that we can be critically reflective about what our data does and does not have the power to represent and being cognisant of the extent to which any findings based on it can be generalised.

2.2.3 Size and balance in corpus design

Two key concepts underpinning the issue of representativeness are size and balance. One of the most common questions that can arise during the process of building a corpus relates to how large that corpus ought to be. There are no strict rules regarding how large a corpus should be, and, instead, the size of a corpus is likely to be determined by a number of factors. First, the size of a corpus can be determined by practical considerations. As we mentioned earlier, some types of (healthcare) contexts and the language that is produced within them can be difficult for researchers to access. This can necessarily limit the amount of language use we will be able to sample for our corpus.

Additionally, the size of our corpus can be constrained by the resources available to us, in terms of personnel, time, and money.

A challenge for compilers of corpora concerns the amount of digital language data that is produced and which then becomes available for corpus analysis every day. Indeed, the amount of digital health data made available through social media (and other platforms) is seen by Moreno-Ortiz and García-Gámez (2023) as presenting both opportunities and challenges for researchers looking to index and process large amounts of language data as corpora. Twitter data, in particular, is lauded for hosting content consisting of 'high velocity granular data which includes metadata that allows the analysis of a phenomenon's evolution over time' (Moreno-Ortiz and García-Gámez 2023, online first), but this amount of information can prove to be inscrutable and slow to process. In response to this challenge, Moreno-Ortiz and García-Gámez (2023) explore different sampling strategies for navigating large social media datasets, referring to Chen et al.'s (2020) corpus of 31 billion English-language tweets collected to explore talk about COVID-19. They discuss the procedures involved in extracting the data that Chen et al. (2020) have made available, summarising the decisions both they and the original research team have made to streamline data extraction and processing at the expense of some content and metadata (e.g., discounting retweets and removing hyperlinks and certain Unicode characters known to cause formatting issues). Moreno-Ortiz and García-Gámez (2023, online first) report success with their sampling approach, suggesting that smaller samples can be 'both representative and relevant for [...] qualitative researchers, as well as easier to process from a computational perspective'.

In addition to such practical issues, the size of a corpus can also be determined by certain theoretical considerations. One of these relates to the linguistic feature(s) that the corpus is intended to be used to study. Kennedy (1998) avers that for studying prosodic features (e.g., rhythm, stress, and intonation in speech), a corpus of 100,000 words will usually be sufficiently large to allow generalisations to be made. For studying morphological features, he suggests that we would require a corpus closer to half a million words in size. And then for describing how words are used (as we might do in a discourse analysis), Kennedy suggests that a corpus of around a million words should be sufficient. These are only general guidelines, though, and there is no consensus on ideal or adequate corpus size. Indeed, there is certainly no 'one-size-fits-all' approach (McCarthy and Carter 2001). One clear advantage of building a smaller corpus is that the human analyst is likely to be able to account for a larger proportion of the uses of even the most frequent words and, in some cases, to account for every use of a word of interest. Additionally, a more manageable amount of data can make it easier to investigate function and meaning in a corpus, as well as to interrogate the contexts in which the texts in the corpus were produced, which can support researchers in identifying links between these insights and their analytical findings.

In addition to the linguistic feature(s) we might be studying, another factor that can dictate how large our corpus ought to be relates to the type of language that the corpus is intended to represent. Baker (2023) advises that the more varied the type of language under study is, the larger the corpus will need to be. This is one reason why general language corpora tend to be very large; because they aim to represent language use on a broad scale, they typically contain many different types of texts. For example, the 100 million-word BNC2014 contains both spoken and written language. Then within that, the written section contains texts belonging to 24 genres, including academic essays, novels, personal letters, newspapers, and religious texts. Because specialised corpora are not designed with the aim of representing language use on such a broad scale, they tend not to have to represent as much variation in terms of text type, which is one of the reasons they tend to be much smaller than general corpora.

This brings us to the concept of balance. Because we want our corpus to be as representative as possible of the variety or context that we are interested in, we want, as noted above, to make sure that we represent all the variability in the clearly defined 'population' of language use that we want to study. But as well as including all the variability in the population, we also need to make sure that we represent these variables in a balanced way so that one group or variable is not over-represented relative to another. If we return to our example of a corpus of healthcare interactions from earlier, we want to make sure that our samples of healthcare interactions are fairly balanced in terms of size so that no variable (area of provision, type of practitioner, geographical zone, health concern, type of patient, or any other variable) was over- or under-represented in the corpus.

Balancing our corpus applies not only to the individuals represented in it but also to other factors, such as the type of texts we include and when and where they are produced. It is important to remain critical of the concept of balance and how we operationalise it in our corpus and to report clearly on any sampling frame we use when designing a corpus. For example, Brookes and Baker (2021, p. 28) discuss how the structure of their corpus of obesity coverage in the UK press enabled them to carry out 'systematic comparisons of articles according to their format (i.e., broadsheets vs. tabloids), political leaning (i.e., left-leaning vs. right-leaning) and date of publication'. However, one of the aspects they had to navigate was the (im)balance across publications, both in terms of number of articles and word count. They report that 30% of the articles in the corpus come from the *Daily Mail* and explain that '[t]his imbalance represents the real-life press landscape and specifically the corresponding imbalance in terms of how much obesity coverage is provided in each newspaper' (Brookes and

Baker 2021, p. 28). This demonstrates that researchers may have to deal with the over-representation of certain contributors to public and media discourses, if this reflects actual differences in their publication output. In response, Brookes and Baker (2021) factor into their analysis the relativisation of occurrences and contextualisation of examples depending on which publication they come from.

Ensuring that our corpus is balanced in terms of such variables can help to protect against one group or variable being over-represented relative to another. Returning again to our example of a corpus of healthcare interactions, if we disregarded the issue of balance and ended up with a corpus that was (overly) skewed towards practitioners from a certain geographical location, first language, or age or sex group, for example, this would hinder the extent to which any findings based on our corpus could be generalised to our target population (i.e., all healthcare encounters in the UK).

Balancing a corpus can, however, be challenging. It is often the case, for example, that texts representing some variables are lengthier than others. This is a challenge that has been confronted by many corpus developers over time. A popular approach to this issue is to assemble a corpus of size-matched samples of texts to ensure a balanced representation. As an example, we can consider the BE21 corpus (Baker 2023) – a 1-million-word corpus comprising 500 text samples (each 2,000 words in length) representing a range of genres of contemporary written British English. This corpus was built according to the Brown sampling frame (so named because it was originally developed in the design of the Brown corpus of written American English during the 1960s (Kučera and Francis 1967)). An advantage of designing a corpus according to a sampling frame is that the resulting corpus can then be relatively easily compared against other corpora built using the same sampling frame (indeed, there are a number of corpora, known as the 'Brown family', that have been built according to the Brown sampling frame – see McEnery and Brookes 2022).

We can imagine how this issue of variable text length might impact the design of a corpus of health communication. For instance, if we return to our example of a corpus of healthcare interactions, we might find that doctors in London have much shorter consultations than ones in Lancaster, with the latter then contributing more words than the former. In such cases, sampling the same number of interactions from London- and Lancaster-based doctors would introduce an imbalance due to the differing lengths of their respective interactions. Rather than collecting entire texts (in this case, interactions), one way around this is to sample the same number of words from the texts for inclusion in the corpus. So, rather than having 100 consultations from each set of doctors, we might have 100 samples of 1,000 words from each set of doctors. We would, of course, have to decide from where in the interactions we would take our 1,000-word samples. However we decide to approach this, what is most important is that we apply that approach consistently; if we decide to sample the first 1,000 words from the interactions, we should apply this consistently across all the texts we sample, across all variables.

Of course, designing a corpus in a balanced way requires us to know the full range of variability in our target population. However, in most cases it is not possible (or at least realistic) for us to know the full extent of this variability. For this reason, true 'balance' (if such a thing exists) can be difficult and, in some cases, impossible to achieve. Nevertheless, it is important to be mindful of the effects of imbalance on our corpus, and to reflect critically on how any imbalances in our corpus might influence our findings and, in turn, what we can claim on the basis of these. In cases in which we do not know the full range of variability in our target population, it can be up to the researchers themselves to decide what variables are likely to influence the findings and then to balance their corpus according to these.

2.3 Collecting texts

Once we have designed our corpus, in terms of deciding what texts we want to include and in what sizes and proportions, we can then turn our attention to collecting those texts. At this point in particular, the distinction between corpora of spoken and written (including digital and computer-mediated) language becomes especially important. We begin by considering the processes involved in collecting spoken language data, which is arguably the most challenging type of text to collect, at-scale, for a corpus.

2.3.1 Collecting spoken recordings

The collection and processing of spoken language for corpora is generally costlier and more time-consuming than it is for written corpora. This is because, whereas written texts are increasingly available in the kind of machine-readable format that is necessary for them to be analysed using computational corpus techniques, in the majority of cases speech must first be recorded and then transcribed before it can be included in a corpus. Although assistive speech-to-text technologies have become increasingly sophisticated, a 'fully accurate and sophisticated automated approach to spoken corpus construction has still not been developed' (Knight and Adolphs 2021, p. 21). As such, the process of recording and transcribing speech remains 'largely manually driven' (ibid.).

The two stages in corpus construction which distinguish the development of spoken corpora from their written (including computer-mediated) counterparts are recording and transcription. These two stages are intertwined, with each influencing the other, while both are further influenced by the type of analysis for which the resulting corpus is intended. As Knight and Adolphs (2021, p. 21) point out, '[t]he data recording stage is determined by the type of analysis planned, which in turn determines the granularity and detail of transcription, coding and mark-up and the participants and/or contexts in which recordings take place'. For this reason, they advise that '[i]t is therefore important to plan the development of a corpus carefully and to consider all practical and ethical issues that may arise' (ibid.). Overall, this should lead to an iterative approach, whereby the process of corpus of construction is itself evaluated and, if necessary, modified throughout.

Beginning with the recording stage, which can be considered the data collection phase, there is no standard approach to this. Rather, the approach taken should be determined by the eventual purposes to which the corpus will be put (i.e., the type of analysis that will be carried out on it). However, the approach taken should be ethical (you will need to obtain formal, written, informed consent from participants *before* recording them – see Section 2.6 on ethical considerations). In terms of the recording equipment, any device can be used, provided that it can support high-quality recordings (e.g., phones, voice recorders, or other mobile devices). It is a good idea to test the equipment before embarking in lengthy recording sessions, to check both that the equipment works and that it can provide recordings that are of sufficient quality for the kind of analysis you want to conduct. It is important to bear in mind that the collection of naturally occurring speech for a spoken corpus cannot be 'redone' (i.e., the same speech cannot be reuttered in an authentic way at a later stage, even if we can keep many of the variables of the interaction the same). It is also good practice to keep multiple copies of your recordings, as files can become damaged or corrupt, or become otherwise unusable. Having just a single copy of a recording would mean that such events lead to a loss of data.

In addition to the actual interaction that you want to analyse, during the process of recording it is also important to gather information about the participants and the context of the interaction. This could include, for example, demographic information about the participants, details of the circumstances in which the interaction took place, and any other details that you consider relevant to the interaction and which could be drawn upon in your analysis. This information, which is about the data, is known as 'metadata'. The type of metadata we gather, and how much, will depend on what we believe will be required for the purposes for which our corpus is intended. It is important to state our intention to collect such metadata when applying for ethical approval for a project and then when informing participants about it for the purposes of obtaining their consent (see Section 2.6 on ethical considerations). This metadata can then be included in the corpus to facilitate more sophisticated types of analysis (see Section 2.5). It is important to document this information at the point of data collection, as it is difficult, and often impossible, to rectify the loss or omission of metadata further down the line. Therefore, the process should be principled and yield data and metadata that provides information which is sufficiently rich to facilitate in-depth linguistic inquiry. Summarising the importance of this issue, Knight and Adolphs (2021, p. 24) advise that researchers strive to

[C]ollect data which is as accurate and exhaustive as possible, capturing as much information from the discursive environment as possible. This involves documenting information about the participants, location and overall context in which the event takes place, as well as the type of recording equipment being used and the technical and physical specifications applied to the recording itself.

2.3.2 Transcribing spoken texts

Once the speech has been recorded, it will need to be transcribed into a written, machine-readable format in order to render it amenable to computational corpus analysis. The process of transcription can be time consuming (it is estimated that one hour of recorded speech can take around ten hours to transcribe). It is sensible, then, not to gather and attempt to transcribe very much more speech than is required for the corpus. Yet at the same time, just how long it takes to transcribe spoken language depends, in no small part, on the level of detail with which we carry out the transcription. Knight and Adolphs (2021, p. 26) caution that, because 'there are so many layers of detail that carry meaning in spoken interaction, this task can easily become a black hole [...] with a potentially infinite amount of contextual information to record'. The reason for this, they point out, is that 'spoken interaction is essentially multi-modal in nature, featuring a careful interplay between textual, prosodic, gestural and environmental elements in the construction of meaning' (ibid.) (see also Adolphs and Carter 2013).

When building a specialised spoken corpus to be used for a specific project or programme of research, the type of transcription used can be driven by the kind of analyses we intend to perform. This can then inform the planning of the transcription stage. Knight and Adolphs (2021, p. 28) assert that

> it is advisable to identify the spoken features of interest at the outset and to tailor the focus of the transcription accordingly. For example, a study of discourse structure might require the transcription to include overlaps but not detailed prosodic information.

There are many frameworks that can be followed for transcription (see Knight and Adolphs 2021). For many projects, simple orthographic transcription will suffice, particularly if you are interested in lexical and grammatical choices. However, if you are interested in features such as overlapping speech, interruptions, and prosody, then such features will need to be accounted for in the framework you use. Any existing framework can be selected or adapted according to your purposes. Most importantly, the framework you adopt should be suitable for the research questions you intend to ask of your corpus, it should be applied consistently to all recordings within the corpus, and it should be clearly documented in any corpus manual produced or any publications based on it.

Indeed, researchers working with spoken corpora – and generating their own transcripts – will certainly benefit from careful consideration of the conventions they want to use and the way in which they want to record various aspects of spoken language prior to beginning the process of transcription, not least of all to minimise the chance that the transcripts need to be revised or corrected. Gut (2021, p. 239) notes that '[a]ll spoken corpora contain orthographic transcriptions' but that 'they can vary considerably in terms of the orthographic conventions chosen'. In addition to known lexical variation (e.g., color vs colour), differences in transcription can arise in the case of communicative units that have no standard form, such as sounds of hesitation ('erm').

When transcribing talk, we have to decide whether we are going to document audible variations that will help to discern contracted forms such as 'wanna' from the more standard 'want to' or even plain errors or mispronunciations such as 'hotspital'. We might also want to document paralinguistic features that contribute to how meaning is communicated but which are not standardised in any codified form. Bonsignori (2019, p. 119), for example, describes a multimodal approach in which hand/arm gestures, gaze direction, facial expressions, head movements, body posture, and intonation were analysed alongside linguistic features such as specialised vocabulary and speech acts in an attempt to give 'a holistic description of oral communication in situated and specialised contexts'. Documenting these features typically requires the development of a set of codes that can be applied consistently and which account for the full variation of forms in the data.

For the purposes of compiling a corpus, decisions about notation have consequences for automatic tagging procedures such as tokenisation, POS-tagging, and lemmatisation, as well as for the continued use of the corpus, since the level of annotation provided in one study may not be sufficient for another study when, for example, it is no longer possible to recover the audible aspects of prosody from the original recording.

It is often the case that the substantial work of collecting spoken health communication data is carried out by an interdisciplinary team and/or for the purposes of conducting various kinds of analysis. Thomas and Wilson (1996, p. 94) report the difficulties they experienced when combining methodologies in relation to data formatting. Their transcripts were prepared for conversation analysis and did not have punctuation, which they indicate was required for their automatic content analysis.

Collins and Hardie (2022) offer some recommendations for applying a transcript protocol that streamlines the re-operationlisation of transcripts produced for, say, qualitative ethnographic study, for an indexed corpus. These recommendations are the product of a study in which such a conversion was required and, noting the variable notation across the transcripts, Collins and Hardie (2022) suggest a regularised system that poses minimal disruption to routine transcribing practices but which establishes unique functions for brackets and other notations that are used to signal content meaning (such as redactions, unclear content, non-lexical vocalisations, etc.). The recommendations, therefore, are designed 'to generate minimal ambiguity when qualitative-research transcription data is mapped to [eXtensible Markup Language] or other structured format and operationalised as a searchable corpus' (Collins and Hardie 2022, p. 132). Furthermore, regardless of whether or not the transcripts are intended for corpus analysis, the conventions help to 'future-proof' the data, should the opportunity or desire to reconfigure the data as a corpus arise further down the line. For a more detailed account of spoken corpus construction, see Adolphs and Carter (2013) and Knight and Adolphs (2021).

2.3.3 Studies on spoken corpora of health communication

As we will see in Chapter 4, a number of studies have compiled corpora from television shows, as another type of simulated medical talk. Medical encounters, as depicted in television shows, are generally more accessible and may even be readily available as transcripts. Campos Silva (2021) describes the step-by-step process by which users can build a corpus of data from the medical drama *Grey's Anatomy*, based on transcripts that have been uploaded to a dedicated TV script website, using the online corpus compilation and analysis tool *Sketch Engine*. Subsequently, readers are guided on how to produce teaching materials based on the corpus data, for communicative tasks such as talking patients and relatives through difficult situations, e.g., organ donation (Campos Silva 2021). Law (2019, p. 140) similarly discusses the practical benefits of using fan scripts – which are often checked for accuracy through a form of 'peer review' when posted to fan websites – in the compilation of a corpus of scripts from the medical drama series *House, M.D.* Law (2019) still undertook a process of manual checking against the broadcast shows, as well as reformatting the files to remove all non-dialogue elements, such as fade-ins, scene headings, action sequences, scene transitions, mood brackets, parentheticals, commercial tags and character name tags. Nevertheless, much of the work of transcription had already been done.

Similar to television scripts, Partington (2002) explains how transcripts of government press briefings are often available online and researchers are also likely to be able to locate the recorded videos in order to check their quality. In reference to transcripts from White House press briefings, Partington (2002, p. 2) discusses how what is published online might differ from the audible delivery in that brief repetitions or recapitulations are omitted and intercalations are missing, the effect of which is that 'moments of hesitation, of tentativeness, tend to be hidden from the transcript reader'

(Partington 2002, p. 2). This matter can be further compounded when such texts are made more widely available through translation; Fu and Wang (2022) have found, through a corpus analysis, that in addition to a general pattern of simplification in translation, there is evidence for modifications in hedging strategies that align with rhetorical conventions for Chinese and American political press briefings, respectively. Furthermore, once these aspects of the data are omitted, they are very difficult or even impossible to recover. Cortes (2015, p. 52) describes working with a corpus of 43 machine-readable files that were 'converted to text format and manually cleaned of all non-linguistic annotation (pause markings, paralinguistic annotations such as laughter or coughing annotations, etc.)'. These files were not collected for the express purpose of conducting a corpus analysis but, rather, for a larger project in which various qualitative and quantitative approaches were applied to the same collection of texts representing medical interviews with patients to discuss diabetes management (see Antón and Goering 2015).

TASK 2.1

Imagine you are going to transcribe a video recording of a medical consultation for inclusion in a corpus. As an example, you might search for and watch a video recording of such an interaction online. Then consider the following questions:

- Beyond the use of words, what features of the communication seem to be contributing to the interaction (this might include paralinguistic features such as tone of voice, laughter and so on, as well as non-linguistic features such as gesture and body language)?
- How would you represent these features in your transcription, and do you foresee any challenges with this?
- On the basis of the above, what aspects of the communication might be lost from your analytical view when you represent this interaction in a corpus?

2.3.4 Collecting written texts

Turning our attention now to written texts, including digital and computer-mediated ones, it is fair to say that corpora representing these modes are generally far easier to build than those representing speech. The internet has undoubtedly transformed the process of corpus building, especially for studying written and computer-mediated language, as it can provide ready access to an unfathomable number of downloadable texts that already exist in an electronic format. These texts do not just constitute e-language, as many of them were originally 'written' (in the more traditional sense) but have since been made available on websites or through online archives. Such resources provide much more convenient means for corpus building than their original paper forms. For example, websites such as *LexisNexis* can be used to download the text from large numbers of news articles according to user-determined criteria. The Project Gutenberg website provides downloadable copies of literary texts which can then be stored and analysed as corpora. Meanwhile, if we are interested in studying academic texts, for example medical journals, we can use a tool such as *AntCorGen* (Anthony 2022a) to download texts in the health sciences and other disciplines. If we decide to download texts from online sources such as these, we may have to convert them into a format that is suitable for the tool we are using. This might mean that we need to convert some texts from one format to another, e.g., from a PDF into plain UTF8 text. There are numerous software tools that can perform such tasks quickly and effectively, such as *AntFileConverter* (Anthony 2022b).

If we want to collect data from a large number of websites or from websites which have a large number of pages, this process can be made easier using website copiers such as HTTrack or BootCat (Baroni and Bernardini 2004). Such tools can scrape all text and, in the case of the former, images and hyperlinks from user-determined webpages with impressive efficiency. Online texts can also be retrieved in a less structured manner using BootCat, which can compile a relatively unstructured corpus of texts in terms of registers by trawling the Web on the basis of a series of user-specified search terms.

To exemplify how online sources can be gathered for the construction of a corpus of health communication, Davies (2021) describes the procedures for building the News on the Web (NOW) corpus and its subsidiary Coronavirus corpus, which he reports comprised 900 million words. Referring to the compilation of the larger NOW corpus, Davies (2021, p. 584) explains that some of the restrictions imposed by the target sources (which had previously been Google News) render them uncollectable, which limits the possible completeness of the data. Davies (2021) explains that processes such as searching for articles, collecting URLs, downloading the materials and metadata, removing duplicates, cleaning the data, and part of speech (POS) tagging, can be performed automatically and that these procedures run continuously to update the NOW corpus and, likewise, the Coronavirus corpus, daily. To create the standalone Coronavirus corpus, Davies (2021, p. 588) established a comprehensive list of search terms derived from an initial keyword analysis of texts in which 'coronavirus', 'COVID', or 'COVID-19' occurred at least three times. A series of manual checks of samples of the resultant texts found that between 96%–99% of the collected articles were acceptably 'about' the COVID-19 pandemic (Davies 2021, p. 588). The Coronavirus corpus (Davies 2021), therefore, constitutes a very useful resource for exploring news coverage from the onset of the COVID-19 pandemic, not least because its compilation is the result of computational programming and processing power that is likely beyond the skills of most researchers in corpus linguistics.

The ubiquity of digital technologies likely means that other modes are influenced by communicative practices established in digital spaces, and, similarly, the universality of a health issue such as the global COVID-19 pandemic can make it difficult to establish a focus on any other health topic in the 'COVID context'. Jones et al. (2023, p. 3) set out to collect tweets about the pandemic but came to the realisation that 'it is hard to draw the line between messages exclusively "about" the coronavirus and those about continuing UK public health concerns such as cancer, stroke, cardiovascular disease, mental health, diabetes and so on'. Nevertheless, they maintained an inclusive approach to data collection with the understanding that the impact of the COVID-19 pandemic could be felt in relation to the delivery of services for other health concerns. By way of example, references to 'additional' measures and the context of 'the current situation' demonstrate that even when the pandemic was not mentioned in explicit, searchable terms, there were, nevertheless, allusions to its influence (Jones et al. 2023).

If the texts we want to include in our corpus are not readily available in an electronic format, or they do exist electronically but as graphics files that are not amenable to corpus processing, then these will have to be converted into a format that is suitable for corpus analysis. This can be done by keying those texts in by hand or, if their print is of sufficient quality, by scanning them using optical character recognition (OCR) software. In most cases, scanning texts is more efficient than keying them in by hand, which can be extremely time-consuming. However, scanning also presents issues, as OCR software can struggle to process certain types of texts, particularly those with an unconventional layout, such as websites and newspaper articles which have vertically parallel columns (for which the OCR software finds it difficult to determine where one line ends and another begins). OCR software can also be prone to error, especially when processing texts that are damaged or have low print quality. This issue can be particularly apparent when compiling corpora of historical written texts, for which the results will usually have to be corrected by hand. The manual correction of OCR output for any type of text can be very time-consuming and generally becomes more painstaking the larger our corpus is (and, of course, the poorer the quality of the output is). This process is relevant to the next step in corpus construction: cleaning.

2.4 Cleaning

The texts we collect for a corpus often require further processing before we can start analysing them, as some of their features can adversely influence the accuracy of the analytical procedures we intend to carry out. One issue that frequently arises in the compilation of corpora containing online and some other types of written texts relates to the presence of so-called 'boilerplate' text. This refers to the language that occurs within a text but which is likely to constitute 'noise' in the context of a linguistic or discourse analysis and which can, therefore, hinder our research. For example, if we download news articles from the *LexisNexis* website mentioned earlier, the text files we receive will include labels which indicate, among other things, the 'headline', 'byline', and the name of the 'author' of the article. When occurring in every text in the corpus, such elements can accumulate quickly and become problematic for frequency-based analytical measures. There are some tools that can help with this. For example, *WordSmith Tools* (Version 7 onwards) now includes a 'boilerplate removal' function which is much faster than manually removing such elements by hand. However, rather than simply removing such elements, we may wish to use them as a form of metadata, in which case they can provide the basis for corpus annotation (discussed in the next section). Deciding on what counts as 'boilerplate' material is a subjective judgement which has to be made by the researcher and will depend on our research aims.

Another issue that can arise during the collection of (particularly online, written) texts is the presence of duplicate material. For example, *LexisNexis* can store multiple versions of a single news text, e.g., the online and print versions of an article, as separate downloadable files. This issue is exacerbated further in the case of online news articles that report on developing stories, as such articles are typically updated throughout the day, each time producing a 'new' article, with all updated versions being stored as separate texts in repositories such as *LexisNexis*. As with boilerplate text, duplicated material can skew the results of frequency-based corpus analytical techniques and can also hinder the representativeness of our corpus in a more general sense. Existing corpus analysis tools can, again, provide some assistance here. From Version 7 on, *WordSmith Tools* includes a 'duplicate text' function which allows users to group texts in a corpus according to a user-determined threshold of linguistic similarity. This allows users to check high-similarity results and, if they wish, to remove duplicate texts from the corpus. Another approach that can be used to identify duplicate texts is to search for long strings of words that are used repeatedly, such as recurrent seven-word strings. Because such lengthy strings of words rarely recur in natural language, their repeated use can indicate the presence of duplicate texts. Whatever approach is taken, there is no entirely reliable automated way of identifying and removing duplicate texts, so this is a task that will require some checking by the corpus builder. Furthermore, as with the identification of boilerplate material, deciding on what counts as a duplicate text is up to the corpus compiler to decide and will depend on the aims of our research.

Another consideration that attends to corpus cleaning pertains to the presence of non-standard orthography. Inconsistent orthographic representation is a characteristic feature of much user-generated online language. Such texts can contain typos, abbreviations and spelling mistakes (Barton and Lee 2013). Meanwhile, texts sampled from different geographical locations and historical periods can exhibit distinct spelling conventions even within the same language. One of the reported characteristics of written health documents in clinical contexts is the high frequency of abbreviations, domain specific acronyms, and incomplete sentences (Dalianis 2018). The prevalence of non-standard forms is further emphasised in historical texts, which might use what are now outdated spelling conventions. The preference for non-standard forms can tell us something about the discursive representation of health issues. In their preparation of the RIDGES herbology corpus, for example, Schnelle et al. (2022) discuss the need for manual normalisation and tokenisation prior to manual annotation of references to menstruation, which is made difficult, in part, because of the vagueness of terms such as '(*ihre*) *Zeit*' ('their time'). This highlights a convention for using euphemistic terms.

Unless such variation is to form part of the analysis, we might decide to standardise the spelling in the texts in the corpus in order to improve the accuracy of word frequency counts and other frequency-based measures. Tools such as *VARD* (short for 'Variant Detector' (Baron 2011)) can assist in this process. *VARD* uses techniques from modern spell checkers to detect spelling variants and find candidate equivalents. Using this software, then, users can quickly scan for instances of non-standard orthography in their corpora and decide for each case whether to replace the non-standard uses with an alternative rendering or retain them in their current form. And indeed, although *VARD* was developed for the study of historical texts, we can also see its potential to be applied to modern medical texts. Pakhomov et al. (2005) report that the content of clinical notes from the Mayo clinic comprised 30% non-word tokens, abbreviations, acronyms, misspellings, wrongly used grammar, etc. This represents a significant amount of the data which is unlikely to be recognised according to the standard programming of automatic tokenisers, lemmatisers, and speech taggers. Even in cases in which standard orthographic forms are used, Dalianis (2018, p. 22) notes that accounts of events in patient records tend to be 'short and efficient, and written in telegraphic style', which might disrupt the computation of POS-tags. Decisions relating to regularisation are consequential to how units of analysis are counted and queried, which we need to balance with respect to maintaining the texts' authenticity. This is particularly important given that such features tell us not only about spelling conventions but also about register norms.

Hunt and Harvey (2015, p. 136) recount their deliberations around the appropriate procedures for cleaning up their user query data (taken from a health advice website) in terms of balancing the extent to which they would standardise the text context – thereby optimising the computational analysis – versus preserving the authenticity of users' queries. Smith et al. (2014) determined that 7.6% of tokens in the Teenage Health Freak data used non-conventional or non-standard spelling. While some of these can be interpreted as typographical errors (e.g., 'iam' for 'I am'), other instances appear to be deliberate, expressive modifications, such as 'sooooo' (i.e., elongated 'so'). These authors subsequently carried out a comparison of the keyword lists derived from the 'corrected' and 'uncorrected' data, reporting that while the 'uncorrected' list logically generates more entries, differences in the rank positions of keywords appearing on both lists were small (Smith et al. 2014). This suggests that procedures for obtaining keywords are reasonably robust and that prevalent terms can be identified without corrective processes or regulation of non-standard orthography.

Certain factors, however, can mean that rates of non-conventional spelling are higher, resulting in a higher proportion of the data that might otherwise be overlooked without some kind of regularisation. In their analysis of below-the-line comments attached to news articles on obesity, Brookes and Baker (2021) remind us that one of the drivers behind creative orthography in digital spaces is to circumvent moderation practices, with users typing 'cr#p' in place of 'crap', for instance. Their response was to introduce a degree of standardisation, which they executed using the aforementioned *VARD* tool. In this case, *VARD* allowed the researchers to collate variants of words for the purposes of frequency-based analyses, without losing sight of the variations of the lexical form.

Whether we decide to standardise the spelling in our corpus will likely depend on the aims of our analysis, then. If we decide to standardise the spelling, it is important to describe this process as fully as possible when documenting the design and construction of the corpus, and it can be a good idea to retain the original spellings in some form (e.g., in separate, 'unedited' version of the corpus files, or using some form of annotation – introduced in the next section). Even if this information does not appear to be immediately relevant or useful, it is good practice to 'future-proof' your corpus, and retaining such information can help to expand the kinds of analyses that can be carried out on the corpus at a later point in time.

2.5 Annotation

Once they have been assembled, corpora can be encoded – or 'annotated' – with additional information relating to the texts or language(s) they contain (Leech 1997). This information can allow for more sophisticated types of analyses to be carried out on a corpus. This information can take several forms. McEnery and Hardie (2012) identify three types of information that we might want to include in annotation: metadata, textual mark-up, and linguistic annotation. The first type, metadata annotation, refers to information about the text itself. For a spoken text, such as our earlier example of a corpus of healthcare interactions, this might include details about the context in which the interaction took place and demographic information about the participants. For a written text such as a newspaper article, this might include information about the article's author, the newspaper it was published in, and its date of publication (it is at this point where the kind of 'boilerplate' text we discussed earlier can come into use). Such information can help us to focus on particular groups (e.g., healthcare interactions involving female doctors) or particular types of texts (e.g., tabloid newspapers rather than broadsheets), or to divide our corpora up in ways that allow us to make comparisons according to these and other variables.

The second type of annotation, textual mark-up, is typically used to represent paralinguistic features of the texts in the corpus. For a corpus of spoken healthcare interactions, this might involve marking out features such as laughter or the use of accompanying modes such as gestures (to capture the latter we would, of course, need to use video as well as audio recording at the point of data collection). For a written text, such as a newspaper article, we might use textual mark-up as a way of indicating the presence of certain format features, such as the use of bold or italicised text, or to mark where paragraphs start and end or where images might occur.

Finally, linguistic annotation can be used to mark the language in the texts in our corpus for certain kinds of (implicit) linguistic information that will be helpful for our analysis. For example, we can linguistically annotate our corpus with information about parts of speech, lemmas, grammatical structures, and semantic categories, among other features. Whether we annotate our corpus, and the types of information we include if we *do* decide to annotate it, will depend on the kinds of analysis that we intend to carry out, as well as the resources that are available to us.

Resources for annotating corpora with linguistic information are developing all the time. As well as online systems which provide such features as part of speech and semantic annotation, tools such as *#LancsBox* (Brezina et al. 2015) and *Sketch Engine* (Kilgarriff et al. 2014) provide annotation for parts of speech in a range of languages. A popular semantic tagging system is the University Centre for Computer Corpus Research on Language (UCREL) semantic analysis system (USAS) (Wilson and Thomas, 1997). This tag set comprises 21 major fields which include, for example, 'General and Abstract Terms', 'The Body & the Individual', 'Arts & Crafts' and 'Emotional Actions, States & Processes', among many others. Words allocated to these fields can also be assigned to more specific sub-fields. For example, the field 'The Body

& the Individual' sub-divides into the more specific categories: 'Anatomy and Physiology', 'Health and disease', 'Medicines and medical treatment', 'Cleaning and personal care', and 'Clothes and personal belongings'.

Metadata, textual mark-up, and linguistic annotation are all typically encoded in corpora using eXtensible Markup Language (XML). XML is standard not only in the annotation of corpora but also for tasks such as reliably transferring webpages and word processor documents. Using XML, tags are contained within angular brackets and surround the text to which they refer (e.g., <tag> *text* </tag>). Collins and Hardie (2022) discuss the use of XML to document paralinguistic aspects of interactions between patients and health professionals in emergency departments. In the extract below, we can see how utterance boundaries are marked (<u>, </u>) and attributed to different speakers using alphanumeric IDs (SP001, SP002, etc.). Furthermore, we can incorporate transcriber notes for textual mark-up, indicating where there are other audible sounds originating with a participant (cough) or another source in the surroundings (machine beeping), uncertainties regarding the perceptibility of the spoken content (<unclear>) and delineating pauses of varying duration (i.e., short).

```
<u who="SP001">
        Hello <unclear>how</unclear> are you
</u>
<u who="SP002">
        Quite well <voc desc="cough"/> thank you
</u>
<event desc="machine beeps"/>
<u who="SP001">
        I'm very <pause dur="short"> glad
        to hear it
</u>
```

The use of angular brackets makes the tags and the text between the open and closed tags searchable when using corpus analytical software but also allows the words within the brackets (i.e., the tags themselves) to be excluded from analytical procedures. This ensures that the tags applied to the texts in the corpus will not appear as part of the sample and will not interfere with analytical processes and skew frequency-based measures.

Brookes et al. (2022, p. 12) were interested in narratives that occurred as part of patient feedback on the National Health Service (NHS) across a range of ratings (1–5). The research team manually tagged a sample of 500 comments (comprising a random selection of 100 comments for each rating) using XML mark-up for the narrative components outlined by Labov and Waletzky (1967). Their markup enabled them to investigate not only the presence of narratives in the feedback comments but also the position and frequency of distinct narrative elements. Following this, Brookes et al. (2022) qualitatively analysed the persuasive properties of the narratives, discussing how they function to construct a version of events that is imbued with evaluations. Thus, while the process requires meticulous annotation – and cross-checking for consistency – the tagging facilitated a corpus-assisted analysis of more complex discourse-level phenomena (in this case, elements of a narrative), compared with standard corpus querying.

We can annotate the texts in a corpus automatically, semi-automatically, or manually. Automatic annotation is fast and convenient, which naturally makes it appealing. For some tasks, automatic annotation can be carried out with a high degree of accuracy. For example, the CLAWS tagger annotates texts for parts of speech with a rate of accuracy of approximately 97%. However, some types of texts can be particularly challenging for automated taggers. For example, because taggers tend to be trained on edited texts containing standard language use, these tools can struggle to parse texts that contain unpredictable or non-standard spelling and grammar, such as unedited user-generated social media posts. Automated taggers also struggle to process texts that contain more than one language; indeed, McEnery and Hardie (2012, p. 31) note the general 'patchiness' of taggers for languages other than English as a challenge to the field of corpus linguistics. Whatever approach we take, and regardless of the type of text we are annotating, it is always advisable to manually check (at least a sample of) automatic tags in order to assess the tagger's performance and, if necessary, to correct errors in the wider corpus.

Leech (1993) proposed seven maxims for good practice in annotation, which should be followed as closely as possible (McEnery and Wilson 2001, pp. 33–34):

1. it should be possible to remove the annotations and revert back to the raw corpus;
2. it should be possible to extract the annotations themselves from the texts for storage elsewhere;
3. the annotation scheme should be based on guidelines that are available to the end user of the corpus;
4. it should be made clear how and by whom the annotation was carried out;
5. the end user should be made aware that the annotations are not infallible;
6. annotations should be based, as far as possible, on widely agreed upon and theory-neutral principles; and
7. no annotation scheme has the *a priori* right to be considered as a standard; standards, where they exist, emerge through practical consensus.

(As summarised by McEnery and Brookes 2022, p. 44)

Annotation can add value to a corpus, making it easier to organise corpora (and within that, sub-corpora) into contextually meaningful categories as well as enabling linguistically meaningful patterns to be identified and searched for more easily. It is, of course, possible for the researcher to manually check and correct erroneous tags assigned to a corpus by a computational tagger, and above we have advised that users follow this practice. However, we should also bear in mind that the larger the corpus we are dealing with, the more laborious and less practical this process of manual checking becomes. Overall, annotation can be time-consuming and resource-draining, even with computational assistance. It only makes sense, then, to apply tags to a corpus if you can envisage ways in which the resultant tags could enrich either your own analysis or the analysis of those with whom you might share the corpus in the future. Ultimately, annotation is not essential for corpus analysis, and it is not good practice to annotate a corpus just for the sake of it.

2.6 Ethical considerations

Ethical considerations are a crucial part of any corpus study; while we have placed our discussion of them towards the end of this chapter, in reality, such considerations pervade all aspects of a corpus study and should be borne in mind right from the beginning of it. Ethical standards and principles in corpus building are, as in other areas of linguistics, widely debated and there is no "gold standard" for researchers to follow when building corpora. While research ethics can be viewed from a range of perspectives (see De Costa 2016), the 'protection of human subjects, including obtaining participant consent [...] and maintaining confidentiality of research data, is perhaps the prototypical concern in research ethics and certainly an important one' (Isbell et al. 2022, p. 173). Professional organisations and institutional review boards typically advise that informed consent should be obtained from participants in any study *before* their language is collected. This now represents standard practice not only in corpus linguistics research, but in applied linguistics research generally.

Some researchers argue that for ethical purposes, we should draw a distinction between texts that exist within public and private domains – with the implication that because texts existing within private domains are likely intended for private audiences, informed consent from their authors is required before these can be collected and studied. However, this is a general guide, and the mode and medium of the language collected can also influence our ethical considerations when building a corpus. When collecting written texts, it can be important to obtain the informed consent of those who composed the texts in question. This concern becomes particularly acute when the texts in question were not originally intended for public consumption (e.g., private letters or emails). For written texts that have been produced for public consumption (e.g., novels, newspapers, and academic journal articles), informed consent is not typically required. However, in such cases, copyright restrictions might mean that permission has to be sought from the copyright holder before a text can be included in a corpus. When compiling corpora of written texts, it is standard practice in the field to obtain informed consent from participants *after* the text has already been written but *before* it is included in the corpus, unless there is legal provision that does not require that (Brookes and McEnery 2021). In the UK, for example, the provisions of copyright legislation in the UK permits the use of electronic texts for research as of right, with professionally published texts being produced in full knowledge of these legal provisions, making the seeking of further permission unnecessary (McEnery and Brookes 2022).

For the compilation of spoken language corpora which contain recordings or transcripts of speech, informed consent will have to be obtained from the participants prior to the recording taking place. As with the collection of written language, the distinction between public and private domains is an important one; spoken language produced for a mass public audience (for example, in a film or television programme) typically does not require informed consent to be obtained from those who produced that speech. However, again, copyright restrictions may have to be taken into consideration when collecting such texts.

Perhaps the most ethically challenging textual mode for corpus linguists to collect is online, computer-mediated communication. Any practical benefits of having such born-digital language readily available in an electronic, corpus-friendly format are often swiftly counterbalanced by the lack of standardised ethical practice regarding the collection of such data. In view of the variability in the forms and contexts of what might fall under the broad moniker of 'online communication', there is an increasing movement within the field (and beyond) to reject so-called 'blanket policy' approaches in favour of more process-driven ones. Within such process-driven approaches, ethical decisions are made on a case-by-case basis and should respond to each stage of a study (identifying a potential research field, accessing the site, gathering data, publishing results, etc.) (see Hunt and Brookes 2020).

A challenge we are particularly likely to face when designing and assembling corpora of online language concerns the – at best, blurry – distinction between private and public domains. As we have noted, the former is widely accepted to be more likely to require informed consent be sought from participants. However, discerning between private and public domains can be difficult when it comes to online contexts. Users can capitalise on the broadcast functions of social media, for example, but simultaneously engage in very personal conversations with their close friends through the same platform. Similarly, users might withhold personal details in a digital space, remaining a silent observer of a discussion of a pertinent health topic or conversing in generalities; alternatively, they might provide specific details about very personal experiences as part of a strategy for establishing legitimacy as an 'expert patient' (Fox et al. 2005). At the same time, there are indications that users recognise the flexibility afforded by digital platforms for managing these options themselves. Kinloch (2018, p. 67) describes her efforts to collect informed consent for her study on infertility blogs as follows:

> Bloggers were contacted via email and given the opportunity to remove their data from the study prior to data collection [...] No bloggers actively withdrew from the study, however 5 blogs changed their security settings from public to password protected and I chose to remove these from the study, as I no longer felt them to be public domain from an ethical viewpoint.

This example suggests that at least some users are familiar with security settings and the mechanisms through which they can manage their own visibility and inclusion. Nonetheless, we should continue to be transparent about our procedures and reasoning around our inclusion of participants.

The example of Kinloch's study also brings us to another concern which further complicates the public–private distinction when it comes to online contexts of communication; namely, users' expectations and understandings of how their online information will be used, even if this information exists in a publicly accessible space. This is because, as Hunt and Brookes (2020, p. 72) put it,

> From a technical perspective, many online contexts – and particularly websites whose content is predominantly user-generated – are freely accessible to the public, with their content comparable to a publicly authored digital book [...]. From this perspective, web users have opted to communicate in a public setting and their data can be used for research purposes without their notification or consent. However, even while technically public, web users may nevertheless perceive their interactions as at least partially private and can suffer harm when information that they perceived to be private is published in different contexts.

As a means of overcoming this challenge, some researchers have drawn on Nissenbaum's (2010) model of 'contextual integrity' when trying to understand the norms and expectations that are likely to be held by members of online communities regarding the use and flows of their information (see, for example, Mackenzie 2017). However, others have raised doubts regarding just how feasible it is for corpus compilers to achieve 'contextual integrity' when the size and scope of their corpora are likely to mean that their data represent a likely larger number of unknown (and in many cases, unknowable) participants compared to the types of datasets that are typically used in more ethnographically oriented studies of online communication (see Collins 2019).

TABLE 2.1 Dimensions of research and level of risk (adapted from Giaxoglou 2017)

Dimensions of research	Low risk	High risk
1. Types of data	Large scale or 'big' data obtained via computerised programmes (e.g., java, API protocols)	'Small' data obtained via ethnographic observation methods, interviews, surveys, online ethnographies
2. Methodology	Quantitative	Qualitative
3. Site/platform	Sites/platforms with privacy settings (e.g., Facebook)	Sites/platforms without privacy settings (e.g., early days of MySpace)
4. Research focus	Focus on large-scale trends Focus on discourse patterns Focus on texts	Focus on persons and their lives

Beyond the public–private distinction, we should also consider the potential risks of carrying out the research, in terms of the harm that might be brought to those whose texts we are collecting. Weighing up the benefits of the research against the potential for harm is, of course, not straightforward, and decisions in this regard are not to be taken lightly. Giaxoglou (2017), following Page et al. (2014), offers a matrix for determining the level of risk that a study's design is likely to pose to participants (summarised in Table 2.1).

A study situated closer to the higher risk characteristics along these dimensions of research should, it is suggested, necessitate greater researcher precaution. However, as Hunt and Brookes (2020) point out, corpus studies might not fit neatly into these dimensions, as corpus analyses typically involve both quantitative and qualitative elements, and some corpora contain texts produced across different sites of online interaction, each with different privacy settings.

Existing frameworks guiding linguistic research are perhaps more ideally suited to qualitative (often ethnographic) studies than to corpus studies. The guidelines and principles described above can, therefore, provide a useful guide when compiling a corpus, but it is advisable to be flexible and to pursue a 'process-driven' approach, alongside becoming as familiar as you can with the online environment you are researching, in order to make informed and contextually sensitive decisions regarding ethical requirements. To get a sense of what such an approach might look like in the context of a corpus study of health communication, we can consider Hunt and Brookes's (2020) research on the discourse around mental illness in online support groups. Hunt and Brookes (2020) gathered data from websites which they deemed represented 'public' more than 'private' spaces on the basis of the following criteria:

- did not require registration or permission to access;
- contained visually prominent user guidelines which emphasised the public nature of the forum and/or the breadth of people that may read users' contributions and did not prohibit research from taking place on the site;
- had a large number of members (ranging, in their case, between several hundreds and tens of thousands of users), which is argued to correlate with contributors' perceptions that their messages will have a wide-ranging audience (see Eysenbach and Till 2001); and
- offered a facility for users to communicate more privately (e.g., direct messages and password-protected sub-fora).

Following Giaxoglou (2017), who recommends analysing online contributors' discourse to understand their orientation to the context as more private or public, Hunt and Brookes (2020) also observed how the contributors in their study typically oriented to a wider audience, indicated in uses of plural first-person pronouns to speak on behalf of the forum, as well as the presence of thread-initial posts addressed to 'anyone' or 'everyone'.

As corpus compilers, our commitment to the participants in our study should extend beyond considerations around informed consent, and another consideration which cuts across corpora of all modes pertains to participant anonymity. If the texts in the corpus are not publicly available, then they may need to be anonymised. This will certainly need to be done if this was what was agreed with the participants as part of the informed consent process and/or if an ethics review board requires it. Generally speaking, though, even if the texts in the corpus are available in the public domain, approaches to corpus compilation increasingly emphasise the importance of protecting the identities of the participants involved. As a consequence, corpora of written, spoken, and digital interactions are typically subjected to a process of de-identification. In this process, references to names and other personally identifying information are manually modified or removed. This process is particularly important if the corpus is to be made publicly available. However, for corpora which are not to be shared beyond the immediate research team, it can be sufficient just to anonymise data extracts reproduced for public consumption (e.g., in research articles) rather than having to anonymise the corpus itself.

Modifying or removing identifying information from written texts can be labour-intensive but is not particularly complicated. This is also the case for corpora which contain spoken transcripts or recorded speech. However, preserving participants' anonymity becomes a much more complex task when dealing with audio or video recordings of conversations. Knight and Adolphs (2021, p. 27) point out that this is because

Audio data is 'raw', existing as an 'audio fingerprint' of vocalisations that are specific to an individual [...]. A similar problem arises with the use of video data. Although it is possible to shadow, blur or pixelate video data in order to conceal the identity of speakers, these measures can be difficult to apply in practice (especially with large datasets).

Knight and Adolphs (2021) argue that it is important to discuss such anonymisation issues with participants *prior to* recording to ensure that participants understand what will be captured by the recordings and how this will be used (and possibly distributed).

Regarding the compilation of corpora of online language, even if we judge a particular online communicative context to constitute a public rather than private domain, corpus compilers should be mindful that many of the people contributing to such platforms are unlikely to have envisaged their language being reproduced as data extracts within academic publications. One way of protecting participants' identities can be to use pseudonyms to refer to the sites or online communities from which the texts in the corpus were sampled as well as removing references to participants' (online and offline) identities in quoted extracts from the data. Yet here, the searchability of online texts presents an additional challenge and one which may become even more pronounced when sampling language that is produced around sensitive topics or by groups that might be perceived as vulnerable (as is often the case in health communication research). One way to approach this is to sample texts from websites which, at least at the point of data collection, are not indexed on search engines in a way that means they can be reached by typing in a stretch of text from, say, a forum post contained within it. This measure can help to ensure that participants' online profiles cannot be easily identified using quoted data.

As well as thinking about the participants in a corpus, ethical considerations should also address the role of the researcher, both in terms of how their involvement might impact the participants and the research and how the researcher might be impacted by the research process itself. Beginning with the latter, it is important to reflect critically on how the data and the research process itself might impact the researcher(s) involved in a project and to anticipate how this might influence the research and the findings and to try to minimise or avert any risk of harm to the researcher(s). Such concerns might become particularly pronounced when researching vulnerable groups and sensitive health topics. It is a good idea to undertake a risk assessment as part of any application for ethical approval and to identify support mechanisms that can be accessed throughout the research process, including to respond flexibly to any unanticipated risk of harm.

Another way in which ethical issues can relate directly to corpus builders concerns the (perceived) impact that they might have on members of the communities they are accessing for the purposes of data gathering, particularly when this involves obtaining informed consent. When researching online discussions of sensitive topics, including those relating to health, researchers should be responsible, respectful, and sensitive in their approach to collecting, using, and reporting on the language produced by such groups. Such considerations, while important, can introduce additional complexities when compiling a corpus. Elgesem (2015) urges those researching online communities concerned with sensitive health-related topics to weigh the need for informed consent against the implications of obtaining it. With this in mind, in the aforementioned study by Hunt and Brookes (2020), the researchers judged that requesting informed consent from a large number of mental health forum users might risk disrupting the fora and undermining their primary role as recovery-oriented communities (see also Nosek et al. 2002). They judged this risk to be greater than the potential harm that would likely be brought about by the passive observation they undertook of the fora, though as discussed above, they did take additional steps to preserve the anonymity of the forum participants who featured in their corpora.

In this section, we have addressed some of the main ethical issues which underpin corpus compilation but which importantly also go beyond it. Such considerations are, we hope to have demonstrated, likely to be influenced by the kind of language under study, the real-world contexts in which that language occurred, and, perhaps most importantly, the researcher's subjectivity and own ethical position. For this reason, we hope the discussion we have provided here will be of greater use to readers making such considerations when designing their own corpora and corpus studies, rather than simply issuing blanket guidelines which will not realistically be able to reflect the wide and ever-growing range of modes, contexts, and groups that are represented in corpus research on health communication. In general terms, ethics procedures should seek to minimise – and where possible, remove – the harm that research could do to both the researcher and the researched. The guidance and procedures put in place by institutional ethics boards and subject associations (such as, for example, the British Association for Applied Linguistics) are designed to help researchers navigate this process and, ultimately, to undertake ethically sound research. We would, therefore, encourage readers embarking on corpus studies of health communication to consult all available guidelines, to engage with discussions around ethical considerations in previous research in their field, and to liaise with their institutional ethics review boards.

TASK 2.2

Now we want to consider how we might go about designing a corpus that is suitable for studying a particular kind of health communication data. Imagine that, broadly, you want to explore how people talk about vaccinations. Consider the following questions:

- What would you like your corpus to represent in terms of language(s), geographical zone(s), context(s), individual(s), type(s) of text, topic(s) relating to vaccination, and time period(s)?
- Considering your answer to the above, what practical challenges do you anticipate with collecting data to account for any of these variables (e.g., will any of the languages, individuals, contexts, or time periods be particularly difficult to represent in your corpus)?
- What ethical considerations will have to be made, and what would be your approach to each of these? For example:

  - Would you favour interactions that are more public or more private?
  - What are the implications of this for the kinds of views that you will likely capture and represent in your corpus?
  - How would you go about seeking informed consent to include these contributions in your research?
  - What might be the consequences of publishing these perspectives, e.g., if they contain misinformation?

2.7 Chapter summary

In this chapter, we have explored some of the main theoretical and practical considerations that underpin corpus design and construction, focusing in particular on specialised, purpose-built corpora. The structure of the sections of this chapter broadly reflect the order in which much corpus design and construction occurs. However, as noted in the introduction, this is not hard and fast, and it is quite normal for corpus construction to be iterative. For example, it can be a good idea to undertake analysis on a small, 'pilot' version of a corpus before committing to constructing the corpus in its entirety. This can help researchers to identify problems and modify their corpus design accordingly. Ethics is an important aspect of the research process which pervades all its parts and which should certainly come into our thinking during the early stages of designing a corpus linguistics research project. There are also some potentially important aspects of corpus design and construction that we have not explored in much detail here, such as ways of sharing corpus data and evaluating representativeness following construction (for a discussion, see Egbert et al. 2022). Moreover, we have largely described the process of designing monolingual corpora, and it should be borne in mind that projects requiring multilingual corpora, or so-called 'parallel' corpora of different languages, will necessitate additional considerations regarding how such corpora are designed and then analysed (for a discussion, see Curry 2021).

This exploration has demonstrated how the decisions made throughout this process are shaped, first and foremost, by the aims of our research and the other purposes that we intend for our corpus. Beyond this, such decisions will be shaped by factors such as the mode and context of the communication we want our corpus to represent, ethical considerations, and practical constraints both in terms of the language (and volume of language) that is available to us and the resources we have available to collect and process it. Importantly, whatever choices we make, we should document these and the rationale behind them in a detailed and comprehensive manner. Doing so will make it easier during a project write-up, which will make it easier for others to evaluate, replicate, and potentially use our corpus in the future (should we decide to make it available to others).

Corpora of spoken language tend to be more taxing to construct – the speech must first be recorded and transcribed before it is included in the corpus. Written texts tend to be easier to collect, especially if they are readily available in a machine-readable format, otherwise we might need to use OCR software or key them in by hand before they can be analysed. Computer-mediated texts are usually the easiest type of text to collect for a corpus as they are often 'born-digital', which means that they are readily available in machine-readable format. Such texts can, therefore, be collected relatively quickly and usually will not have to be reformatted before they can be processed by corpus analytical software. However, these texts can present other challenges, particularly if they exist online first. User-generated texts such as social media posts can present particular ethical challenges and, because the language use they contain is generally unedited, non-standard spelling can skew the accuracy of frequency-based measures, while non-standard spelling and grammar can adversely affect the performance of automatic taggers. Such texts might therefore need to be 'cleaned' before use to standardise their spelling. Meanwhile, corpora containing texts obtained from repositories, such as newspaper articles, might need to be cleaned to remove duplicate results. All these processes can be carried out more efficiently using the tools introduced throughout this chapter.

Designing and building a corpus can be a lengthy, labour-intensive, and resource-sapping process. Planning is essential to minimise the risk of errors and wasted effort. The value of any corpus, essentially, lies in whether or not it is suitable for the purposes for which it is intended. Being clear about these purposes and about what we want our corpora to *represent* is, therefore, key to planning, and it is important to have a sense of these from the outset of the process of corpus design and construction. As part of the initial planning, it is also a good idea to survey existing resources; if there is an existing, publicly available corpus that suits our purposes, then we might be able to save ourselves considerable time and work by using that rather than constructing a new corpus from scratch.

Further reading

- Baker, P. (2023). *Using corpora in discourse analysis* (2nd edition). Bloomsbury.

Chapter 3 describes the processes underpinning the design, construction, and annotation of a corpus for discourse-based research. It includes discussion of critical considerations, for example relating to how large a corpus ought to be.

- Collins, L. (2019). *Corpus linguistics for online communication: A guide for research*. Routledge. https://doi.org/10.4324/9780429057090

Chapter 2 of this book provides a similar discussion to Baker's but focuses in particular on corpora composed of texts from online contexts. The chapter also provides a detailed discussion of ethical considerations attending to the collection of such texts.

- Egbert, J., Gray, B., & Biber, D. (2022). *Designing and evaluating language corpora: A practical framework for corpus representativeness*. Cambridge University Press. https://doi.org/10.1017/9781316584880

This book provides a detailed and critical discussion of considerations attending to the design and construction of corpora. It also describes how corpora can be evaluated in terms of their representativeness.

References

Adolphs, S., Brown, B., Carter, R., Crawford, P. & Sahota, O. (2004). Applied clinical linguistics: Corpus linguistics in health care settings. *Journal of Applied Linguistics, 1*(1), 9–28. https://doi.org/10.1558/japl.v1.i1.9

Adolphs, S. & Carter, R. (2013). *Spoken corpus linguistics: From monomodal to multimodal*. Routledge. https://doi.org/10.4324/9780203526149

Anthony, L. (2022a). *AntCorGen* (Version 1.2.0) [Computer Software]. Waseda University. https://www.laurenceanthony.net/software

Anthony, L. (2022b). *AntFileConverter* (Version 2.0.2) [Computer Software]. Waseda University. https://www.laurenceanthony.net/software

Antón, M. & Goering, E.M. (Eds.). (2015). *Understanding patients' voices: A multi-method approach to health discourse*. John Benjamins. https://doi.org/10.1075/pbns.257

Atkins, S. (2019). Assessing health professionals' communication through role-play: An interactional analysis of simulated versus actual general practice consultations. *Discourse Studies, 21*(2), 109–134. https://doi.org/10.1177/1461445618802659

Baker, P. (2023). A year to remember? Introducing the BE21 corpus and exploring recent part of speech tag change in British English. *International Journal of Corpus Linguistics*, online first. https://doi.org/10.1075/ijcl.22007.bak

Baroni, M. & Bernardini, S. (2004). BootCaT: Bootstrapping corpora and terms from the web. *Proceedings of LREC 2004* (pp. 1313–1316). ELDA.

Barton, D. & Lee, C. (2013). *Language online: Investigating digital texts and practices.* Routledge. https://doi.org/10.4324/9780203552308

Biber, D. (1993). Using register-diversified corpora for general language studies. *Computational Linguistics, 19*(2), 219–241.

Biber, D. (2004). Representativeness in corpus design. In G. Sampson & D. McCarthy (Eds.), *Corpus linguistics: Readings in a widening perspective* (pp. 174–97). Continuum.

Bonsignori, V. (2019). A multimodal analysis of spoken medical English in expert-to-expert interaction in TV programmes. *Ibérica, 37*, 115–140.

Brezina, V., McEnery, T. & Wattam, S. (2015). Collocations in context: A new perspective on collocation networks. *International Journal of Corpus Linguistics, 20*(2), 139–173. https://doi.org/10.1075/ijcl.20.2.01bre

Brookes, G. (2019). Insulin restriction, medicalisation and the Internet: A corpus linguistic study of the discourse of diabulimia in online support groups. *Communication & Medicine, 15*(1), 14–27. https://doi.org/10.1558/cam.33067

Brookes, G. & Baker, P. (2021). *Obesity in the news: Language and representation in the press.* Cambridge University Press. https://doi.org/10.1017/9781108864732

Brookes, G., McEnery, A., McGlashan, M., Smith, G. & Wilkinson, M. (2022). Narrative evaluation in patient feedback: A study of online comments about UK healthcare services. *Narrative Inquiry, 32*(1), 9–35. https://doi.org/10.1075/ni.20098.bro

Campos Silva, S. (2021). Exploring hospital interactions with Grey's Anatomy: Building and exploiting a TV series corpus for nursing vocational schools. In E. Le Foll (Ed.), *Creating corpus-informed materials for the English as a foreign language Classroom. A step-by-step guide for (trainee) teachers using online resources* (third edition). Open Educational Resource. https://elenlefoll.pressbooks.com. CC-BY-NC 4.0. https://dx.doi.org/10.5281/zenodo.4992504

Chen, E., Lerman, K. & Ferrara, E. (2020). Tracking social media discourse about the COVID-19 pandemic: Development of a public coronavirus Twitter data set. *JMIR Public Health and Surveillance, 6*(2), e19273. https://doi.org/10.2196/19273

Collins, L.C. (2019). *Corpus linguistics for online communication: A guide for research.* Routledge. https://doi.org/10.4324/9780429057090

Collins, L.C. & Baker, P. (2023). *Language, discourse and anxiety.* Cambridge University Press.

Collins, L.C. & Hardie, A. (2022). Making use of transcription data from qualitative research within a corpus-linguistic paradigm: Issues, experiences and recommendations. *Corpora, 17*(1), 123–135. https://doi-org.ezproxy.lancs.ac.uk/10.3366/cor.2022.0237

Cortes, V. (2015). Using corpus-based analytical methods to study patient talk. In M. Antón & E.M. Goering (Eds.), *Understanding patients' voices: A multi-method approach to health discourse* (pp. 51–70). John Benjamins. https://doi.org/10.1075/pbns.257.04cor

Curry, N. (2021). *Academic writing and reader engagement: Contrasting questions in English, French and Spanish corpora.* Routledge. https://doi.org/10.4324/9780429322921

Dalianis, H. (2018). *Clinical text mining.* Springer. https://doi.org/10.1007/978-3-319-78503-5_4

Davies, M. (2021). The coronavirus corpus: Design, construction and use. *International Journal of Corpus Linguistics, 26*(4), 583–598. https://doi.org/10.1075/ijcl.21044.dav

De Costa, P. (2016). *Ethics in applied linguistics research: Language researcher narratives.* Routledge.

Egbert, J., Gray, B. & Biber, D. (2022). *Designing and evaluating language corpora: A practical framework for corpus representativeness.* Cambridge University Press. https://doi.org/10.1017/9781316584880

Elgesem, D. (2015). Consent and information – Ethical considerations when conducting research on social media. In H. Fossheim & H. Ingierd (Eds.), *Internet research ethics* (pp. 14–34). Cappelen Damm Akademisk. https://doi.org /10.17585/noasp.3.1

Eysenbach, G. & Till, J.E. (2001). Ethical issues in qualitative research on internet communities. *British Medical Journal, 323*(7321), 1103–1105. https://doi.org /10.1136/bmj.323.7321.1103

Fox, N., Ward, K. & O'Rourke, A. (2005). The 'expert patient': Empowerment or medical dominance? The case of weight loss, pharmaceutical drugs and the Internet. *Social Science and Medicine, 60*(6), 1299–1309. https://doi.org/10.1016 /j.socscimed.2004.07.005

French, L. & Lapointe, S. (2016). Creating and exploring spoken corpora of health communication for second-language training purposes. In L. Pickering, E. Friginal & S. Staples (Eds.), *Talking At work: Corpus-based explorations of workplace discourse* (pp. 255–280). Palgrave Macmillan. https://doi.org/10.1057/978-1-137 -49616-4_11

Fu, R. & Wang, K. (2022). Hedging in interpreted and spontaneous speeches: A comparative study of Chinese and American political press briefings. *Text & Talk, 42*(2), 153–175. https://doi.org/10.1515/text-2019-0290

Giaxoglou, K. (2017). Reflections on internet research ethics from language-focused research on web-based mourning: Revisiting the private/public distinction as a language ideology of differentiation. *Applied Linguistics Review, 8*(2–3), 229–250. https://doi.org/10.1515/applirev-2016-1037

Gut, U. (2021). Spoken corpora. In M. Paquot & S. Th. Gries (Eds.), *A practical handbook of corpus linguistics* (pp. 235–256). Springer.

Hamilton, C., Adolphs, S. & Nerlich, B. (2007). The meanings of 'risk': A view from corpus linguistics. *Discourse & Society, 18*(2), 163–181. https://doi.org/10.1177 /0957926507073374

Hunt, D. & Brookes, G. (2020). *Corpus, discourse and mental health.* Bloomsbury.

Hunt, D. & Harvey, K. (2015). Health communication and corpus linguistics: Using corpus tools to analyse eating disorder discourse online. In P. Baker & T. McEnery (Eds.), *Corpora and discourse studies: Integrating discourse and corpora* (pp. 134–154). Palgrave Macmillan. https://doi.org/10.1057/9781137431738_7

Iedema, R., Merrick, E.T., Kerridge, R., Herkes, R., Lee, B., Anscombe, M., Rajbhandari, D., Lucey, M. & White, L. (2009). Handover–Enabling Learning in Communication for Safety (HELiCS): A report on achievements at two hospital sites. *The Medical Journal of Australia, 190*(S11), S133–S136. https://doi.org /10.5694/j.1326-5377.2009.tb02620.x

Isbell, D.I., Brown, D., Chen, M., Derrick, D.J., Ghanem, R., Gutiérrez Arvizu, M.N., Schnur, E., Zhang, M. & Plonsky, L. (2022). Misconduct and questionable research practices: The ethics of quantitative data handling and reporting in applied linguistics. *The Modern Language Journal, 106*, 172–195. https://doi.org /10.1111/modl.12760

Jones, C., Oakey, D. & O'Halloran, K.L. (2023). 'I will say the picture of the background is not related to the words': Using corpus linguistics and focus groups to reveal how speakers of English as an additional language perceive the effectiveness of the phraseology and imagery in UK public health tweets during COVID-19. *Applied Corpus Linguistics, 3*(1), 100053. https://doi.org/10.1016/j. acorp.2023.100053

Kennedy, G. (1998). *An introduction to corpus linguistics.* Longman. https://doi.org /10.4324/9781315843674

Kilgarriff, A., Baisa, V., Bušta, J., Jakubíček, M., Kovář, V., Michelfeit, J., Rychlý, P. & Suchomel, V. (2014). The Sketch Engine: Ten years on. *Lexicography, 1*, 7–36. https://doi.org/10.1007/s40607-014-0009-9

Kinloch, K. (2018). A corpus-assisted study of the discourses of infertility in UK blogs, news articles and clinic websites. Doctoral thesis, Lancaster University. https:// www.proquest.com/dissertations-theses/corpus-assisted-study-discourses -infertility-uk/docview/2150556146/se-2.

Knight, D. & Adolphs, S. (2021). Building a spoken corpus: What are the basics? In A. O'Keeffe & M. McCarthy (Eds.), *The Routledge handbook of corpus linguistics* (pp. 21–34). Routledge. https://doi.org/10.4324/9780367076399-3

Kučera, H. & Francis, W.N. (1967). *Computational analysis of present-day American English.* Brown University Press.

Labov, W. & Waletzky, J. (1967). Narrative analysis. In J. Helm (Ed.), *Essays on the verbal and visual arts* (pp. 12–44). University of Washington Press.

Law, L. (2019). Creativity and television drama: A corpus-based multimodal analysis of pattern-reforming creativity in House M.D. *Corpora, 14*(2), 135–171. https:// doi.org/10.3366/cor.2019.0167

Leech, G. (1993). Corpus annotation schemes. *Literary and Linguistic Computing, 8*(4), 275–281. https://doi.org/10.1093/llc/8.4.275

Leech, G. (1997). Introducing corpus annotation. In R. Garside, G. Leech & T. McEnery (Eds.), *Corpus annotation: Linguistic information from computer text corpora* (pp. 1–18). Longman.

Mackenzie, J. (2017). Identifying informational norms in Mumsnet Talk: A reflexive-linguistic approach to internet research ethics. *Applied Linguistics Review, 8*(2–3), 293–314. https://doi.org/10.1515/applirev-2016-1042

Mahlberg, M., Smith, C. & Preston, S. (2013). Phrases in literary contexts: Patterns and distributions of suspensions in Dickens's novels. *International Journal of Corpus Linguistics, 18*(1), 35–56. https://doi.org/10.1075/ijcl.18.1.05mah

McCarthy, M., & Carter, R. (2001). Size isn't everything: Spoken English, corpus, and the classroom. *TESOL Quarterly, 35*(2), 337–340. https://doi.org/10.2307 /3587654

McEnery, T. & Brookes, G. (2022). Building a written corpus: What are the basics? In A. O'Keeffe & M. McCarthy (Eds.), *The Routledge handbook of corpus linguistics* (second edition, pp. 35–47). Routledge. https://doi.org/10.4324 /9780367076399

McEnery, T. & Hardie, A. (2012). *Corpus linguistics: Method, theory and practice.* Cambridge University Press. https://doi.org/10.1017/CBO9780511981395

McEnery, T. & Wilson, A. (2001). *Corpus linguistics: An introduction* (second edition). Edinburgh University Press. https://doi.org/10.1515/9781474470865

Mishan, F. (2004). Authenticating corpora for language learning: A problem and its resolution. *ELT Journal, 58*(3), 219–227. https://doi.org/10.1093/elt/58.3.219

Moreno-Ortiz, A. & García-Gámez, M. (2023). Strategies for the analysis of large social media corpora: Sampling and keyword extraction methods. *Corpus Pragmatics.* Online first. https://doi.org/10.1007/s41701-023-00143-0

Nissenbaum, H. (2010). *Privacy in context: Technology, policy, and the integrity of social life.* Stanford University Press.

Nosek, B.A., Banaji, M.R. & Greenwald, A.G. (2002). E-Research: Ethics, security, design, and control in psychological research on the Internet. *Journal of Social Issues, 58*, 161–176. https://doi.org/10.1111/1540-4560.00254

Page, R., Barton, D., Unger, J.W. & Zappavigna, M. (2014). *Researching language and social media: A student guide.* Routledge. https://doi.org/10.4324/9781315771786

Pakhomov, S., Pedersen, T. & Chute, C.G. (2005). Abbreviation and acronym disambiguation in clinical discourse. *Proceedings of the AMIA annual symposium* (pp. 589–593). American Medical Informatics Association. https://www.ncbi.nlm.nih.gov/pmc/articles/PMC1560669/.

Partington, A. (2002). *The linguistics of political argument: The spin-doctor and the wolf-pack at the white house.* Routledge. https://doi.org/10.4324/9780203218259

Schnelle, G., Odebrecht, C., Lüdeling, A., Perlitz, L. & Fisher, C. (2022). "Die Blumenzeit der Frau": A corpus-based study of the development of medical references to menstruation in historical texts in herbology. In T. Hiltunen & I. Taavitsainen (Eds.), *Corpus pragmatic studies on the history of medical discourse* (pp. 153–176). John Benjamins. https://doi.org/10.1075/pbns.330.07sch

Slade, D., Manidis, M., McGregor, J., Scheere, H., Chandler, E., Stein-Parbury, J., Dunston, R., Herke, M. & Matthiessen, C.M.I.M. (2015). *Communicating in hospital emergency departments.* Springer. https://doi.org/10.1007/978-3-662-46021_4

Smith, C., Adolphs, S., Harvey, K. & Mullany, L. (2014). Spelling errors and keywords in born-digital data: A case study using the Teenage Health Freak Corpus. *Corpora, 9*(2), 137–154. https://doi.org/10.3366/cor.2014.0055

Thomas, J. & Wilson, A. (1996). Methodologies for studying a corpus of doctor–patient interaction. In J. Thomas & M. Short (Eds.), *Using corpora for language research.* (pp. 92–109). Longman.

Widdowson, H.G. (2000). On the limitations of linguistics applied. *Applied Linguistics, 21*(1), 3–25. https://doi.org/10.1093/applin/21.1.3

Wilson, A. & Thomas, J.A. (1997). Semantic annotation. In R. Garside, G. Leech & T. McEnery (Eds.), *Corpus annotation: Linguistic information from computer text corpora* (pp. 53–65). Longman.

3
ANALYSING A CORPUS

3.1 Introduction

In the previous chapter, we explored some of the considerations that attend to constructing or selecting a corpus for the study of health communication. Yet on its own, a corpus is not particularly useful for undertaking analysis of language. As we saw in the previous chapter, corpora are typically stored in a machine-readable format so that they can be analysed using computer software. Corpus analysis software can assist our analyses by helping us to carry out various procedures which would be impossible, or at least very impractical, to perform by hand. Such procedures, which are introduced in this chapter, allow us to search for every occurrence of a given word or combination of words; generate frequency information about words, chains of words, or grammatical types; perform statistical tests on those frequencies to measure the significance or strength of relationships between linguistic phenomena; and present the language in the corpus in ways that render it more amenable to manual, qualitative analysis.

We begin this chapter by looking at the different types of software tools that are available for storing and analysing corpora and by exploring some of the considerations that might guide our decision regarding which tool(s) we want to use. Following that, we introduce some of the main analytical procedures or techniques that such software tools allow us to perform on our corpus. Specifically, we explore frequency analysis, keyword analysis, collocation analysis, cluster analysis, and concordance analysis. Each technique is introduced in turn, with worked demonstrations based on a corpus of health communication data. As we work our way through these techniques, we broadly move from the more quantitative towards the more qualitative. There is no

DOI: 10.4324/9781003099659-3

'standard' approach to corpus analysis, and the techniques to be introduced in this chapter can be combined in various ways and used selectively or in conjunction with other techniques not considered here. Such decisions will depend on the type of analysis we want to carry out. Yet, as we will see, whatever approach we take, the human analyst is required to make a number of methodological choices which will shape the kinds of outputs the analytical software gives us. Then, importantly, those outputs must be interpreted by the human analyst (the computer cannot do it for us!).

3.2 Selecting a software tool

Before we can analyse our corpus, we must first decide what software tool we want to use. As noted in the previous section, corpora are generally queried using specialist software tools also known as 'concordancers'. Anthony (2022a) identifies three types of corpus software tools: (i) online tools, (ii) offline tools, and (iii) do-it-yourself (DIY) tools. These tools allow us to analyse our corpora and, in some cases, to compile, clean, and store corpora, too. We will now consider tools belonging to each of these types in turn, before briefly considering some of the main strengths and limitations of each. In keeping with the theme of this chapter, we focus here just on how these tools can support the *analysis* of corpora (rather than, for example, with text gathering, cleaning, and processing). Newcomers to corpus linguistics will likely find it easier to use tools belonging to the first two types (online and offline tools), as these do not require any programming skills on the part of the user. Moreover, the developers of such tools typically provide instructional videos and guides on how to use them. DIY tools, meanwhile, will likely appeal most to those with advanced programming skills.

Online tools typically exist in the 'cloud', which means that they 'reside on one or more remote servers and are developed, managed and updated remotely' (Anthony 2022a, p. 103). Examples of popular online tools include *CQPweb* (Hardie 2012) and *Sketch Engine* (Kilgarriff et al. 2014). Online tools are accessed through standard Web browsers, requiring an internet connection. Some are free to use, while others require the payment of a licence fee or subscription.

Offline tools, on the other hand, will need to be purchased as a standalone package or downloaded and manually installed onto a computer hard drive. Use of these tools, therefore, requires 'a computer with an operating system, hard disk space, and random access memory (RAM) that matches the requirements of the software' (Anthony 2022a, p. 103). Unlike online tools, offline tools are not managed by their creators. Therefore, it is up to the users of offline tools to make sure that they check for and install updates and use the most recent versions available. Popular examples of offline tools include *AntConc* (Anthony 2022b), *#LancsBox* (Brezina et al. 2015), and *WordSmith*

Tools (Scott 2020). Some offline tools are free to download (e.g., *AntConc*), while others require the payment of a one-off licence fee (e.g., *WordSmith Tools*).

Finally, DIY tools typically come in the form of 'scripts'. These are 'text files containing a list of commands that need to be executed by a scripting programming language, such as Python or R' (Anthony 2022a, p. 103). Such scripts are typically given as appendices or supplementary files accompanying research papers, or are published on personal websites or repositories such as GitHub.[1] Anthony (2022a, pp. 103–104) points out that 'DIY tools are often in a state of constant flux, with tools frequently created, updated, renamed, moved and deleted'. He offers two examples of DIY corpus tool repositories that are 'relatively stable but sit at the opposite ends of the scale in terms of size and scope' (ibid.). The first is the large library of Python scripts that constitute the Natural Language Toolkit.[2] The second is the more specialised series of R scripts provided alongside the book, *Quantitative Corpus Linguistics with R* (Gries 2016). Using DIY tools will, of course, require some knowledge of programming, and if you have more advanced programming skills, you might even choose to write your own script to suit the needs of your analysis. To read more about DIY tools and programming in corpus linguistics, see Anthony (2020).

Online, offline, and DIY tools each have particular strengths and limitations which are important to bear in mind. In some cases, such considerations can help to guide our decisions about which tool(s) to use for a study.

Beginning with online tools, these have the distinct advantage of being able to store very large corpora. Indeed, some corpora are too large to be feasibly stored on a personal computer, while some very large corpora are only available through interfaces built into online software tools. Online tools can also rapidly process such large corpora, for which the same procedures can take considerably longer to carry out using offline tools (and, in the case of exceptionally large corpora, can even cause offline tools to crash). Another advantage of using online tools is that these are maintained and updated by their developers, which means users can be sure that they are always using the latest version of the tool and will not have to check for or install updates. A disadvantage of online tools is that they can come to resemble something of a 'black box' technology – in many cases, it is not possible for users to access the raw corpus files (if using corpora hosted within the tools), and it is not clear what texts are included in the corpus and how these have been collected and cleaned. Another disadvantage is that many online tools do not allow users to upload their own corpus data. This can be particularly problematic for corpus research on health communication, which, as we discussed in Chapter 2, tends to utilise specialised, purpose-built corpora. Fortunately, more and more online tools are introducing the facility for users to upload and analyse their own corpora (this includes *CQPweb* and *Sketch Engine*, mentioned earlier).

An advantage of offline tools is that they facilitate direct access to the data. As Anthony (2022a, p. 107) observes, with offline tools, the corpus data 'can be viewed in its raw form, loaded into the tool and probed in various ways. In this way, offline tools are more transparent than online tools'. This, in many ways, is the inverse of the 'black box' problem associated with some online tools and might represent an advantage that offline tools have over their online counterparts. Likewise, some of the strengths of online tools correspond to weaknesses in offline ones, namely that the limited memory and processing power of personal computers means that the offline tools used on them can be sluggish and even crash when trying to process very large corpora. Of course, if the corpus we are analysing is small or moderately sized, this is unlikely to be an issue.

The main advantage of using DIY tools is that they allow users to work more flexibly with their corpora and to introduce innovative forms of visualisation and even potentially to develop new analytical approaches within corpus linguistics. Of course, the disadvantage of DIY tools is that users will have to acquire programming skills, even to implement existing scripts. To yield the full benefits of DIY tools and create innovative ways of analysing and visualising corpus data requires more advanced programming skills. While DIY tools are becoming increasingly popular in corpus linguistics, it remains the case that most users employ online or offline tools rather than carrying out programming themselves. This situation is liable to change in the future as the general level of proficiency in programming languages develops. Subsequently, DIY tools will likely play an ever-increasing role in corpus linguistics research.

Whether we use an online, offline, or DIY tool will depend on a number of factors, not least of which is the data we are analysing (some corpora are only available through the interfaces of online tools or might be too large to be stored offline). Another important consideration is the kinds of analytical techniques we want to use, as the available tools do not all offer the same analytical techniques and statistical measures. It is to such analytical techniques that we now turn our attention, beginning with frequency analysis.

3.3 Frequency analysis

Frequency essentially provides us with a list of all the words that are present in our corpus and tells us how often each word occurs. Many techniques in corpus linguistics are based on frequency, and generating frequency information about the words that occur in a corpus can provide a good starting point for an analysis, affording a rapid overview of the linguistic landscape of the data. Frequency information can be generated for individual words or recurrent sequences of two or more words. Many software packages also afford the possibility to obtain lemmatised frequency lists. If our corpus is annotated, for example reflecting the grammatical or semantic properties of the language in the corpus (see Section 2.5), some tools also allow us to assess the frequency of those tags. An example of a study of health communication based on assessing the frequency of tags is Cortes (2015), who collected a corpus of interviews with patients to consider what grammatical features were associated with those who were adherent to their treatment recommendations, compared with those who were not. Differences in the frequencies of categories of personal pronouns and present progressive tense markers, for example, directed Cortes (2015) to the ways that patients expressed attitudes about their health and the treatment that related to their motivations for compliance (this study is discussed further in Chapter 4). In most cases, frequency information is generated for individual words occurring in the corpus, and it is in this sense that terms such as 'frequency', 'frequency information', and 'frequency lists' tend to be used.

To demonstrate what frequency information looks like, Table 3.1 displays the ten most frequent words in a specialised corpus of newspaper articles on the topic of dementia. This corpus, which we will refer to as the *Daily Mail Dementia News Corpus*, contains articles published by the British tabloid newspaper the *Daily Mail* (including its Sunday and online editions), between 2013 and 2022. The corpus contains 1,970 articles which mention the word 'dementia' at least once in their headline and/or three or more times throughout the 'body' of the main article. This corpus amounts to 1,994,225 words. We generated this word frequency list using the previously mentioned software tool, *WordSmith Tools* (Version 8) (Scott 2020).

Table 3.1 contains four columns. The first shows the rank of the words in the corpus in terms of their frequency. The second column displays the word, while the third shows each word's frequency. The final column shows the number of texts in which each word is found, which can be useful if we want to assess a word's distribution in the corpus. In theory, this table could

TABLE 3.1 Top ten words in the *Daily Mail Dementia News Corpus*, ranked by frequency

Rank	Word	Frequency	Texts
1	*the*	95,734	1,970
2	*to*	56,955	1,967
3	*and*	49,440	1,965
4	*of*	49,028	1,965
5	*a*	44,473	1,969
6	*in*	38,046	1,961
7	*that*	20,750	1,893
8	*for*	20,457	1,928
9	*is*	20,353	1,892
10	*it*	18,532	1,839

extend to include every word-type found in the corpus. Focusing on the first row, we can see that the most frequent word in the corpus is 'the', which occurs 95,734 times across 1,970 texts. This is, in fact, the total number of texts in the data, meaning that the word 'the' occurs in 100% of the texts in the corpus.

If we consider the words themselves, we can see that this table is dominated by what might be referred to as grammatical or 'function' words, such as 'the', 'to', 'and', 'of', and so on. Indeed, the most frequent words in most corpora are such grammatical words, and this reflects their high density in general language (Leech et al. 2009). Studying the frequency and use of these kinds of grammatical items can be helpful for learning about the genre and register features of the texts in a corpus (Scott and Tribble 2006; Biber and Conrad 2009). However, such words reveal much less about the thematic content of the texts in the corpus and are likely to be less useful for studying discourse (Baker 2010), which is often the focus in corpus studies of health communication. For such a focus, it can often be more useful to focus on lexical or 'content' words (i.e., nouns, verbs, adjectives, and lexical adverbs). We can use a word list to study lexical words – indeed, Table 3.1 includes one ('dementia'). However, doing so usually requires us to filter our results and look further down the word list to extract such words manually. This is what we did to generate the list of the 20 most frequent lexical words in the corpus in Table 3.2.

As we can see, the most frequent lexical words in this corpus do, indeed, help us to learn more about the thematic content of the texts in the corpus, on the basis of which we might be able to develop hypotheses and hunches about how dementia is represented in this corpus and the discourses that surround it. Such topics include dementia and types of dementia ('dementia', 'alzheimer's', 'disease'), 'people' with dementia, the 'care' they receive and where they receive it ('(care) home'), the anatomical characteristics

TABLE 3.2 Top ten lexical words in the *Daily Mail Dementia News Corpus*, ranked by frequency

Rank	Words	Frequency	Texts
1	dementia	15,437	1,970
2	people	8,710	1,575
3	said	8,471	1,696
4	care	7,588	903
5	brain	5,164	981
6	alzheimer's	4,836	1,157
7	years	4,171	1,364
8	disease	4,168	1,185
9	home	3,990	846
10	risk	3,587	821

of dementia ('brain'), and factors which might influence people's 'risk' of developing the syndrome. We can also, perhaps, infer that there is evidence of a focus on time ('years') and the use of quoted speech to bring the perspectives of different social actors into the coverage ('said'). These are, as we have said, hypotheses or hunches about how these words are likely to be used based on our knowledge of the language and the genre of news texts. To substantiate these hypotheses and test them out, we would need to analyse more qualitatively how these words are, in fact, used in the texts in our corpus. We will see later in this chapter how corpus techniques can help in this process.

How we use frequency information will depend on the aims of our study. Word lists can be helpful to identify the frequencies and distributions of particular words of interest. Alternatively, we could use frequency in the kind of inductive way that we have above – scanning the word list and extracting lexical items for analysis and disregarding grammatical words in the process. However, in general, corpus linguists tend to be reluctant to *prima facie* disregard any word in the corpus, particularly if that word is especially frequent. A more statistically robust way of identifying words which reveal the thematic content of the texts in our corpus is to use keywords.

3.3 Keyword analysis

Keywords are words that occur statistically more frequently in the corpus we are analysing when compared against another corpus (Scott 1997). For the purposes of this comparison, we refer to the corpus we are analysing as the 'target' corpus, while the corpus that we compare it against is referred to as the 'reference' corpus. The reference corpus is usually equal in size to or larger than the target corpus and should represent a norm or 'benchmark' for the type of language being studied. For example, Adolphs et al. (2004) used the Cambridge and Nottingham Corpus of Discourse in English (CANCODE), which comprises 5 million words of general English, as a reference corpus against which to compare their 61,981-word corpus of telephone interactions between health advisors and patients (this study is discussed further in Chapter 4). By virtue of their markedly high frequency (relative to the reference corpus), keywords can be interpreted as reflecting language use that is characteristic of the texts in the target corpus.[3] For this reason, keywords are used as a way of quickly and reliably surveying the thematic content of a corpus, providing an inductive 'way in' to the corpus that typically precedes and guides more qualitative analysis (Baker 2023a; Mahlberg 2014).

Although keywords are calculated computationally in modern corpus linguistics, the procedure, nevertheless, requires the researcher to make a number of important decisions which will influence the kinds of keywords that are produced. One decision that we have already alluded to relates to the choice of reference corpus. As noted, the reference corpus serves as a norm or benchmark against which we can compare our target corpus. As such, the keywords generated will represent what is distinctive about the texts in our target corpus relative to that benchmark. When using keywords to study discourse, the reference corpus should, ideally, represent language that is matched to that in our target corpus in terms of register (i.e., speech, writing, computer-mediated language) and genre (i.e., casual conversation, newspaper articles, emails). This helps to ensure that the keywords will flag up what is lexically characteristic of the texts in our target corpus rather than generating keywords that arise due to variables at the level of genre and register (unless, of course, we are interested in studying such variables). Essentially, we should aim to use a reference corpus that is matched to our target corpus in terms of any variables that we would like to control in our analysis.

As well as selecting the reference corpus, we also have to decide what statistical measure we will use to determine the 'keyness' of each word in the corpus. There are a number of statistical tests available for measuring keyness. Gabrielatos (2018, p. 230) points out that '[a] core distinction made in any current introductory book on statistics is between effect-size and statistical significance'. Effect size indicates 'whether the difference or relationship we have found is strong or weak' (Mujis 2010, p. 70). Statistical significance, on the other hand, indicates 'the high probability that the difference between two means or other findings based on a random sample is not the result of sampling error but reflects the characteristics of the population from which the sample was drawn' (Sirking 2006, p. 306). Different software tools provide different options regarding statistical measures, so this might be a consideration when deciding which tool to use.

In the context of keyword analysis, then, effect size measures help us to focus on words with large (i.e., statistically marked) differences in frequencies between our target corpus and the reference corpus, whereas measures of statistical significance help us to ensure that the observed frequency differences are dependable. Effect size measures should be used to rank keywords, while statistical significance measures provide thresholds that can be used to provide a more robust 'cutoff' point for isolating keywords for closer analysis (see, for example, Hunt and Brookes 2020). Cutoffs can also be applied in relation to other factors. Most corpus software tools will ask users to stipulate a minimum frequency for keywords (a standard cutoff is five), and some researchers stipulate that keywords should occur in a minimum proportion of the texts in their data (ibid.). Such measures can be combined with statistical analyses; for example, in the aforementioned study by Hunt and Brookes (2020), the researchers stipulated that in addition to meeting the threshold for statistical significance, their keywords should also occur in at least 5% of the texts in their data.

To demonstrate what a keyword analysis might look like, we have generated keywords for the *Daily Mail Dementia News Corpus* introduced in the previous section. For our reference corpus, we used a corpus called BE21 (Baker 2023b), which contains just over 1 million words of written British English published in the year 2021. We stipulated that for a word to be considered 'key', it should occur at least 5 times in the target corpus and at least once in the reference corpus.[4] Keyword analysis can be more robust if we combine measures of significance with effect size. The significance measure we used was Log Likelihood (Dunning 1993). The threshold for the Log Likelihood score can be adjusted to establish a greater degree of confidence; a Log Likelihood score of 3.84 indicates a confidence level of 95% (standard in social sciences (McEnery 2006)), while a score of 6.63 indicates a confidence level of 99%. When generating the keywords in Table 3.3, we stipulated that keywords should have a Log Likelihood score of 15.13, which indicates a confidence level of 99.99%, i.e., the chance of a keyword resulting from a sampling error is 0.01%. Having generated a set of keywords that met our conditions for confidence, we then ranked them using the Log Ratio effect size measure (Hardie 2014; McEnery and Baker 2016, p. 23). This score reflects the size of the observed difference in relative frequency of each keyword between the target and reference corpus, with bigger differences producing higher Log Ratio scores. This combination of measures, therefore, uses Log Likelihood as a cut-off to ensure that keywords are significant, while the use of Log Ratio allows us to rank qualifying keywords according to how unusually high, or 'marked', their frequency is in the target corpus. For a discussion of the statistical measures that can be used in keyword analysis, see Gabrielatos (2018).

The top 20 keywords, ranked by Log Ratio score, are displayed in Table 3.3. In this table, we have also provided the relative frequencies of the keywords (normalised per million words (PMW)) in both the target and reference corpus because, as we will discuss later, it is the comparison of these frequency figures which underpins keyword analysis.

Before commenting on the keywords, it is useful to first clarify how these words have become keywords. Although frequency is a crucial factor in identifying keywords, high frequency alone is not enough for a word to be judged as 'key'. What is most important in determining whether or not a word is a keyword is the relative frequencies of the word between the two corpora being compared. For example, the top keyword in this table, 'dementia', occurs 7,740.85 times PMW in the *Daily Mail Dementia News Corpus*. This is much greater than its normalised frequency of 19.64 times PMW in the BE21 corpus. Therefore, the word 'dementia' is a keyword in our target corpus when its frequency is considered not simply on its own, but against the reference corpus, which is taken to represent some norm of usage.

TABLE 3.3 Top ten keywords in the *Daily Mail Dementia News Corpus* compared to BE21, ranked by Log Ratio score

Rank	Keywords	Target corpus		Reference corpus		Log Likelihood score	Log Ratio score
		Frequency	Frequency (PMW)	Frequency	Frequency (PMW)		
1	dementia	15,437	7,740.85	20	19.64	12474.07	8.62
2	alzheimer's	4,759	2,386.39	8	7.86	3825.65	8.25
3	charlton	307	1,53.944	1	0.98	242.01	7.29
4	plaques	255	127.87	1	0.98	199.48	7.02
5	cholesterol	245	122.85	1	0.98	191.31	6.97
6	inflammation	345	173.00	2	1.96	264.38	6.46
7	sufferers	515	258.25	3	2.95	394.53	6.45
8	barbara	994	498.44	6	5.89	759.78	6.40
9	footballer	156	78.23	1	0.98	118.77	6.32
10	footballs	138	69.20	1	0.98	104.17	6.14

As Table 3.3 shows, the keyword procedure has reliably filtered out the high frequency grammatical items which dominated our word frequency list in Table 3.1. Instead, what has been brought to the fore are words that are most characteristic of the language used in our corpus and which are more revealing in terms of the content, or 'aboutness' (Scott and Tribble 2006, pp. 59–60), of the dementia-related newspaper articles it contains.

One way we could go about analysing these keywords would be to group them into semantic categories reflecting the most characteristic themes in the corpus. Expectedly, we get keywords that are used to refer directly to dementia ('dementia') and more specific reference to the most common type of dementia, Alzheimer's Disease ('alzheimer's'). Other keywords are technical terms denoting parts of the anatomy that are linked to dementia ('plaques', 'cholesterol'), as well as relevant biological processes ('inflammation'). We can also see reference to people with dementia, in general terms ('sufferers') and in terms of public figures. Specifically, there is evidence of reference to the retired football player, Bobby Charlton ('charlton'), whose diagnosis was reported in the corpus, as well as actress, Barbara Windsor ('barbara'), whose life and death with dementia are reported on. Perhaps less expectedly, stories about Bobby Charlton belong to a wider genre of news articles in the corpus that are about the marked prevalence of dementia in retired football players, with the development of the syndrome being linked to the action of heading footballs. It is for this reason that 'footballer' and 'footballs' are also keywords.

Manual categorisation of keywords, such as the brief one we have presented here, should be based not just on 'eyeballing' the decontextualised words in the keyword list but by inspecting how those words are actually used within the wider contexts of the texts in the corpus. This is because words can be polysemous and perform multiple (sometimes unexpected) functions within and across texts. These various meanings and functions only become visible to us, as analysts, once we engage with how words are used within and across the texts of our corpus. It is through such qualitative engagement that we have been able to confidently group the keywords above into semantic categories, and later in this chapter we will introduce some of the techniques that can support this part of the analysis.

Because keywords are, as noted, relatively more frequent in the target corpus than in the reference corpus, they reflect what is lexically characteristic of language used in the target corpus compared against the language used in the reference corpus. The choice of reference corpus, therefore, shapes the keywords that will be produced, and using different reference corpora is likely to produce keywords that highlight lexical distinctiveness in different ways. To demonstrate this, the keywords in Table 3.3 show us words that are characteristic of the articles in the *Daily Mail Dementia News Corpus* relative to general written British English, as represented by the BE21 corpus. However, if we wanted to compare the coverage of dementia in the *Daily Mail* against other newspapers, we would require a different reference corpus.

To show what such an analysis might look like, we created a different corpus to use as a reference corpus – one that contains articles about dementia published in another British newspaper, *The Times*. We will call this corpus the *Times Dementia News Corpus*, and we gathered the texts for it in the same way as we did for the *Daily Mail Dementia News Corpus*, using the same parameters. The *Times Dementia News Corpus* contains 1,933 articles (1,412,609 words). Like the *Daily Mail*, *The Times* is a right-leaning newspaper. However, they differ in format; where the *Daily Mail* is a tabloid, *The Times* is a broadsheet. Therefore, keywords produced by comparing the *Daily Mail* (tabloid) against *The Times* (broadsheet), aside from telling us what kinds of language use distinguish these two newspapers' respective coverage of dementia, might also begin to give us a sense of what distinguishes tabloid coverage of dementia from broadsheet coverage of the same topic. Table 3.4 gives the top 10 keywords for the *Daily Mail Dementia News Corpus* when the *Times Dementia News Corpus* is the reference corpus. Note that these keywords were produced using the same parameters as for those in Table 3.3.

The keywords in this table are entirely different to those in Table 3.3, and this is all down to the different reference corpus we have used. Compared to *The Times*, the *Daily Mail* might be more likely to report on violent crime perpetrated against people with dementia ('assault'), and the sentences that are passed to the perpetrators ('jailed'). While the keywords in this table differ entirely to those in Table 3.3, a thematic 'echo' can be seen: a couple of the keywords, again, reflect the *Daily Mail's* interest in Barbara Windsor; 'eastenders' is a British soap opera in which Windsor starred for many years, and 'babs' is an affectionate shortening of 'barbara'. The keyness of the more familiar sounding 'babs' might also reflect more informal tabloid style (Conboy 2006). This also helps to explain why 'gran' is a keyword; due to its more formal style, *The Times* prefers to use the term 'grandmother' (75 cases, compared to just 5 for 'gran').

The *Daily Mail* is also more likely to explicitly evaluate the people and events in its stories – the crimes it reports on are often labelled as a 'disgrace', and people are reported to have 'tragically' been diagnosed with dementia and to have died 'peacefully' with the syndrome. This kind of overt evaluation is, again, a feature of tabloid discourse (ibid.) and is a way in which the *Daily Mail* constructs the 'newsworthiness' of the events being reported on (Bednarek and Caple 2017). Another likely feature of tabloid coverage of illness is a marked reliance on (particularly militaristic) metaphor. This is reflected in the keyness of 'frontline' and 'battled', which are used to metaphorically characterise, respectively, attempts to develop a cure for the syndrome and lived experiences of it, in militaristic terms (see also Brookes 2023).

TABLE 3.4 Top ten keywords in the *Daily Mail Dementia News Corpus* compared to the *Times Dementia News Corpus*, ranked by Log Ratio score

| Rank | Keywords | Target corpus | | Reference corpus | | Log Likelihood | Log Ratio |
		Frequency	Frequency (PMW)	Frequency	Frequency (PMW)	score	score
1	disgrace	54	27.08	1	0.71	49.60	5.26
2	babs	60	30.09	2	1.42	50.11	4.41
3	tragically	39	19.56	2	1.42	29.31	3.79
4	jailed	65	32.59	3	2.12	50.31	3.94
5	frontline	46	23.07	3	2.12	31.98	3.44
6	peacefully	45	22.57	3	2.12	31.04	3.41
7	battled	46	23.07	4	2.83	28.43	3.03
8	eastenders	264	132.38	5	3.54	241.80	5.22
9	assault	87	43.63	5	3.54	63.14	3.62
10	gran	46	23.07	5	3.54	25.36	2.70

TASK 3.1

Below, we have presented two sets of keywords for a corpus of articles about the topic of obesity published by the British tabloid newspaper, the *Daily Mail*. The keywords in List A were obtained by comparing this corpus against the BE21 as a reference corpus. The keywords in List B were obtained by comparing the corpus against a comparable corpus of articles about obesity published by the British broadsheet newspaper, the *Guardian*.

Keyword List A: *Daily Mail* obesity articles vs. BE21

'Weight', 'obesity', 'fat', 'cent', 'diet', 'per', 'obese', 'sugar', 'food', 'diabetes', 'health', 'eating', 'healthy', 'overweight', 'body', 'disease', 'cancer', 'calories', 'eat, 'children'

Keyword List B: *Daily Mail* obesity articles vs. the *Guardian* obesity articles

'Weight', 'her', 'she', 'body', 'study', 'found', 'risk', 'dr', 'researchers', 'said', 'diet', 'size', 'stone', 'fat', 'after', 'my', 'calories', 'obese', 'eating', 'your'

Look at the keywords in both lists and consider the following questions:

- Can the keywords in List A and List B be grouped into thematic or semantic categories?
- What might the keywords in List A tell us about the language used in the *Daily Mail's* coverage of obesity relative to general written British English?
- What might the keywords in the List B tell us about how the *Daily Mail* reports on the topic of obesity compared to the way the *Guardian* does?
- Which of the keywords in List B are likely to reflect differences between the tabloid and broadsheet formats (and why)?
- While the *Daily Mail* is politically right-leaning, the *Guardian* is politically left-leaning. Which keywords in List B are likely to reflect this difference (and why)?

Keywords have formed an important part of many corpus studies of health-related discourse in which comparisons against general language reference corpora, such as we made in Table 3.3, afford thematic overviews of corpora which serve as an inductive 'way in' to the data, or as Adolphs et al. (2004, p. 25) put it, as a way to '"take the pulse" of the [texts] under investigation so as to guide subsequent qualitative work.' Meanwhile, keyword comparisons against other specialised corpora provide a way of systematically contrasting health-related language across different contexts, registers, and genres, as we did in Table 3.4, as well as over time and between cultures. We will see in more detail examples of studies using keyword analysis in Chapter 5, in which we discuss Brookes and Baker's (2022) comparison of keywords in UK newspapers' coverage of obesity according to their format (tabloid vs broadsheet) and editorial stance (right-leaning vs left-leaning), and Chapter 6, in relation to Harvey et al.'s (2007) use of a keyness analysis to identify the prevailing topics in adolescent health queries to an online advice service. While we have focused on keywords in this section, it is also worth noting that the concept of keyness has been applied to other elements, such as clusters (introduced later) and semantic tags (introduced in the previous chapter). We will see an example of how keyness can be applied to the study of semantic tags in Chapter 4, when we discuss Thomas and Wilson's (1996) investigation of the different communicative approaches taken by doctors providing cancer care.

Keyword analysis can provide a rapid and replicable overview of key themes in the corpus, as these are reflected in the most characteristic words within it. However, looking at words in isolation – as in a frequency list or a keyword list – is limiting, as it provides a decontextualised view of the corpus and reveals nothing about how those words are actually used in the texts in which they appear. To gain such insight, we need to take a more contextualised view of the words and keywords of interest and examine their use *in situ*. There are techniques that can support this more qualitative analysis of a corpus, which we introduce now, beginning with collocation analysis.

3.4 Collocation analysis

Collocation is the 'process whereby words keep company with one another and thereby convey meaning via co-occurrence' (McEnery 2006, p. 18). Following Firth's (1957, p. 6) dictum that 'you shall know a word by the company it keeps', we can learn more about a word's meanings and patterns of use by analysing the words with which it often co-occurs or 'collocates'. In corpus linguistics research, collocation analysis is typically guided by the use of a word association measure that indicates how often two or more words occur alongside each other across the texts of a corpus. With the help of statistical techniques, we can also determine whether this association is notable as a sizeable effect (in other words, whether the collocating words have a measurably strong preference to occur together as opposed to being randomly associated).

As with keyword analysis, deriving collocates requires the human analyst to make a series of procedural decisions that will ultimately shape the amount and type of words that are flagged as collocates by the software tool. We first have to decide on the collocational span – that is, the number of words to the left and/or right of the search word within which we want to search for candidate collocates. Tighter spans will produce a smaller number of collocates which occur within closer proximity to the search word, while wider spans will produce a higher number of collocates, some of which might not occur in such close proximity to the search word. The span chosen will depend on the research questions being answered, but in corpus studies of discourse, a span of five words to the left and right of the search word (otherwise expressed as L5 > R5) has been judged to provide a 'good balance between identifying words that actually do have a relationship with each other (longer spans can throw up unrelated cases) and giving enough words to analyse (shorter spans result in fewer collocates)' (Baker et al. 2013, p. 36).

We also have to decide whether we want to impose a minimum frequency threshold for collocational pairings. Lower thresholds will produce larger numbers of collocates, many of which are likely to only occur alongside the search word sparingly, whereas higher thresholds will produce a smaller number of more selective collocates. Most corpus analysis tools operate with default thresholds between a minimum of three and five. However, this can be adjusted by the user. The threshold we choose will likely depend on the size of the corpus, the frequency of the search word (higher thresholds can be used with more frequent search words), and how selective we, as analysts, want to be.

Once we have settled on a span and frequency threshold, we then have to decide how we will rank, score, or 'cutoff' the candidate collocates. We can do this by either ranking collocates according to the frequency with which they co-occur with the search term or using a statistical measure. Software tools offer a range of statistical techniques for measuring the strength of a collocational pairing, and many of these are based on the notion of exclusivity (i.e., the extent to which two words do not frequently co-occur simply as a result of them both being frequent in the corpus). Popular statistical measures in collocation analysis include Mutual Information (MI), MI^3, Z-score, Log Likelihood, Log Log, and Log Ratio (see Gablasova et al. 2017 for a discussion of collocation statistics and how each measure determines the amount and type of collocates produced).

To demonstrate how a collocation analysis might proceed, in Table 3.5 we show a series of collocates of the word 'dementia' in our *Daily Mail Dementia News Corpus*. We used a collocation span of five words to the left and right of the search word (L5 > R5) and, because our search word is highly frequent (it is the most recurrent noun in the corpus, with 15,437 cases), we stipulated that collocation pairings should occur at least 100 times. Even this very high threshold gave a large number of collocates, which we ranked using the cubed version of the MI statistic (MI^3). MI determines collocation strength by comparing the observed frequency of each collocational pairing

TABLE 3.5 Top ten collocates of 'dementia' in the *Daily Mail Dementia News Corpus*, ranked by MI^3 score

Rank	Word	Frequency	Texts	MI^3 score
1	*with*	3,702	1,363	28.49
2	*of*	5,110	1,546	28.39
3	*to*	4,004	1,435	27.12
4	*risk*	1,339	463	26.37
5	*people*	1,705	785	26.13
6	*living*	578	386	24.07
7	*patients*	739	370	24.04
8	*diagnosed*	563	387	23.88
9	*have*	1,103	670	23.75
10	*vascular*	291	171	23.33

against what would be 'expected' based on the relative frequency of each word and the overall size of the corpus. The computer then derives an MI score based on the difference between the observed and expected frequency of co-occurrence, with higher scores assigned to stronger collocational pairings (Gablasova et al. 2017). While traditional MI tends to favour exclusive and low-frequency collocational pairings, MI^3 favours collocational pairings which have a higher frequency of co-occurrence (Evert 2008) and which are 'more established in the discourse' (Brezina et al. 2015, p. 160).

The MI^3 statistic has reliably produced a mixture of grammatical and lexical collocates which, when analysed more qualitatively, can gesture towards the various ways in which dementia is grammatically framed in the corpus as well as the kinds of topical contexts in which it tends to be reported on. Many of the collocates cohere around a focus on people affected by dementia ('people', 'patients'), and their relationships to dementia are grammatically encoded in various ways: as people 'with' dementia, people 'living with' dementia, and people who 'have' dementia. There is a lot of focus on incidence statistics, including how many people have been 'diagnosed' with the syndrome, as well as dementia 'risk'. There is also some evidence of specification about different types of dementia ('vascular'). In a full collocation analysis, we would examine all the collocates meeting our frequency and statistical thresholds to provide a more complete picture of the linguistic patterns in which our search word, 'dementia', occurs in the corpus. As part of this, and to test and substantiate any hypothesis we might generate about why particular words collocate with each other, we need to examine *how* these words are actually used together in context. Such a perspective on the language use in the corpus is not afforded by collocation analysis alone but requires the use of other corpus analysis techniques (particularly concordance, introduced later).

TASK 3.2

Below, we have presented a list of collocates of the word 'obesity' in the corpus of *Daily Mail* articles we considered in Task 3.1. These collocates occur within a window of five words to the left and right of the search word and are the 20 strongest collocates when ranked by MI^3.

Collocates of 'obesity' in the *Daily Mail's* coverage of obesity

'childhood', 'epidemic', 'crisis', 'diabetes', 'rates', 'tackle', 'rising', 'linked', 'levels', 'combat', 'disease', 'tackling', 'problem', 'heart', 'rise', 'fuelling', 'fight', 'high', 'child', 'smoking'

Look at the collocates in this list and consider the following questions:

- What might the collocates tell us about what might be framed as causing or being caused by obesity?
- What evidence is there for the use of metaphor, and what aspects of obesity are these likely to be used to represent?
- What might the collocates, including metaphorical ones, tell us about how obesity and people with it are evaluated in the *Daily Mail*?

Using collocation analysis, then, we can rapidly and reliably highlight the relationships between words in a corpus, measure the distance between those words when they do co-occur, assess the frequency and exclusivity of these relationships, and ascertain whether or not the relationships are statistically significant. In this way, collocation analysis has provided researchers examining health communication data the opportunity to learn more about words' meanings and patterns of use by inspecting their relationships with other words in the corpus. In Chapter 5, we discuss Lehto (2022) as an example of the use of collocation analysis to investigate attitudes towards patients as expressed by health professionals in late modern English medical texts.

3.5 Cluster analysis

Collocation analysis takes us beyond the solitary linguistic items displayed in frequency and keyword lists and, as such, offers a logical 'next step' following those inductive analytical procedures. However, even with collocation, we are still dealing with a relatively decontextualised view of the data. A technique that can help us to get a more contextualised view of the language in the corpus is cluster analysis. A cluster is a recurrent fixed sequence of two or more words. A multitude of terms have emerged to describe this phenomenon – including lexical bundles, chunks, fixed expressions, formulaic sequences, multiword sequences and n-grams – and while their meanings are similar, they are sometimes used in more nuanced ways (for a discussion, see Mahlberg 2013; Jones 2022). For the purposes of this chapter, we will refer only to clusters, using the definition given above.

Studies of clusters have found that fixed sequences of words are often repeated because they are associated with particular functions that are relevant to the types of texts and contexts in which they recur, as well as the needs of the individuals or groups that created those texts (Mahlberg 2013). Psycholinguistic research has provided evidence that frequently repeated clusters require less cognitive processing effort than infrequent sequences (Conklin and Schmitt 2008). As well as reducing the cognitive effort for both those producing and processing language (Wray 2002), repeated patterns, such as those that can be identified in a cluster analysis, can also perform particular textual and ideological functions (Mahlberg 2013, p. 50).

When undertaking a cluster analysis, an important decision we have to make pertains to any frequency threshold that we might want to impose on the results. The minimum frequency of the clusters we analyse can be determined by the analyst, and while this decision will be driven by the research aims and the size of the corpus, a common cutoff seems to be 20 occurrences PMW. Any decision regarding a frequency threshold for the clusters we consider becomes particularly important when we consider that longer clusters tend to be less frequent than shorter ones, and the drop off in frequency can be quite dramatic. For example, Carter and McCarthy (2006) found 45,015 two-word clusters in their 5-million word-corpus of spoken interactions but only 31 six-word clusters with 20 or more occurrences.

As well as setting a minimum frequency threshold for the clusters we identify, another decision that researchers often take is to restrict the length of clusters. Again, the length of the clusters we consider will depend on our aims and the corpus we are analysing. However, in general, highly frequent two-word and three-word clusters are often disregarded in favour of longer sequences. Hyland (2008) decided to focus on four-word clusters because he found them to be easier to interpret than three-word clusters and because there are more of them than there are five-word clusters.

To show what the output of a cluster analysis looks like, Table 3.6 displays the ten most frequent four-word clusters containing the word 'dementia' in our *Daily Mail Dementia News Corpus*.

Building on our observations of the collocates of 'dementia' in the previous section, we can see how recurrent clusters might help to give us a sense

TABLE 3.6 Top ten four-word clusters containing 'dementia' in the *Daily Mail Dementia News Corpus*, ranked by frequency

Rank	Cluster	Frequency	Texts
1	*the risk of dementia*	213	158
2	*people living with dementia*	200	155
3	*risk of developing dementia*	163	127
4	*dementia in the uk*	152	111
5	*likely to develop dementia*	126	92
6	*been diagnosed with dementia*	94	73
7	*was diagnosed with dementia*	93	80
8	*dementia and alzheimer's disease*	92	52
9	*increased risk of dementia*	59	50
10	*dementia is an umbrella*	53	45

of how some of the word pairings indicated in Table 3.5 function in the context of broader patterns. For example, we can see how risk is framed in relation to dementia in the clusters ranked at number #1, #3, and #9. The latter also implies a scalar view of risk, and a focus on what might bring about an increase in the risk of developing dementia. These clusters also contain repeated uses of the strong grammatical collocate 'of' that we saw in Table 3.5, while cluster #5 contains the strong grammatical collocate 'to' and also expresses risk – albeit less directly – in referring to the likelihood of developing dementia. The clusters in this table also help to confirm our hypotheses about how strong collocates such as 'living' (#2) and 'diagnosed' (#6 and #7) are used. Cluster #4 provides evidence of a particular focus on dementia in a domestic context, which might be particularly characteristic of tabloid coverage (Conboy 2006). Finally, the remaining clusters gesture towards patterns which we could examine to learn about how dementia is defined in the corpus; Cluster #8 suggests a grouping together of dementia with its most common sub-type, Alzheimer's Disease, while Cluster #10 suggests an understanding of dementia as an 'umbrella term' that comprises many sub-types.

TASK 3.3

Below, we have presented a list of clusters containing the word 'fat' in the corpus of *Daily Mail* articles about obesity that we explored in Tasks 3.1 and 3.2. As a reminder, this word was a keyword in this corpus, relative both to general language and another newspaper's coverage of obesity.

Clusters containing the word 'fat' in the *Daily Mail's* coverage of obesity

'grams of saturated fat'
'fat around the waist'
'lower fat and sugar'
'low fat mediterranean diet'
'can make you fat'
'fat cells around the'
'makes your children fat'
'i was too fat'
'i was a fat'
'accused of fat shaming'

Look at the clusters in this list and consider the following questions:

- What different senses or meanings of the word 'fat' can you observe from this list of clusters?
- How might these different senses of 'fat' contribute to the representation of obesity in the articles?
- How do your observations based on these clusters compare with the initial impressions of the word 'fat' you developed when inspecting it as one of the keywords earlier in Task 3.1? Is 'fat' used in ways you expected, or were there any surprising results?

We can see from the above how cluster analysis, in showing us longer repeated strings in which a given word occurs in our corpus, can help to take us beyond collocation analysis, thereby enabling a better appreciation for the *in situ* patterns in which that word occurs. However, like with the interpretation of frequency, keyword, and collocation output, we need to support our interpretations of the patterns revealed through cluster analysis with recourse to a yet more contextualised view of the language in the corpus. For this, and all the other techniques introduced in this chapter, we can use concordance lines. It is to concordance analysis that we turn in the next section.

3.6 Concordance analysis

The final technique we wish to introduce here, concordance analysis, allows us to examine every occurrence of a user-determined word or phrase within its contexts of use in the corpus. With the search word running down the centre of the computer screen and a few words of context displayed to the left and right, the concordance output can be very useful for spotting patterns that might be less obvious during more linear, left-to-right readings of the data. The rows of text are known as 'concordance lines', and these can be displayed in various ways to support researchers in observing the data from different perspectives. For instance, sorting concordance lines by the order in which they occur within the corpus permits a more linear reading of the data. Displaying the concordance lines in a random order can help researchers to more objectively obtain a sample for closer analysis and minimise the influence of the corpus structure, e.g., favouring occurrences that appear in the earliest part of a diachronic corpus. Finally, sorting alphabetically according to the words surrounding the search word can help to make recurrent patterns more visible. For a yet more contextualised view of the data, the user can also access each original text in its entirety, usually by simply clicking the highlighted search word in the centre of the concordance line. Concordance analysis, therefore, essentially provides a means for adopting a different perspective on the language in the corpus, providing the opportunity for human analysts to undertake closer, more qualitative examination of words or phrases in the corpus and to develop theory-informed observations based on extended patterns of use.

To demonstrate the general appearance of a concordance output, Table 3.7 displays a sample of concordance lines for uses of the word 'dementia' in the *Daily Mail Dementia News Corpus*, sorted alphabetically according to the word in the L1 position (this word is highlighted on each line). When sorting the concordance lines in this way, the recurrence of references to 'football's dementia crisis' becomes more apparent.

The analysis of concordance lines can proceed in a number of ways. Sometimes it is possible to read and analyse all the instances of a particular search term, particularly if it is not too frequent in the corpus. However, searches of highly frequent phenomena generate large numbers of concordance lines, and it is often not feasible for an analyst, or even a small team, to closely examine many thousands of concordance lines. Indeed, there are 15,437 occurrences of the top noun in our *Daily Mail Dementia News Corpus*. Therefore, approaches to concordance analysis often require a principled way of down-sampling to a more manageable number of concordance lines that can be analysed by hand. Various approaches have emerged to deal with this issue. For example, Baker et al. (2019) recorded patterns that could be observed by analysing random samples of 100 texts accessed through concordance output. Sinclair (2003) recommends analysing a random sample of 30 concordance lines, recording observable patterns, and then repeating the process until new patterns cease to emerge (and so a 'saturation point' is judged to have been reached).

Once the researcher has settled on a way of down-sampling (if that is necessary) and sorting concordance lines, they can then set about analysing them. How the concordance output is interpreted will depend entirely on the research questions being answered, as well as any theoretical or analytical framework the analyst might be following. Whatever the approach

TABLE 3.7 Sample of concordance lines of 'dementia', sorted alphabetically according to the word in the L1 position

#	Left context	Search word	Right context
1	The 75-year-old has been accused of neglecting **football's**	dementia	crisis Gordon Taylor – the outgoing PFA boss accused of
2	began an operation to learn the extent of **football's**	dementia	crisis Players' union want to discover how many ex-
3	chief, especially as he was accused of neglecting **football's**	dementia	crisis while in charge. The 76-year-old's annual
4	the campaign urging football's powers to tackle **football's**	dementia	crisis. At that time, Robson was receiving no help
5	to be hauled before a parliamentary hearing into **football's**	dementia	crisis. In a significant development, the Department for Digital,
6	have expected Taylor to face a grilling under **football's**	dementia	crisis, it was the MPs who came under fire –
7	As part of SportsDaily Mail's campaign to tackle **football's**	dementia	crisis, we are calling on teams to limit headers
8	organisation had been 'asleep at the wheel' during **football's**	dementia	crisis, which has claimed lives of ex-players MPs
9	brain function. But as SportsDaily Mail campaigns to tackle **football's**	dementia	crisis, the hope is this technology will detail exactly
10	Taylor - the outgoing PFA boss accused of neglecting **football's**	dementia	crisis – will soon enjoy the perks of retirement after
11	new campaign urging football's powers to tackle the **football's**	dementia	crisis. At that time, Robson was receiving no help
12	Every day there is a new story in **football's**	dementia	CRISIS. But the shambolic players' union fail to act
13	in professional training in a bid to tackle **football's**	dementia	crisis. Charlotte Cowie, the Football Association's head of
14	SportsDaily Mail's call for immediate action to tackle **football's**	dementia	crisis. Lampard wants stricter limits on young players heading
15	yesterday which will again turn the spotlight on **football's**	dementia	crisis. News of Law's plight comes nine months
16	Nobby Stiles have shone further light on English **football's**	dementia	crisis. The authorities stand accused of sweeping the issue
17	training ball' to protect players' brains amid **football's**	dementia	crisis. The West Ham boss is already being really
18	funding and research programmes to help deal with **football's**	dementia	crisis. To compound matters, SportsDaily Mail has also been told
19	Tuesday about the players' union's handling of **football's**	dementia	crisis. It comes after family members of former footballers
20	SportsDaily Mail's call for immediate action to tackle **football's**	dementia	crisis. Lampard wants stricter limits on young players heading

chosen, it is often necessary to go beyond the window offered by the con-cordance line and view the wider textual context from which each line origi-nates. In many corpus analysis tools, concordance lines are hyperlinked to the texts from which they originate, meaning that the researcher can usu-ally access the text simply by double-clicking the search word located in the centre of the line.

Through analysing the concordance lines displayed in Table 3.7, we can get a sense of the range of ways in which football's purported dementia crisis is represented in the *Daily Mail*. The most common pattern in this sam-ple seems to be reference to the newspaper's own campaign to address, or 'tackle', the football dementia crisis (see concordance lines 4, 7, 11, 14, 18, and 19). This includes the newspaper endorsing the development of a new light-weight football to help reduce the risk of players developing dementia in the future (Lines 13 and 17). The *Daily Mail* also reports on and makes accusations that the football players' union, the Players Football Association (PFA), and its Chief Executive, Gordon Taylor, have neglected the issue (Lines 1, 3, 8, 10, and 12). Relatedly, there are reports that Taylor will face a parliamentary inquest over the matter (Lines 5, 6, and 9), as well as articles which set out to expose the full extent of the purported crisis (Lines 2, 15, 16, and 19). On the basis of these observations, then, we can get a sense that the *Daily Mail's* interest in the issue of dementia prevalence in football play-ers has much to do with accountability; the 'crisis' frequently described in the coverage has less to do with individual crises or the impacts of dementia on the personal lives of footballers diagnosed with the syndrome; rather, the texts focus on the purported neglect on the part of the players' union. The newspaper makes its stance on this issue clear, both in terms of its frequent reference to its own campaign, as well as its explicit criticism of the PFA and Gordon Taylor. The fact that the *Daily Mail* targets the players' union for blame – rather than, say, the governing body of football in England, the 'Football Association' – might reflect a broader anti-trade union sentiment that characterises the UK's right-leaning press (Fowler 1991). However, sub-stantiating this interpretation would require further analysis and, perhaps, necessitate a comparison of how this issue is reported in this newspaper relative to others that have a more sympathetic stance towards trade unions.

The concordance function exists within all corpus analysis tools, and it can usually be accessed with relative ease. As well as searching for a word or string of words of interest by typing these into the concordance interface, it is usually possible to generate a concordance output showing uses of a particular word or pattern arrived at through another technique. For example, double-clicking a keyword or cluster will, in most tools, show the concordance lines for that keyword or cluster. Meanwhile, double-clicking a collocate will bring up concordance lines showing instances of the given co-occurrence of the

TABLE 3.8 Sample of concordance lines of collocation of 'dementia' with 'risk' in the *Daily Mail Dementia News Corpus*

#	Left context	Search word	Right context
1	in later life is linked to an increased **risk** of	dementia.	Researchers from the University of Amsterdam studied the health
2	that those diagnosed with depression were at increased **risk** of	dementia,	they looked at the association with mild cognitive impairment.
3	This is the first time a link between champagne and	dementia	**risk** reduction has been found. A lot more research
4	Italians could also lower an individual's **risk** of developing	dementia,	a study reveals. The diet enjoyed by countries in
5	are already thought to help lower the **risk** of developing	dementia.	including Alzheimer's. But amlodipine is the first to
6	brain function scores actually translate into a reduced **risk** of	dementia.	But she added: This small study indicates a possible
7	used to treat diabetes could cut the **risk** of developing	dementia	by 20 per cent, a study has found. Almost 15,000 people
8	to protect the ageing brain by reducing the **risk** of	dementia.	While the link between adherence to a Mediterranean diet
9	While the link between adherence to a Mediterranean diet and	dementia	**risk** is not new, ours is the first study
10	is evidence it could be putting youngsters at **risk** of	dementia	in later life. Youngsters in Scunthorpe, Lincolnshire – where supplies
11	anaesthetic in later life could raise the **risk** of developing	dementia	by a third, warn researchers. Brain changes caused by
12	The latest study found a 35 per cent higher **risk** of	dementia	in older people having surgery under general anaesthetic compared
13	and other medical conditions which might raise the **risk** of	dementia.	Altogether 19 per cent had undergone a general anaesthetic and 14
14	steak, spinach, liver and nuts could cut the **risk** of	dementia	in later life, say researchers. A study has found
15	study had a nearly 41 per cent higher **risk** of developing	dementia	than those who were not anaemic. The link remained
16	causes dementia. The best way to reduce your **risk** of	dementia	is to lead a healthy lifestyle. Enjoy a balanced
17	previous observations of a link between anaemia and a higher	dementia	**risk**, but it hard to say with any certainty
18	the condition.' While age is the biggest **risk** factor for	dementia,	current research suggests that lifestyle choices may have an
19	clean and hygienic could lead to a higher **risk** of	dementia,	researchers have warned. Their study pinpointed a significant
20	has found regular exercise can cut your **risk** of developing	dementia,	while other studies suggest keeping the brain active by

collocate and the search word. To demonstrate this, Table 3.8 displays uses of 'dementia' when it collocates with 'risk'.

The concept of risk has emerged already in our foray into this corpus, as it was one of the strongest collocates of 'dementia'. Through the prism of concordance, we can see more clearly how this concept is invoked in relation to dementia. The cases in this table of concordance lines can be broadly divided into two categories: the presentation of factors that increase the risk of developing dementia and the presentation of factors that reduce the risk of developing dementia. We can see that factors attributed to an increase in dementia risk include poor lifestyle choices (Line 18), poor hygiene (19), co-morbidities such as depression (2) and anaemia (15 and 17), and requiring anaesthetic later in life (11, 12, and 13). Factors that are reported to reduce risk include leading a generally healthy lifestyle (16), exercising (20), eating a varied diet (14) and a 'Mediterranean' diet (4, 8, and 9), drinking champagne (3), playing brain-training games (6), and receiving certain treatments for other conditions (7). We also note that what is presented as raising or reducing dementia risk focuses on factors that individuals (readers) can address themselves and not on broader factors that might fall within the remit of the government (Harvey 2005; Brookes 2022). As such, we might interpret this as evidence of a neoliberal framework of personal responsibility, which is perhaps most explicit in Line 20, in which readers are addressed personally through use of the second-person form 'you' and advised on how to 'cut *your* risk of developing dementia'.

TASK 3.4

During our analysis of the clusters in Task 3.3, we encountered the term 'fat shaming'. To explore this concept further, the sample of concordance lines in Table 3.9 displays some of the uses of this term in *Daily Mail* articles about obesity. Read these concordance lines and consider the following questions:

- What attitudes or stances are expressed towards the idea of fat shaming in these concordance lines?
- How do the various ways in which fat shaming is discussed compare with your initial impressions of the term when we encountered it within the clusters in the previous task?
- Are any of the concordance lines more difficult to interpret than the others? Do any of them contain ambiguous elements which might be resolved by looking at more of the extended contexts in which these lines originally occurred?

TABLE 3.9 Sample of concordance lines of 'fat shaming' in *Daily Mail* articles about obesity

#	Left context	Search word	Right context
1	The former Fat Families star is an advocate of constructive	fat shaming	and believes we need to get tougher on
2	of the plus-size community saying the scheme amounts to	fat shaming	and bullying. Steve floated the idea of Warn
3	sales of irresponsible manufacturers who are profiting at our expense	Fat shaming	and name calling isn't the answer
4	her body weight after turning down gastric surgery has condemned	fat shaming	and says obese people are misunderstood.
5	labelled "nasty" for his blunt approach, but he says constructive	fat shaming	is an effective weight loss method. Steve, who
6	alarming because if we continue to have social environments where	fat shaming	is the norm, these kids will continue to suffer
7	develop unhealthy concerns about their weight. It's clear that	fat shaming	can have devastating consequences on a woman's
8	per cent) and 'being physically attacked' (12per cent). Not surprisingly,	fat shaming	children can cause them to gain MORE weight
9	obesity campaigns. The impact of stigma:	Fat shaming	card, that's a cowardly response.' He continued:'
10	great. When people run away from it and play the	fat shaming	

3.7 Chapter summary

In this chapter, we have introduced some of the most established techniques that can be used to analyse the language in a corpus, and we have focused on their specific application to the study of health communication. As we have seen, there is a range of techniques available which, when brought together, can provide complementary insights into the linguistic patterns making up the texts of the corpus. Some of these techniques provide more quantitative information about the language used in a corpus, while others enable more qualitative analyses to be undertaken. The order in which we have introduced these techniques here moves from the more quantitative and towards the more qualitative. Corpus studies of health communication typically involve bringing together a variety of these techniques, with those at the more quantitative end of the spectrum providing an inductive 'way in' to the corpus data, which is then followed up with more qualitative interpretation of frequent or statistically salient linguistic patterns in context. As we have noted, there is no single way of undertaking a corpus analysis, and the techniques introduced here can be used selectively and brought together in different ways, according to the type of analysis researchers want to carry out. Moreover, studies in corpus linguistics have applied additional techniques and the suggested further reading provides instruction in applying such methods, in addition to offering further examples of the procedures we have introduced in this chapter.

In introducing a selection of the most established analytical techniques in corpus linguistics, we have provided, by way of a case study, somewhat cursory analysis of a specialised corpus of newspaper articles about dementia. Through this case study, we have demonstrated something of a cyclical approach which reflects the way in which many contemporary corpus studies of health communication proceed. Specifically, this involves (1) using the frequency analysis and keyword analysis functions to identify general themes in the data, (2) using collocation analysis and cluster analysis to develop a sense of the immediate textual contexts within which a (key)word or theme of interest typically occurs, and (3) closely reading concordance lines containing words or broader patterns of interest in order to confirm or revise our hypotheses and to develop a more deeply contextualised understanding of those words and/or patterns. This final stage is arguably the most important and should always underpin the interpretation of the patterns we identify. During this final stage, researchers will benefit from 'going beyond' the corpus itself to draw on knowledge of the institutional contexts in which the texts in the corpus were originally produced and the wider sociocultural contexts of which those texts are both reflective and constitutive. Doing so will enrich any explanation for the patterns observed through examination of the corpus data.

Which analytical techniques we use, how we use them, and how we combine them will depend on the aims of the analysis. Whatever the approach taken, it is important to acknowledge and embrace your role as the human researcher in this process. The human user of any software tool is required to make multiple decisions throughout the process of a corpus analysis. These include, but are not limited to, deciding what tools to use, what parameters and cutoffs to use, and what statistical measures to use. It is important to make these decisions carefully and consistently within a study and for our decision-making to be guided by the questions that underpin the research. It is also important to fully document the decisions made and to report these when writing up the results, including how they were determined and with some critical reflection on how the decisions might have influenced the results. The role of the human researcher is also crucial in the interpretation of the output from software tools. Lists of words, keywords, collocates, and clusters are not, in and of themselves, analysis. Rather, and like concordance lines, they provide different ways of viewing the language in a corpus and particularly favour perspectives that help researchers to identify and quantify patterns. The computer will not interpret these patterns for us; this is the role of the human researcher. Therefore, the positionality of the researcher, and how this is likely to influence the results, is something that should be acknowledged and embraced, and is something that researchers should be mindful of when undertaking a corpus study.

Notes

1 https://github.com/
2 https://www.nltk.org/
3 The study of keywords tends to focus on what are known as 'positive' keywords – that is, words that occur with a significantly higher frequency in the target corpus compared to a reference corpus. However, it is also possible to study negative keywords, which are words that occur with a significantly lower frequency in the target corpus compared to the reference. As the inverse of positive keywords, negative keywords are judged to be 'underused' in the target corpus relative to the norm represented by the reference corpus. In this chapter, and throughout this book, when referring to 'keywords' we are referring to positive keywords specifically (unless stated otherwise).
4 Note that we also stipulated that for a word to be considered as a keyword it should also occur at least once in the reference corpus. This can help to guard against words arising as key simply due to differences in style or formatting conventions (e.g., whether percentages are expressed using *percent, per cent,* or *%*). This decision should be made carefully, and it is a good idea to manually check the keywords that taking such a step would remove in case this inadvertently results in the removal of keywords that could be relevant to your analysis.

Further reading

- Baker, P. (2023a). *Using corpora in discourse analysis* (2nd edition). Bloomsbury.

This book provides accessible and worked examples of how the analytical procedures introduced in this chapter can be used to study discourse. Additionally, Chapter 2 covers study design, including software tool selection.

- Brookes, G. (2020). Corpus linguistics in illness and healthcare contexts: A case study of diabulimia support groups. In Z. Demjén (Ed.), *Applying linguistics in illness and healthcare contexts* (pp. 44–72). Bloomsbury. http://dx.doi.org/10.5040/9781350057685.0023

This chapter provides a more detailed, worked demonstration and critical discussion of how the techniques introduced in this chapter can be applied to the analysis of health communication data. It uses an analysis of a corpus of messages posted to online support groups as an example.

- Taylor, C. & Marchi, A. (Ed.). (2018). *Corpus approaches to discourse: A critical review.* Routledge. https://doi.org/10.4324/9781315179346

This edited book brings together chapters which critically review the use of corpus analytical techniques for discourse-based research. There are contributions covering the techniques introduced in this chapter as well as considerations relating to the use of statistical measures.

References

Adolphs, S., Brown, B., Carter, R., Crawford, P. & Sahota, O. (2004). Applied clinical linguistics: Corpus linguistics in health care settings. *Journal of Applied Linguistics, 1*(1), 9–28. https://doi.org/10.1558/japl.v1.i1.9

Anthony, L. (2020). Programming for corpus linguistics. In M. Paquot & S.Th. Gries (Eds.), *A practical handbook of corpus linguistics* (pp. 181–207). Springer. https://doi.org/10.1007/978-3-030-46216-1_9

Anthony, L. (2022a). What can corpus software do? In A. O'Keeffe & M. McCarthy (Eds.), *The Routledge handbook of corpus linguistics* (second edition, pp. 103–125). Routledge. https://doi.org/10.4324/9780367076399

Anthony, L. (2022b). *AntConc* (Version 4.2.0) [Computer Software]. Waseda University. Available from https://www.laurenceanthony.net/software.

Baker, P. (2010). *Sociolinguistics and corpus linguistics.* Edinburgh University Press.

Baker, P. (2023a). *Using corpora in discourse analysis* (second edition). Continuum.

Baker, P. (2023b). A year to remember? Introducing the BE21 corpus and exploring recent part of speech tag change in British English. *International Journal of Corpus Linguistics*. Online first. https://doi.org/10.1075/ijcl.22007.bak

Baker, P., Brookes, G. & Evans, C. (2019). *The language of patient feedback: A corpus linguistic study of online health communication*. Routledge. https://doi.org/10.4324/9780429259265

Baker, P., Gabrielatos, C. & McEnery, T. (2013). *Discourse analysis and media attitudes: The representation of Islam in the British press*. Cambridge University Press. https://doi.org/10.1017/CBO9780511920103

Bednarek, M. & Caple, H. (2017). *The discourse of news values: How news organizations create newsworthiness*. Oxford University Press. https://doi.org/10.1093/acprof:oso/9780190653934.001.0001

Biber, D. & Conrad, S. (2009). *Register, genre, and style*. Cambridge University Press. https://doi.org/10.1017/CBO9780511814358

Brezina, V., McEnery, T. & Wattam, S. (2015). Collocations in context: A new perspective on collocation networks. *International Journal of Corpus Linguistics*, 20(2), 139–173. https://doi.org/10.1075/ijcl.20.2.01bre

Brookes, G. (2022). Empowering people to make healthier choices: A critical discourse analysis of the tackling obesity policy. *Qualitative Health Research*, 31(12), 2211–2229. https://doi.org/10.1177/10497323211027536

Brookes, G. (2023). Killer, thief or companion? A corpus-based study of dementia metaphors in UK tabloids. *Metaphor & Symbol*, 38(3), 213–230. https://doi.org/10.1080/10926488.2022.2142472

Brookes, G. & Baker, P. (2022). Fear and responsibility: Discourses of obesity and risk in the UK press. *Journal of Risk Research*, 25(3), 363–378. https://doi.org/10.1080/13669877.2020.1863849

Carter, R. & McCarthy, M. (2006). *Cambridge grammar of English*. Cambridge University Press.

Conboy, M. (2006). *Tabloid Britain*. Routledge.

Conklin, K. & Schmitt, N. (2008). Formulaic sequences: Are they processed more quickly than nonformulaic language by native and non-native speakers? *Applied Linguistics*, 29(1), 72–89. https://doi.org/10.1093/applin/amm022

Cortes, V. (2015). Using corpus-based analytical methods to study patient talk. In M. Antón & E.M. Goering (Eds.), *Understanding patients' voices: A multi-method approach to health discourse* (pp. 51–70). John Benjamins. https://doi.org/10.1075/pbns.257.04cor

Dunning, T. (1993). Accurate methods for the statistics of surprise and coincidence. *Computational Linguistics*, 19(1), 61–74. https://aclanthology.org/J93-1003.pdf.

Evert, S. (2008). Corpora and collocations. In A. Ludeling & M. Kyto (Eds.), *Corpus linguistics: An international handbook* (pp. 1212–1248). Mouton de Gruyter. https://doi.org/10.1515/9783110213881.2.1212

Firth, J.R. (1957). *Papers in linguistics 1934–1951*. Oxford University Press.

Fowler, R. (1991). *Language in the news: Discourse and ideology in the press*. Routledge.

Gablasova, D., Brezina, V. & McEnery, T. (2017). Collocations in corpus-based language learning research: Identifying, comparing, and interpreting the evidence. *Language Learning*, 67(S1), 155–179. https://doi.org/10.1111/lang.12225

Gabrielatos, C. (2018). Keyness analysis: Nature, metrics and techniques. In C. Taylor & A. Marchi (Eds.), *Corpus approaches to discourse: A critical review* (pp. 225–258). Routledge. https://doi.org/10.4324/9781315179346

Gries, S.Th. (2016). *Quantitative corpus linguistics with R*. Routledge. https://doi.org/10.4324/9781315746210

Hardie, A. (2012). CQPweb - Combining power, flexibility and usability in a corpus analysis tool. *International Journal of Corpus Linguistics, 17*(3), 380–409. https://doi.org/10.1075/ijcl.17.3.04har

Hardie, A. (2014). Log Ratio – An informal introduction. *ESRC Centre for Corpus Approaches to Social Science Blog*. https://cass.lancs.ac.uk/log-ratio-an-informal-introduction/.

Harvey, D. (2005). *A brief history of neoliberalism*. Oxford University Press.

Harvey, K. Brown, B., Crawford, P., Macfarlane, A. & McPherson, A. (2007). 'Am I normal?' Teenagers, sexual health and the internet. *Social Science & Medicine, 65*, 771–781. https://doi.org/10.1016/j.socscimed.2007.04.005

Hunt, D. & Brookes, G. (2020). *Corpus, discourse and mental health*. Bloomsbury. http://dx.doi.org/10.5040/9781350059207

Hyland, K. (2008). Academic clusters: Text patterning in published and postgraduate writing. *International Journal of Applied Linguistics, 18*(1), 41–62. https://doi.org/10.1111/j.1473-4192.2008.00178.x

Jones, C. (2022). What are the basics of analysing a corpus? In A. O'Keeffe & M. McCarthy (Eds.), *The Routledge handbook of corpus linguistics* (second edition. pp. 126–139). Routledge. https://doi.org/10.4324/9780367076399

Kilgarriff, A., Baisa, V., Bušta, J., Jakubíček, M., Kovář, V., Michelfeit, J., Rychlý, P. & Suchomel, V. (2014). The Sketch Engine: Ten years on. *Lexicography, 1*, 7–36. https://doi.org/10.1007/s40607-014-0009-9

Leech, G., Hundt, M., Mair, C. & Smith, N. (2009). *Change in contemporary English: A grammatical study*. Cambridge University Press. https://doi.org/10.1017/CBO9780511642210

Mahlberg, M. (2013). *Corpus stylistics and Dickens's Fiction*. Routledge. https://doi.org/10.4324/9780203076088

Mahlberg, M. (2014). Corpus linguistics and discourse analysis. In K. Schneider & A. Barron (Eds.), *Pragmatics of discourse* (pp. 215–238). De Gruyter. https://doi.org/10.1515/9783110214406-009

McEnery, T. (2006). *Swearing in English: Bad language, purity and power from 1586 to the present*. Routledge. https://doi.org/10.4324/9780203501443

McEnery, T., & Baker, H. (2016). *Corpus linguistics and 17th-century prostitution: Computational linguistics and history*. Bloomsbury.

Mujis, D. (2010). *Doing quantitative research in education with SPSS* (second edition). Sage.

Scott, M. (1997). PC analysis of key words – And key key words. *System, 25*(2), 233–245. https://doi.org/10.1016/S0346-251X(97)00011-0

Scott, M. (2020). *WordSmith tools* (Version 8) [Computer Software]. Lexical Analysis Software.

Scott, M. & Tribble, C. (2006). *Textual Patterns: Key words and Corpus Analysis in Language Education*. John Benjamins. https://doi.org/10.1075/scl.22

Sinclair, J. (2003). *Reading concordances*. Longman.

Sirking, R.M. (2006). *Statistics for social sciences* (third edition). Sage.

Thomas, J. & Wilson, A. (1996). Methodologies for studying a corpus of doctor-patient interaction. In J. Thomas & M. Short (Eds.), *Using corpora for language research*. (pp. 92–109). Longman.

4

SPOKEN HEALTH COMMUNICATION

4.1 Introduction

In their influential text investigating health consultations, Roter and Hall (2006, p. 4) describe talk as the 'fundamental instrument by which the doctor-patient relationship is crafted and by which therapeutic goals are achieved'. Hunt (2021, p. 133) also tells us that 'much of the business of healthcare consists of spoken interactional routines such as ward rounds, diagnostic history-taking and general practice consultations'. It is talk that brings together the medical expertise of health professionals and the patient's expertise relating to their own history, values, institutions, and experience – talk 'organizes the history and symptoms and puts them in a meaningful context for both the patient and the physician' (Roter and Hall 2006, p. 4). We can infer from an individual's engagement with healthcare services a desire to talk and to find meaning for physical discomfort and/or mental anguish. It has conventionally been through spoken interaction that patients and health professionals express their expectations of each other and reach a common understanding of the purpose of the medical visit.

Having established the concepts and techniques on which corpus linguistics is based in the previous chapters, we focus now on examples in which those methods have been applied in the study of various kinds of health communication. In this chapter, we briefly reflect on concerns shared by researchers in language-based research approaching spoken health communication before discussing what can be gained from using corpus linguistics methods. We consider the variety of forms of health communication that provide us with opportunities for investigating spoken data. We then focus in more detail on the specific words and phrases that have been reported in

DOI: 10.4324/9781003099659-4

those studies, highlighting themes that are of particular relevance in spoken domains, such as interactivity and the representation of different social actors in medical talk. Throughout the chapter, we will refer to the specific corpus methods that have been used to generate insights into how various aspects of health are spoken about and discuss in detail two case studies that exemplify how researchers have navigated from one stage to the next when conducting corpus research on spoken health communication.

4.2 Investigating language in spoken health communication

In this section, we map out some of the fundamental concerns for researchers interested in analysing the language of spoken health communication. Spoken health communication data can be particularly challenging to collect, and we consider the implications of this challenge for data for determining what we can analyse and the suitable methods for doing so.

4.2.1 Data collection

Individuals seeking support for their health concerns may find them-selves engaging in spoken interactions with various health professionals. Recognising the potential impact and influence of such interaction on these individuals, researchers have duly set out to investigate the language aspects of health-related exchanges, whether that involves doctors (Bigi 2016), nurses (Crawford et al. 1998), physiotherapists (Parry 2004), or pharmacists (Pilnick 1999). Understanding how patients translate the physical and/or cognitive manifestations of illness through talk can contribute to optimising how health professionals support patients in getting appropriate care. Yet investigations of spoken corpora, generally, are relatively few in number compared with those of written corpora. Gut (2021) attributes this to the greater costs and demands on time and resources involved in compiling and annotating spo-ken corpora (see also McEnery and Brookes 2022). The practical challenges involved in recruiting participants for collecting examples of authentic spoken interaction are compounded in relation to health data, as this will typically involve discussions of individuals' private health status and concerns (Slade et al. 2015), can involve invasive physical examinations, and can also involve multiple spoken languages (Zhang et al. 2021). As such, it is not common for researchers interested in language to have the opportunity and the means to collect large samples of spoken health data from contexts such as medical con-sultations. Cortes and Connor (2016, p. 236) speculate that issues with data sampling can account for why corpus linguistics methodologies have not been widely used in this context – in other words, that available samples of medical discourse often may not fulfil the size and representativeness requirements necessary to apply corpus linguistics methodologies in a reliable way.

When researchers have been able to collect and analyse spoken health-care interactions using corpus methods, Gut (2021) emphasises the importance of the corpus compilers' influence on the communicative context in which raw data was collected. This influence can range from 'no control at all' to 'highly controlled data elicitation methods' (Gut 2021, p. 237). In subsequent sections in this chapter, we will discuss both examples of health corpus studies that have involved direct elicitation of contributions, for the purposes of reflexive practice or user feedback, for example, and studies based on more naturally occurring speech data in healthcare. In Chapter 1, we established the importance of collecting 'naturally occurring' data for corpus analysis, and in Chapter 2, we extended this discussion to consider different degrees of 'authenticity'. Thus, it is important to acknowledge that data collected through (semi-structured) interviews *can* still be considered naturally occurring, albeit as interview data, as opposed to data reflective of a more conventional healthcare context (such as a medical consultation).

The relative 'authenticity' or 'naturalness' of the open dialogue of a focus group is highlighted when we compare such data with the direct elicitation methods associated with clinical linguistics (Crystal 1981) and experimental studies (e.g., Corona-Hernández et al. 2022), which have value in helping investigators to target specific features of spoken communication. In clinical linguistics, the manner and output of our speech can be treated as indicative or even symptomatic of illness (Crystal 1981; Cummings 2008) and, thereby, a key part of speech-language pathology. Subsequently, interactional tasks might be engineered in order to create opportunities for participants to produce speech features known to be associated with certain communicative disorders.

In their review of experimental approaches to measuring the complexities of 'co-present' (i.e., face-to-face) communication, Barnes and Bloch (2019, p. 223) remark upon the popularity of rating scales and report measures that allow for the relatively straightforward integration of findings into research paradigms. However, they warn that 'the short-term gains offered by pragmatically eliding the complexity of co-present communicative interactions will be offset in the longer term by the persistence of conceptual confusion, category error and indirect and imprecise measurement'. Instead, they recommend that we embrace the complexity of face-to-face interaction and the measurement of 'standard phenomena', which they suggest can be made observable through 'the interactional systems for organising turn-taking, sequences and repair' (Barnes and Bloch 2019, p. 231). Correspondingly, researchers have realised this potential and applied techniques from conversation analysis (CA) as part of a more discursive approach to the analysis of the (spoken) language of healthcare interactions between patients and health professionals (see Maynard and Heritage 2005).

4.2.2 Analytical approach

Health communication research, as we outlined in Chapter 1, has more generally been concerned with the discursive routines that constitute health and illness, with consideration for how the local interactional context as well as the wider sociocultural context can be related to the language features that we see people choose to use in order to discuss health concerns. Through such microanalytic approaches – that focus on the interactive aspects of, primarily, physician–patient interactions – researchers have highlighted how participants appear to pursue distinct, and sometimes conflicting, agendas: with doctors concerned with biomedical evaluation and treatment and patients focusing on everyday life concerns and personal fears (Mishler 1984). Meanwhile, West (1984) has documented communication patterns in doctor–patient interactions that are associated with dominance and subordination, such as physicians interrupting patients (more often than the reverse) and patients asking fewer questions.

These models, which consider how power is negotiated in interaction (Fairclough 2015), have also informed studies in discursive psychology (Edwards and Potter 1992). Wiggins (2009), for example, collected digital audio recordings of 27 discussion-based group meetings between patients and practitioners in a specialist weight-management service in central Scotland and examined how blame was negotiated at the turn-by-turn level, focusing on moments in which patients appear to resist the notion that they are responsible for their weight gain. Wiggins (2009, p. 384) asserts that '[a]t this level of analysis, the "psychologizing" of weight can be more readily understood; we can begin to map out the turn-by-turn movements through which weight is defined, redefined and potentially challenged as a psychological matter'.

Such studies tend to be small-scale and vulnerable with respect to representativeness, reactivity, reliability, and replicability (Heritage and Maynard 2006, p. 361). Nevertheless, Heritage and Maynard (2006, p. 365) argue that because observations of the organisation of talk have been validated qualitatively through reference to the impact of certain discursive choices in the local context of the interaction, they can be subject to quantification 'to yield a more complete picture of a particular dimension of medical practice'. Heritage and Maynard, subsequently, review a number of studies that demonstrate 'robust and sizeable relationships between interactional conduct on the one hand and various kinds of interactional, relational, and medical outcomes on the other' (2006, p. 366). In Wiggins' (2009) study, interactional strategies such as 'resistance' were anchored in specific lexical choices e.g., 'actually'. This suggests that the capacity for corpus software tools to collate instances of important lexical items (such as 'actually') that have been established through preliminary analysis can help to enrich discursive analyses by identifying how often and where they occur across the data.

In the next section, we focus specifically on studies in which corpus methods have been central to the investigation of various forms of spoken health communication. While much of the research in this area has oriented around the clinic, as the quintessential environment for spoken patient–practitioner interaction, we also consider alternative domains that provide opportunities to investigate how health-related topics are spoken about by various participants concerned with issues of health and illness.

4.3 Forms of spoken health communication

We structure our discussion of forms of spoken health communication according to talk about health and illness (i) in the clinic, (ii) in research, and (iii) in the media. The clinical environment offers a variety of contexts in which we can explore the articulation of health-related issues and we start with patient–practitioner interactions before considering interprofessional talk, including training scenarios and reflexive talk on practice. The focus on reflexive talk directs us towards the elicitation of speech as research data, which includes the verbal feedback of health service users participating in focus groups. We then consider the dissemination of reflections on medical practice and research in the form of oral presentations.

The conventions of 'doctor talk' (Skelton and Hobbs 1999) or, more broadly, the discourse of medicine (Staples 2016) that has been established through systematic study of these clinical contexts has also informed fictional representations of medical situations on television, as television producers and scriptwriters pursue their own kind of 'authenticity' (Bednarek 2010). These TV representations can, subsequently, become a pedagogical resource for viewers looking to develop their language for medical purposes as a subdiscipline of language for specific purposes (see Ferguson 2012). We reflect on studies of fictional television texts alongside data collected from press briefings, which became a common feature of public broadcasts in many countries during the COVID-19 pandemic.

4.3.1 Health and illness in the clinic

Clinical encounters offer a clear reminder of how important context is to understanding the ensuing interactions in terms of being located within particular environments and involving particular interlocutors. If we consider the clinical setting, it is a place of work for health professionals and a site of medical services for patients, who can encounter different types of gatekeeping (in terms of booking an appointment and referral, for example) and for whom there can be challenges with respect to accessibility – patients might have to travel to an unfamiliar location in order to access the care they need, if, indeed, it is available. These arrangements place the health professional at a particular advantage in that they are likely to be more familiar with the environment, both in terms of its geographical location and of the fixtures and equipment that furnish the consultation rooms and the institutional practices therein. This, to a large extent, reflects the nature of the practitioner–patient relationship in that patients generally consult with health professionals for their medical expertise. Healthcare providers have superior knowledge of procedures, therapeutic regimens, and clinical information and this, in part, could account for the drive – in many parts of the world – towards a patient-centred model of care that seeks to minimise the power asymmetry between the health professional and patient through shared decision-making (Stewart et al. 2014). Thus, the communication strategies we are likely to see in medical interviews adopting this approach will work to try to understand the 'whole person' and their subjective experience of illness, to 'find common ground' and 'enhance the patient-clinician relationship' (Stewart et al. 2014, p. 7).

Clinicians also need to be aware of different communicative preferences relating to different cultures and recognise the conventions that might be written into the documents that guide consultations. Magaña (2019), for example, conducted a study of video recordings of 23 psychiatric interviews collected in a rural town in California. Focusing on the use of metaphor, Magaña (2019) has shown that conventionalised English-language metaphors – such as mood disorders articulated in terms of the spatial metaphor of feeling up or down – can inhibit communication with Spanish-speaking Mexican-origin patients in the United States who might more typically use alternative framings, such as personifying mental health issues as an opponent or traveller. Thus, while metaphor has the potential for redressing an 'epistemic imbalance' as a framing strategy through which something that is less familiar is represented in terms of something more familiar (Semino et al. 2018), there is potential for further confusion if the selected metaphorical framing does not offer the clarity and familiarity it is intended to provide. In spoken interactions, particularly those that take place face-to-face, audible hesitations and associated paralanguage can signal when there is potential misunderstanding.

It is also the case that there will be limits to health professionals' understanding, for example, when engaged in diagnostic assessment, which are observable in spoken interactions with patients. Contrary to the view that a health consultant with advanced medical knowledge will express their professional point of view with certainty and authority, some of the earliest corpus studies of spoken doctor–patient interaction have shown that 'there is a higher degree of uncertainty in the doctor's language than in the patients'' (Skelton et al. 1999, p. 624), which is understood to be reflective of the somewhat speculative aspects of diagnostic medicine and treatment (Dahm and Crock 2022). In their analysis of 61 transcripts of consultations between a haematologist and various patients, Skelton et al. (1999, p. 624) found that the doctor used evaluative language to 'offer reassurance in the face of uncertainty', such as conveying that they themselves were 'not worried'. They argue that nego-tiating vagueness/specificity is an important aspect of the interaction with a view to achieving 'a degree of accuracy which is psychologically acceptable to the patient and sufficiently precise for the doctor' (Skelton et al. 1999, p. 624). This highlights the interpersonal aspects of the clinical encounter in that health professionals show consideration for the communicative behav-iours of the patient they are in interaction with, alongside attending to the topic of health and illness.

Skelton and Hobbs (1999) have investigated aspects of dominance and support in interactions between doctors and patients taking place in primary care consultations. Through examination of concordance lines of targeted features, they report that doctors in their study consulted in 'an overtly non-directive, negotiated style, which is realised through suggestions and affective comments' (Skelton and Hobbs 1999, p. 576). Their work has contributed evidence of how strategies that form a core part of clinical communication training can be located and investigated in relation to specific language fea-tures. The use of mitigated directives (e.g., 'maybe you could try') and affec-tive question tags ('isn't it'), for example, can provide insights into how a broader empathetic attitude is realised in these interactions. However, they do problematise the simple distinction of a directive as either mitigated or unmitigated and caution against orienting instruction around language fea-tures that are 'surface representations of the overtly non-directive, negotiated style' (Skelton and Hobbs 1999, p. 578). In other words, competence in this area is not simply a case of learning and using the 'right' words.

Similar studies reiterate that identifying high-frequency words marks only the beginning of a corpus linguistics approach and of understanding effec-tive clinical communication. Thomas and Wilson (1996) outline a computer-assisted approach to studying doctor–patient interactions in the context of cancer care and discuss the application of a semantic tagger – the SEMTAG module – which would later form part of the UCREL Semantic Analysis System (USAS) (see Archer et al. 2004). They highlight terms that have a par-ticular sense in the context of their clinical data, such as 'waterworks', which they explain 'is never used in its normal sense of "a public utility"' (Thomas and Wilson 1996, p. 99) but, rather, is used as a euphemism to refer to the urinary system. Similarly, in the context of this cancer-related talk, the term 'lump' is allocated to the same category as 'tumour' rather than a category that captures its more general meaning of describing a shape.

Given the context specificity of meaning, the traditional procedures of (manual) content analysis have warranted the creation of bespoke dictionar-ies for classifying data in relation to each theory or hypothesis (Thomas and Wilson 1996). Developers of automatic semantic taggers such as the USAS have subsequently strived for a level of categorisation that is general enough to be applied in relation to a range of (language) topics and across contexts

(Löfberg and Rayson 2019). Thomas and Wilson (1996) maintain that while manual checking is required, the advantage of their 'Automatic Content Analysis of Market Research Interview Transcripts' tool is that it can be used to determine a set of rules for mapping the automatically identified semantic categories, ultimately streamlining the analytical process.

TASK 4.1

Thomas and Wilson's (1996) work has highlighted that certain terms used in general English can have particular meanings in a clinical context, which has implications for how we apply automatic semantic tagging. Each of the terms listed below would generally be allocated to a sub-category of the semantic field 'emotion' in the UCREL Semantic Analysis System (2008):

- relax;
- funny;
- feel;
- patient;
- tender;
- attack;
- relief; and
- anxiety.

Consider the potential ambiguities that can arise in knowing what these and other related terms mean if you are told that they were used as part of spoken exchange in a clinical context.
  For example:

- Might these 'emotion' terms be used to describe a physical sensation or process?
- Would you be concerned about possible incorrect tagging of the words in the list (e.g., consider the meaning of a 'patient journey')?
- Are there any examples that indicate that the tagger *has* recognised usage in a medical context (e.g., would 'attack' otherwise typically refer to an emotional experience)?

Think about any terms that can refer to a clinically recognised condition distinct from their 'ordinary' sense.

Thomas and Wilson's (1996) work reminds us that we must take account of the context in order to understand what words mean. In addition, they report having to investigate the constituent words within certain key categories in order to make sense of the significance of the semantic classification. For example, the category 'Farming/growing' included the word 'culture', referring to the growth of microorganisms in relation to body tissue. They also found that even when a semantic category (such as 'Body') is used with comparable frequency by two different speakers, the constituent words can highlight differences between a doctor favouring non-technical terms (e.g., 'tummy', 'vagina') compared with the highly technical terms used by another doctor (e.g., 'epithelium', 'low grade endometrial stromal sarcoma'). Looking at constituent terms can also help to distinguish mischaracterised idiomatic terms such as 'horse's mouth'. It is generally advisable to manually review any form of automatic categorisation, understand the process of classification, check for potential misclassifications, and consider any further sub-classification within categories.

As Skelton et al. (1999, p. 621) remark, quantitative methods can be used to identify general patterns in clinical encounters, but these patterns exist in a complex context that can only partly be described quantitatively, and 'quantitative statements should always be accompanied by detailed qualitative analysis'. Furthermore, in order to discern what are features of more specialised language behaviours, such as the forms of expression associated with 'adherent' versus 'non-adherent' patients in their study, it is useful to have a sense of the more general aspects of communication in these contexts. One method that situates 'context' at the heart of a corpus linguistics approach to investigating health discourses is register analysis, which explores language variation on the basis that core linguistic features, such as pronouns and verbs, are functional. From this perspective, it is argued that 'particular [linguistic] features are commonly used in association with the communicative purposes and situational context of texts' (Biber and Conrad 2009, p. 2). In our first case study in this chapter, we will consider research that seeks to establish some of the features of medical interactions and how these may differ according to different contextual factors.

CASE STUDY:

Register features of medical interactions (Staples 2016)

Staples (2016) investigates the distinctive characteristics of provider–patient discourse, conducting a register analysis (see Biber and Conrad 2009) and comparing medical encounters with casual conversations. Through an analysis of doctor–patient interactions, nurse–patient interactions, and informal conversations from the Longman Corpus of Spoken and Written English, Staples reflects on how distinctive characteristics of medical encounters can be considered 'patient-centred', consistent with the focus in Western medical cultures on taking into account patients' needs and interests.

Staples (2016, p. 179) indicates that studies of patient-centred language have tended to be qualitative and focused on microanalyses of individual interactions, employing CA, ethnography, grounded theory, and critical discourse analysis to expose both the context of interaction and provide fine-grained understanding of how communication is facilitated or impeded.

She sets out to demonstrate an approach that allows us to quantify features of medical interactions that have been identified through qualitative approaches as indexing patient-centred language. If we are able to identify specific language features 'used to convey the pragmatic functions associated with patient-centred care' (Staples 2016, p. 180), then corpus linguistics offers a set of procedures that are ideally suited to highlighting patterns in how such features are used and distributed across medical encounters.

To first establish the distinctive characteristics of spoken medical interactions as a register, Staples (2016) conducts a multidimensional analysis, which is a technique that computes rates of occurrences of predefined lexico-grammatical features (Biber and Conrad 2009). Features that are shown to occur with notable frequency are then interpreted in relation to the situational characteristics that determine the context of that language variety, such as speaker roles, setting, the communicative purpose of the event, and the personal relationship between speakers. Informed by previous studies, Staples (2016) focuses on linguistic variables that relate to involvement, narrative features, and stance features that express possibilities, obligations, and predictions.

Staples (2016) conducts a three-part comparison: investigating both nurse–patient and doctor–patient interactions in comparison with a corpus of casual conversational data. Staples (2016) establishes that medical interactions are typically more topic-focused than casual conversations and that the focus is more clearly defined (such as gathering information to determine illness and/or treatment). In addition, in medical interactions, there is a more explicit power asymmetry in that patients generally go to health professionals on the basis of their medical expertise. There may also be finer distinctions depending on whether the health provider is a nurse or a doctor, as nurses and doctors generally provide different kinds of intervention and care.

Staples (2016) then discusses the specific contextual differences that relate to the data she analyses. First, the nurse–patient interactions are taken from the American Nurse Standardized Patient corpus (Staples 2015), taking place in hospital settings in the United States in 2012; the doctor–patient interactions are taken from the BNC1994 (Aston and Burnard 1998); and the casual conversations constitute a sample taken from the Longman Corpus of Spoken and Written English (Biber et al. 1999) which, like the BNC1994, was compiled in the mid-1990s. Second, the doctor–patient exchanges typically reflect interactions between participants who have an ongoing relationship, whereas the nurses and patients in the American Nurse Standardized Patient corpus have no prior relationship. It is important to consider each of these contextual factors when interpreting the observed differences in the language used in each dataset.

Notable differences were found between the two kinds of medical encounter compared with casual conversation, in addition to some more nuanced differences found when comparing interactions involving nurses with those involving doctors. With respect to features of involvement, Staples (2016, p. 190) reports high rates of second-person pronouns used by health professionals and first-person pronouns used by patients. Both types of pronouns were used with a markedly high frequency in the medical encounters compared with the conversational data. A further distinction is drawn between the health professionals, with nurses using an even greater frequency of second-person pronouns compared with doctors, particularly in the phrase 'you know', which Staples (2016) interprets as indicating shared knowledge and rapport-building with patients. This phrase performed a similar function when used by patients in their interaction with doctors. Staples (2016) observes a higher rate of conditionals in the speech of health professionals compared with patients, which are used to allow for patient choice and autonomy in polite directives, such as 'you can still drink alcohol if you want to', or 'I want you to call me if you're having any pain'.

Narrative features were shown to be more characteristic of patient talk compared with the health professionals' contributions, demonstrating how patients report the short- and/or long-term events that led them to their current situation. However, narrative features were less frequent in the medical encounters than in casual conversation. Nurse–patient interactions included high rates of occurrence for past tense features, which, Staples (2016, p. 195) explains, reflects patient history-taking in those interactions as well as recapping procedures that had taken place since the patient entered the hospital.

Staples (2016, p. 199) reports that nurses and doctors used prediction/volition modals especially frequently, 'to foreshadow behaviour within the course of the examination', such as 'What I'm going to do now is to examine...'. This is interpreted as a form of patient-centred care, as it acknowledges the potential discomfort a patient may feel. Furthermore, in providing these indications, practitioners create an opportunity for the patient to prepare for or challenge this intended action. Possibility modals similarly emphasise patient options and were commonly used by nurses and patients to refer to possible treatments or courses of action, e.g., 'we can get the psychiatrist to come and talk to you'. Modal verbs were used by both nurses and doctors to make requests to the patient, i.e., 'Can you describe the pain for me?', as well as in the discussion of possible explanations for symptoms ('could be anxiety'). Staples (2016) notes, however, that while doctors are more conventionally tasked with diagnosis, they expressed uncertainty in this way less frequently.

One feature that was relatively absent in medical encounters when compared with casual conversation was necessity modals (such as 'have to'), which

Staples (2016, p. 203) interprets as indicating that providers tend to avoid overt directives. As such, this is also considered to be evidence of a more patient-centred approach.

In summary, Staples (2016) identifies certain linguistic features that are characteristic of medical encounters when compared with casual conversation and certain elements that distinguish nurse–patient interactions from those involving doctors. The procedures involved in register analysis provided a quantitative basis on which to investigate particular lexico-grammatical features. Subsequently, Staples (2016) drew on her understanding of the different role responsibilities held by nurses and doctors to inform her interpretation of the quantitative differences. She also identified some of the recurrent features that reflect strategies for rapport-building with patients. Her recommendations for engaging health professionals in development programs are to similarly highlight the high frequency of such features and draw on the contextual knowledge that health professionals can provide as a way to collaboratively develop our understanding of communicative strategies for conveying patient-centred care.

Alongside work in which computational linguistics analysis has helped to establish some general trends for 'nurse talk' in comparison with 'doctor talk', Staples (2015) has also carried out corpus studies to investigate differences in lexico-grammatical features used by internationally educated nurses (IENs) and US nurses (USNs) in their interactions with patients. Staples (2015) highlights that one important area of instruction in English for Medical Purposes is developing programs for international medical graduates, given the high number of nurses working in English-language countries whose first language is not English. There can be pragma-linguistic challenges with working in healthcare systems across cultures that relate to key speech tasks in nurse–patient communication, such as expressing empathy, developing rapport, listening reflectively, and reassuring patients.

To facilitate a comparison between IENs and USNs, Staples (2015) generated data based on consultations with 'standardised patients' – actors who are trained to present the same case to multiple healthcare providers and typically employed in the assessment of nurses and doctors and training (see also Chałupnik and Atkins 2020). In this study, the nurses were practising professionals, and the study focused on 102 interactions (52 involving IENs, 50 involving USNs) in which variability according to patient details, health complaint, and, subsequently, health topics was minimised. Broadly speaking, Staples (2015) observes a greater frequency of features that function for rapport-building and face-saving strategies in the talk of USNs compared with IENs, indicating a difference in the extent to which the respective cohorts focus on the interpersonal aspects of the interaction. Specific features identified in this study are discussed in Section 4.4.1.

Alongside the communicative purposes of exchanging information or seeking professional care, the synchronous nature of spoken exchanges, which typically brings practitioners and patients face-to-face, appears to heighten the impetus for communicative practices which serve to maintain the interpersonal relationship. This has also been shown to be the case when participants are speaking to one another remotely. Adolphs et al. (2004) investigated advice- and information-giving interactions taking place over the phone as part of the United Kingdom's NHS Direct service, conducting a keyword analysis to identify salient features of the health practitioners' contributions to these interactions in comparison with general English (represented by the Cambridge and Nottingham Corpus of Discourse in English (CANCODE) corpus). In the health professionals' contributions, they found markers of a highly involved, interpersonal style (indicated, for example, in the regular use of the second-person pronoun, 'you'), alongside efforts to balance direct instructions and imperatives (such as 'try', 'take', and 'avoid') with vague language that provided optionality for the caller and performed important politeness work. Consistent with a patient-centred model of care, the efforts of health practitioners to build relationships with patients contribute to better health outcomes for patients through care that is more carefully tailored to patients' individual needs (Robinson et al. 2008).

Health professionals also engage in spoken exchanges with other health professionals, and effective communication in this context has been shown to be highly influential not only in fostering effective collaboration in healthcare settings (Gharaveis et al. 2018) but also in improving patient outcomes (Mundt et al. 2015). Egan and Jaye (2009) refer to the concept of a 'community of clinical practice' to highlight the importance of participation in informal communication and knowledge-sharing between professionals in clinical contexts. This builds on the principles of Lave and Wenger's (1991) 'community of practice' model of learning, used to explain how, through a shared enterprise – in this case, the work of a clinic – participants develop shared knowledge and repertoires (including language) that reflect and support the collective development of each member of the team.

One of the challenges, however, of investigating how these shared repertoires develop is that they often occur informally, in transitional moments as health professionals move between clinical spaces. Research has shown that 'office layout, floor space dedicated to informal shared spaces, staff proximity, visibility to colleagues, presence of well-trafficked and overlapping pathways are all associated with increased informal communication between colleagues' (Morgan et al. 2021, p. 191), and such factors are a key part of how primary care spaces are designed. Although interactions that take place in such spaces are often brief and opportunistic, they have been shown to be crucial to building relationships and, ultimately, the delivery of effective care (Morgan et al. 2021). While a small number of ethnographic studies have managed to capture some of these types of interactions (e.g., Slade et al. 2015), they remain, largely, understudied in the field of health communication at large.

Opportunities to investigate authentic interprofessional talk are limited, though there are ways in which researchers have capitalised on existing practices that can provide access to interprofessional talk without compromising the delivery of care to patients. The Objective Structured Clinical Examination (OSCE) is one such practice in UK primary care, taking place in clinical settings as a routine part of undergraduate medical training to assess clinical competence (in relation to medical knowledge, interpretation, decision-making, and communication). It is often the case that preparatory assessments are offered as training, using simulated patients in order to facilitate a scenario in which the medical student can demonstrate different dimensions of their clinical competence in response to particular scenarios (De la Croix and Skelton 2009). Although there are concerns about their authenticity as representations of doctor–patient interactions (see Bosse et al. 2010), we can more reliably examine them as naturally occurring instances of interprofessional talk, albeit in an examination scenario.

De la Croix and Skelton (2009) conducted a quantitative and qualitative analysis of 100 OSCEs, focusing on number of words and interruptions and how this correlated with the candidate's performance (specifically, their grade). They report that a higher number of simulated patients' words correlates with a high grade for the trainee. The researchers attribute this, in part, to communicative skills shown by the trainee health professional in eliciting and facilitating dialogue with the patient.

Atkins (2019) also investigated simulated examinations for medical training with a focus on the question of authenticity. One dimension that organisers of such exams have been keen to replicate is the power asymmetry associated with doctor–patient interactions, so Atkins (2019) compared 50 transcribed video recordings of candidates sitting a UK exam for general practice with a corpus of 37 consultations from real-life GP surgeries in London (see Roberts et al. 2004). Atkins's (2019) corpus linguistics analysis reveals a greater amount of talk from the health professionals being examined than the patient role-players in these simulated interactions and that certain formulaic phrases occur much more frequently than in real GP encounters (namely, the word-cluster 'tell me * more about'). A subsequent CA of keyword clusters was carried out in order to investigate how this sequence functions in these interactions. We discuss this in Section 4.4.1. Atkins (2019) emphasises that we should be cautious about assuming that we can learn about 'real-world' doctor–patient interactions from studying these encounters. Nevertheless, what we learn from these investigations does tell us about this particular domain of professional practice. This shift in focus brings us to the next domain of spoken health communication, in which professionals reflect on practice, and (corpus) researchers have facilitated and documented these forms of spoken feedback.

4.3.2 Talk about health and illness in research

Given the challenges of entering the clinic, researchers have created opportunities for interprofessional talk in a more reflective way by inviting healthcare professionals to participate in formats such as focus groups. Inviting health professionals to reflect on their own practice can help to bring to light the priorities of those involved in delivering healthcare. Furthermore, it can offer us an 'inside' view of how procedures in healthcare systems work in practice. In our second case study, we review the work of Hunt and Churchill (2013) who worked with doctors involved in the treatment of anorexia nervosa and show that the beliefs and attitudes towards illness can have implications for the care that patients receive.

CASE STUDY:

Doctors discussing their beliefs about anorexia (Hunt and Churchill 2013)

Eliciting the views of those involved in delivering healthcare can provide key insights into how access to services is contingent upon the interactions between patients and healthcare professionals. Data collection that involves doctors talking about their practice can provide essential materials for the construction of spoken health corpora that can, subsequently, be systematically analysed. Reflecting on their own data collection approach, Hunt and Churchill (2013, p. 464) assert that recording focus group discussions 'provided a valuable means of accessing the language, concepts and norms that are relevant to groups of participants in which the on-going production of talk (i.e. data) is less influenced by the researcher than during interview studies'. They thereby show consideration for maximising the authenticity of their spoken health communication data.

General practitioners play a pivotal role in coordinating care for a range of health issues, and Hunt and Churchill (2013) remind us that the manner of the interaction between patient and GP can have consequences for how patients access care. Furthermore, these interactions form the basis of the therapeutic alliance, i.e., the nature of the relationship between the patient and their care providers, which can influence their engagement with and adherence to treatment.

Anorexia nervosa has a low prevalence compared with other mental health problems, but it also has the highest rate of mortality (Hoek 2006). While treatment is typically delivered by specialist services, the first contact for patients is likely to be their GP. Hunt and Churchill (2013) recruited 12 GPs from three practices in the East Midlands (United Kingdom) for participation in focus groups, presenting their participants with two hypothetical case studies of anorexia scenarios as a prompt for discussion. Vignettes such as these can be effective in offering an appropriate level of detail that reflects the real experiences of patients with whom GPs engage, without requiring them to recall or report the specific details of their own patients. As such, it is useful to involve health professionals in the construction of hypothetical cases to ensure that these depictions are relatable to actual practice, as was the case in this study.

Hunt and Churchill (2013) report that, beyond the case study prompts, the discussions were minimally guided or moderated, allowing participants to refer to their wider experiences as they saw fit. There are advantages in allowing health professionals to direct the conversation in that the content is more likely to reflect what is relevant to practice. However, this can also result in contributions of varying lengths, which can affect the representativeness, balance, and size of any corpus constructed from these contributions. As ever, there is a balance to be struck in terms of how proactive we are in eliciting participant data, managing topic focus, and, to some extent, the length of the contributions. These aspects can, to some extent, be guided through question design. In Hunt and Churchill's (2013) case, they were able to gather sufficient data to carry out keyword analysis and thematic categorisation of the resultant keywords, having transcribed the audio-recorded discussions from their focus groups.

Consistent with conventional keyword analysis procedures, Hunt and Churchill (2013) compared their data with a larger reference corpus, namely the spoken language component of the BNC1994. The authors then describe their process of thematically grouping the keywords, informed by their familiarity with the data, i.e., how particular terms were used in context. We are told, for example, that the term 'mental' repeatedly appears as part of the phrase, 'Mental Health Act'. The term was, therefore, understood to relate to patient management (as opposed to mental illness or cognitive processes, for example). Similarly, the word 'adolescent' typically referred to adolescent psychiatric services rather than patient characteristics. Table 4.1 reflects the themes and constituent keywords reported in Hunt and Churchill (2013, p. 461).

Hunt and Churchill (2013, p. 461) explain that the thematic categorisation of keywords enabled them to present recurrent topics and account for a larger number of individual keywords in their analysis. Their deductive, thematic categorisation demonstrates that the keyword approach can highlight not only what is of topical relevance, including the materials that guided the discussion

TABLE 4.1 Themes and associated keywords reported by Hunt and Churchill (2013)

Theme	Associated keywords
Medical conditions	'eating', 'anorexia', 'disorder', 'overdose', 'depression', 'anorexics', 'bulimia', 'disorders', 'problem', 'depressed', 'bulimic', 'thyroid', 'anorexic', 'anorexia's', 'illness'
Diagnosis and symptoms	'BMI', 'weight', 'impulsive', 'low', 'bloods', 'problem', 'BMI's', 'purging', 'unwell', 'underweight', 'potassium', 'laxatives', 'thin', 'digestion', 'weigh'
Treatment and referral	'Fluoxetine', 'referral', 'referred', 'therapy', 'secondary [care]', 'prescribe', 'antidepressants', 'therapies', 'psych [team]', 'prescribing', 'Sando-K', 'psychoeducation', 'refer', 'adolescent [health team]', 'family [therapy]'
Patient management	'patient', 'problem', 'difficult', 'normal', 'mental [health act]', 'GP', 'patients', 'rapport', 'secondary [care]', 'mum', 'engage', 'denial', 'adolescents', 'family', 'GPs'
Abbreviations	'BMI', 'BMI's', 'ENT'
Modality markers	'maybe', 'kind of', 'probably', 'quite', 'suppose', 'really', 'actually', 'often', 'obviously', 'sort of', 'anymore', 'you'd'
Response tokens	'mm', 'yeah', 'hm', 'mmm'
Scenario-related words	'scenario', 'Julia', 'mum', 'grandmother', 'scenarios'

(scenario-related words), but also the spoken mode of the interaction (modality markers, response tokens). We, as analysts, can then determine the degree of attention they want to pay to aspects that reflect the form of the interaction, in balance with those that more directly attend to the topic of interest, though these different aspects often complement one another.

Hunt and Churchill (2013) articulate their critical discussion of their findings according to the themes of diagnosis, treatment and referral, and patient management, thereby offering a direct response to their aims of investigating how health professionals talk about their perspectives on how patients access care for anorexia nervosa. What is highlighted through this discussion is a degree of uncertainty in relation to the diagnosis of anorexia – particularly as distinct from other eating disorders – and even differentiating eating disorders from more general dieting behaviour. Furthermore, the participants problematised common indicators, such as body mass index (BMI), in terms of offering clear thresholds for diagnosis. This stands in contrast to the binary classification of how clinical decisions are reported to be made, i.e., when it is a case of an eating disorder and when it is not. This level of uncertainty was also reported to be a source of tension when the participants were trying to explain their referral recommendations to patients; the focus group participants reported having to rely on the results of tests as 'rhetorical resources offering objective evidence of physical malfunction to overcome patients' subjective beliefs about their eating' (Hunt and Churchill 2013, p. 463).

The use of corpus linguistics analysis highlighted 'consistent areas of experience between participants and groups across the dataset, and particularly how to broach the "difficult" topic of referral with patients' (Hunt and Churchill 2013, p. 464). Furthermore, the difficulties associated with referral constituted a topic that the participants introduced to the sessions, beyond what was covered in the prompts. Ultimately, the study highlights some of the challenges reported by GPs in managing anorexia, including their own concerns about their levels of specialist expertise and training needs, as well as offering examples of how the focus group participants navigate these challenges. These are factors that determine how patients currently access care and offer possibilities for how this can be improved.

In related work, Hunt (2021) describes a replication of the procedures described in Hunt and Churchill (2013) in a study of GPs' experiences of diagnosing and treating depression. In this study, Hunt (2021) showcases in more detail the procedures of keyword analysis, collocation analysis, and concordance analysis, focusing on focus group data. Concentrating on the keywords 'depressed', 'depression', and 'therapy', Hunt's (2021) analysis demonstrates how quantitative analysis conducted using corpus tools can be combined with linguistically informed, manual analysis to show how concepts of illness are discursively constructed in spoken data. For example, the collocation of 'might' with 'depression' highlighted, to Hunt, (2021, p. 15) the prevalence of expressions of varying degrees of (un)certainty surrounding 'depression'. He subsequently investigated other ways of expressing certainty, including epistemic modality expressed through auxiliary verbs ('might have had depression'), adverbials ('not necessarily'), and premodification ('possible depression'). Hunt (2021) discusses how such formulations point to a tension between 'depression' as a purportedly immutable diagnostic category and the uncertainty with which GPs talk about it.

Health professionals can also be approached for their reflections on practices that involve interprofessional communication. In a series of reports on the 'Discharge Communication Study', Weetman et al. (2019, 2020a, 2020b, 2021) focus on communications between hospitals and primary care in the form of discharge letters. As a form of interprofessional communication, discharge letters are hugely consequential for continuing treatment and patient safety; they contain information relating to the hospital stay, treatment, and what follow-up action is required. We discuss these letters, as a form of written communication, in Chapter 5. In addition to studying the letters, Weetman et al. (2019) held focus groups with professionals and, separately, with patients to elicit views on the practice of issuing discharge letters and on the quality of the information included in them.

The results from the interviews and focus groups with 26 GPs are reported in Weetman et al. (2022b) based on keyword analysis of GP contributions in comparison with the BNC2014 as a reference corpus. The keyword 'follow-up' highlighted the need for a clear action plan, and related keywords alluded to the significance ('necessary') and content ('who', 'what') of such a plan. The GPs showed consideration for the patient as an additional recipient of the letter, expressing apprehension around the specialist language used in discharge letters and, in particular, *acronym(s)*, which was a keyword in their contributions to the data. Nevertheless, discharge letters were described as 'good', 'useful', and 'handy' for patients.

Complementing the perspectives of GPs, Weetman et al. (2020a) also report feedback from 50 patients collected through semi-structured interviews. The research team targeted participants who had recent experience of receiving a discharge letter, identified through the participating clinics through which they also recruited the health professionals. The interviews were structured around eight question prompts, and this directed the researchers to create eight sub-corpora, collating the responses to each question and facilitating a keyword analysis that was focused on the distinct topics established by the question. For instance, within responses to the question, 'How did you feel about the information you were given?', the researchers could target uses of the high-frequency term 'feel' to investigate direct responses. Furthermore, their corpus design meant that they could ensure, by checking dispersion across files, that topics were relevant to a number of participants. Responses highlighted the disparities that can occur between the patient's recollection of the interaction and its documentation for the case file. This highlights the importance of having a record of the exchange but also how that record is influenced by the subjective experience of the person responsible for writing the discharge letter, particularly when this is written according to the stylistic conventions of the format (this is discussed further in Chapter 5). Similarly, one of the recommendations from the project, which was also raised by the GPs, was that the discharge letters should include a section addressed to the patient specifically, summarising the content of the letter in 'ordinary' language (Weetman et al. 2020a, 2020b).

It is important, however, to recognise that language preferences among patients are heterogenous, i.e., that there is no singular system of 'patient language' that can reliably ensure patient comprehension. Cortes and Connor (2016), for example, investigated diabetes self-management among

English- and Spanish-speaking patients in the United States, distinguishing between those who were 'adherent' and 'non-adherent' to their treatment in each language group. The researchers conducted semi-structured interviews with each cohort, in their respective language, which were compiled as corpora and automatically tagged for grammatical features. We discuss these further in Section 4.4.4. In short, while Cortes and Connor (2016) focus primarily on characteristic features that distinguish adherent patients and non-adherent patients, differences between English and Spanish also influenced how participants in the study reported their experiences. This was specifically indicated in the use of second-person pronouns, possessive determiners, and unspecific demonstrative pronouns. Cortes and Connor (2016) show that corpus linguistics methods are effective in highlighting differences in the use of basic grammatical features that can then be examined and interpreted to determine how these contribute to broader strategies of expressing identities and motivations in relation to treatment.

We have seen how focus groups and interviews with health professionals can prompt reflections on practices such as diagnosis and referral, generating contributions to health communication research in the form of spoken responses that can be used to compile corpora. Another way in which professionals reflect on their working practices or on more focused inquiries into medical processes is through research dissemination. Because we are concerned with spoken health communication, we can regard conference talks on health topics as a form of oral presentation that researchers have, in turn, studied as a form of reflexive health communication. Furthermore, we can explore the spoken aspect of these kinds of communication in comparison with written forms of dissemination, such as research articles. Indeed, Webber (2005) conducted a comparative study of presentations delivered at medical conferences with a corpus of research articles matched for topic (diabetology) to investigate features of interactivity in oral presentations (see Section 4.4.3). In many ways, conference presentations were shown to be more 'conversational' than research articles, even though they are conventionally monologic.

Qiu and Jiang (2021, p. 1) used corpus methods to investigate features of stance and engagement in a specific form of oral presentation, the 'Three Minute Thesis' (3MT). This format is designed for postgraduate research students to explain their work to a general audience. Qiu and Jiang (2021) draw on the concepts of stance and engagement to attend to the writer-oriented aim of performing academic persuasion and the aim of engaging the audience. They, subsequently, compiled a corpus of 80 3MT presentations, across a range of disciplines, to investigate the frequency, forms, and functions of stance and engagement features, developing Hyland's (2005) model of stance and engagement for application in a spoken language context. The presence of an immediate audience resulted in a high frequency of first- and second-person pronouns. The presentations also featured a high degree of stance expressions, which the researchers demonstrate were used to foreground the positionality of the propositions in the talk, i.e., that the presenter draws on established knowledge from their discipline that may not be known to members of a general audience. Presenters more frequently referred to their own motivations, expertise, and reasoning, demonstrating a more prevalent first-person perspective compared with research articles. Qiu and Jiang (2021) explain that the frequency of self-mentions simultaneously demonstrates strategies for academic persuasion (i.e., stance) and appeals to the audience (engagement).

Participating in the audience for a (medical) research talk is one of the less common ways in which non-professionals are presented with a view of professional healthcare practices. Indeed, for non-professionals, experiences of clinical health communication are most likely to occur when the individual is in the position of being a patient or, perhaps, vicariously as the relative or carer of a patient. In the next section, we will discuss different media contexts as a form of spoken health communication that is more widely accessible to non-professionals as public information or broadcast entertainment.

4.3.3 Talk about health and illness in the media

Media talk is different from naturally occurring conversation with respect to its communicative context: it is pre-planned, constructed speech that is often the result of collaborative input (Bednarek 2010). Nevertheless, we can investigate broadcast talk in its naturally occurring state – i.e., as broadcast – to consider how features of talk serve to achieve particular communicative goals and attend to imagined audiences.

Television remains a powerful broadcast tool for reaching large audiences, albeit only for those who have the opportunity to be televised. It has, therefore, historically been the reserve of those who belong to powerful media organisations or who otherwise hold a position of social power in some other domain, such as politicians. At times of national health crises, political leaders are responsible for communicating effectively with citizens – in part, to incite behavioural changes that align with policy measures – and political rhetoric can shape collective meaning-making around health challenges (Montiel et al. 2021). Leadership in these moments arguably entails simultaneously 'reading' and 'cueing' public sentiment (Montiel et al. 2021), which can result in wide public support for collective action and inhibit behaviours that would otherwise exacerbate the effects of public health issues.

In their corpus-based investigation of the speeches delivered by the United Kingdom's then-Prime Minister Boris Johnson during press briefings on the COVID-19 pandemic, McClaughlin et al. (2021) demonstrate the use of rhetoric that insists on there being a clear plan for response strategies without offering specific details about practical implementations. Furthermore, there is a shifting emphasis on whose behalf Johnson is speaking, as he refers to decisions that he, individually, has made in contrast with the collective obligation that the incumbent political party and the wider public has in enacting a pandemic response.

Indeed, part of the challenge of mobilising a response to health challenges at a national or global level is that it will involve various stakeholders across sections of society. Cheng et al. (2005) present the Hong Kong Corpus of Spoken English (HKCSE), collected in 2003, as a record of public speech events in response to the severe acute respiratory syndrome (SARS) outbreak. The corpus includes public speeches, question and answer (Q&A) sessions, radio announcements, and forum discussions involving medical professionals, businesspeople, and politicians in Hong Kong. In a subsequent analysis of the data, Cheng (2006, p. 333) finds 'genuine critical self-reflection on how to learn from the tragedy and to better prepare for such crises in the future', reminding us that 'reflections such as these led to the resignations of key officials and the drafting of proposals for institutional reforms'. Cheng (2006) characterises these reflections in terms of the semantic prosodies attached to the highly frequent lexical items 'Hong Kong', 'health', and 'private'. These lexical items are taken to be representative of different social actors, i.e., Hong Kong as a living entity ('Hong Kong has faced many crises'), institutionalised health provision ('health workers', 'health departments') and the 'private sector'. While there is a semantic prosody of 'insufficiency' attached to the existing healthcare system that highlights where improvements need to be made, there is a greater optimism related to the private sector in finding solutions. However, Cheng (2006) cautions that this emphasis on the role of the private sector in finding solutions reflects the composition of the corpus, which is largely made up of contributions from attendees of business events.

Because media events, such as press briefings, tend to involve only representatives of select industries, it is important to recognise that they represent particular kinds of mediated, institutional talk. Press briefings provide us with quite a restricted view of the procedures of political committees, and it is also very difficult to verify that procedures are carried out in the way that they are reported (Partington 2002). What is discussed in press briefings is prepared with acknowledgement of a media audience as well as a wider public audience, and journalists are responsible for asking questions, challenging the prepared statements of the press secretary hosting the briefing, and attempting to reformulate what has been said according to public interest (Partington 2002). This role is facilitated, to varying degrees, by the conventions of the political system; for example, in the United States, members of the press routinely participate in press briefings that take place at the White House, while the governments of many other countries adopt a more monologic approach or might reserve a dedicated portion of the press conference for questions from those in attendance.

De Candia et al. (2013) investigate response strategies to questions from journalists in their corpus-assisted study of White House press briefings and find that, even when the briefing is not strictly focused on a health topic or delivered during the course of a national health crisis, such events can contribute to our investigations of health discourses, as health services are a fundamental concern for governments. However, if health issues are not central to the preplanned messaging, press secretaries and other government officials may want to avoid commenting on such issues, as their response will likely be taken as a governmental position. De Candia et al. (2013) demonstrate this in their investigation of briefings delivered during Barack Obama's presidency, in which the question of health reform arose. They report the strategic use of phraseological wordings such as 'I don't know … but', which was deployed to shift focus from what was perceived to be a contentious issue (or, at least, one on which the press secretary had not been sufficiently briefed) to planned topics, especially those that could readily be presented as achievements.

The careful management of what is said in press briefings in relation to health policy – and other government concerns – shows, in part, an awareness of the significance of broadcast television as a wide-reaching platform. It is on the same basis that Bednarek (2010) makes the case for studying fictional television content, i.e., its wide viewership and significant contribution to popular culture, alongside its value as a resource for language learners to experience their target language. Furthermore, TV shows can influence the language of native speakers by way of providing quotable lines signifying pivotal moments or key characterisation or patterning more consistent speech styles (see Tagliamonte and Roberts 2005).

Fictional television is, to a large extent, defined by its dissimilarity with ordinary life. Cameron and Kulick (2005, p. 118) refer to the creation of a 'pleasurable illusion': the creation of a world and events that transcend the naturalness of the real world and, thereby, become tellable/watchable because of their unordinariness. We can expect, for example, in fictional television to be introduced to quirky characters and dramatic plot developments that allow us to consider extreme and fantastical scenarios. Nevertheless, one of the functions of film and TV dialogue is an 'adherence to the code of realism', and systematic analysis of this dialogue can offer insights into the shared schemata that scriptwriters and audiences have for how ordinary conversation and various professional discourses operate (Bednarek 2010, p. 63).

What we can expect of television dialogue, as a result of a commitment to intelligibility, is a 'tidying up' of dialogue that results in fewer interruptions, false starts, and hesitations. Subsequently, the inclusion of these features is understood to serve some additional purpose, such as for comedic effect, characterisation, or display of emotional states (Bednarek 2010). With these dramatic purposes in mind, Bednarek (2010) demonstrates a corpus stylistic approach to comparing TV dialogue with the Longman Spoken American corpus, which comprises 4.8 million words of everyday conversations (Stern 1997), focusing on frequent words and clusters. The results show a higher degree of emotional/emphatic language in television dialogue, which accords with the potential for argumentation and confrontation that we can expect from the kind of conflict that characterises drama (Bednarek 2010).

TASK 4.2

At english-corpora.org/tv you can search the TV Corpus, which comprises 325 million words of data from 75,000 TV episodes broadcast from the 1950s to the 2010s. We can investigate this corpus to get insights into how aspects of healthcare have been represented in TV shows over the course of 60 years or target our search to specific decades.

Make a list of terms that are likely to denote health professional roles. You can perform a combined search using the following notation: doctor|nurse|patient.

Search for your selected terms in the TV Corpus and note their frequency.

- Which labels appear most frequently in the corpus?
  You can click on each of your terms to review the concordance lines.
- What kinds of TV shows appear regularly among your concordance lines? Note: if you click on the year or location indicated in the concordance line, you will be presented with a brief description of the source that can give you an idea of what the show is about.
- Are there many instances in which a term such as 'doctor' is used in a non-medical context?
- What can you determine about the context of the occurrences? What are the scenarios in which health-related labels are used? Are there other words that suggest a medical context?
- How are the various roles described, and what are they described as doing? Note: You can formalise this process by using the 'Collocates' function from the search tab.
- Finally, having reviewed references to doctors, nurses, etc., to what extent do you consider this TV dialogue to be reflective of 'real-world' (medical) talk? How and why might it differ?

In later work, Bednarek (2018) discusses how television dialogue can function to identify aspects of the 'worlds' that characters occupy, identifying the location as a ward in a hospital, for example. We can also consider how technical language and forms of address – such as 'doctor' – contribute to the cohesion of these imagined worlds. Through investigation of a corpus that encapsulates television dialogue from a range of genres, Bednarek (2018) demonstrates how the frequency and 'ordinariness' of certain words will relate to genre. Using the example of the word 'blood', Bednarek (2018, p. 145) discusses the narrative relevance of the term in supernatural dramas, for example, that might involve vampires; crime dramas that typically involve violence; and medical dramas that deal with injury, surgery, medical tests, etc.

However, it is also the case that, even in non-medical TV shows, characters' exploits and extraordinary experiences can often involve medical treatment, thereby attesting to the breadth and variety of ways in which fictional television offers a representation of healthcare. In instances in which more technical vocabulary is required (for the purposes of the narrative or for realism), scriptwriters may also write in metacommentary that clarifies the meaning for audiences, creating an interaction in which a health professional explains a specialised term to another character (patient, junior doctor), which is, of course, also of benefit to the audience of the show. Bednarek (2018) reminds us that scriptwriters may consult with special advisors, including health professionals themselves, for the purposes of using accurate and appropriate terminology.

Recognising this commitment to authenticity, viewers with an interest in developing their language for medical purposes – principally, medical students – are reported to be capitalising on the benefits of seeing how medical terminology is used in spoken interactions as part of TV dialogue in shows that they may also be enjoying for their entertainment value. This trend stands alongside an increasing need for English language teaching materials in the specialised field of nursing education (Vorbrink 2021). Contributing to this need, Vorbrink (2021) describes the compilation of a corpus of 225 transcripts from the medical television shows *Emergency Room*; *House, M.D*; and *Grey's Anatomy*. The dialogue content of such medical dramas is seen as a resource that can contribute to the development of 'social English' – as a counterpoint to 'technical English' (Miyake and Tremarco 2005) – which Vorbrink (2021) asserts is otherwise lacking in existing training resources. Vorbrink (2021), subsequently, offers worksheets that attend to the communicative tasks of 'giving instructions' and 'informing a patient', for example, on the basis of what is observed in their Social English for Medical Context corpus. This practical activity encourages users to reflect on words and clusters (e.g., 'I have to', 'I need you to') that have been shown to regularly occur in the data, taking into consideration their formality and appropriateness to achieving the communicative goal.

Having discussed a range of sources from which we can compile spoken corpora related to the study of health communication, we now turn our attention to the observations that researchers have made of these corpora through their use of corpus tools. These observations relate not only to the health-related topics of the data but also provide insights into how the spoken mode has shaped the language that is used.

4.4 Features of spoken health communication

In this section, we summarise the observations that researchers have made of spoken health communication corpora. Large-scale investigations of spoken healthcare communication have set out to improve our understanding of 'medical talk', and this can cover a range of areas of discursive representation, such as how health professionals and patients are characterised in talk, as well as how our understanding of specific conditions is influenced by how various participants talk about it. Observations reported from corpus studies also highlight the interpersonal aspects of spoken communication that shape relationships between health professionals and patients or between colleagues, for example. These findings demonstrate that, rather than contributing to a singular view of 'practitioner talk' as a consistent set of language features, there is variation that might be determined by a contributor's commitment to the principles of patient-centred care as well as the changing communicative purposes associated with different stages of a clinical encounter. We begin by discussing observations that relate to the medical agenda of such exchanges.

4.4.1 Medical aspects of spoken health communication

Examining the talk of health practitioners can reveal to us how they attend to their professional responsibilities, guiding the interaction towards medical concerns such as examining symptoms, establishing patient medical histories, and discussing treatment options. More generally, investigations of doctor–patient interactions have highlighted the 'ritualistic aspects of consultations as well as the power asymmetry between doctor and patient as discursively signaled', which is documented through patterns of questioning and topic development, for example (Ferguson 2012, p. 243).

Staples (2016) comments on the use of questions used by nurses and doctors in patient interactions, finding that doctors use more *wh*-questions (who, what, where, why, how) than nurses. She interprets these results in relation to the context in which patients in the data are engaged with health professionals, with nurses focusing more on the health complaint that has been established earlier in the patient journey through triage, compared with doctors in primary care clinics who are the ones to establish the nature of the patient complaint in the first instance.

Collins et al. (2022) similarly attribute the patterns they observe in the distribution and type of questioning utterance used by various health professionals in emergency departments (EDs) to their respective responsibilities. For instance, they attribute the high occurrence of what are termed 'sub-clausal phrasal questions' (e.g., 'High blood pressure?', 'Ibuprofen?') among junior doctors to their involvement in history-taking, in which the practitioner might elide part of the routine questions on their checklist (i.e., 'Do you have any history of …') in order to avoid too much repetition. These question formulations might also function to pick up on – and verify – notable details in the patient's description of the problem ('On your right side?'). They observe that senior doctors have a tendency to produce tag questions that are split over two conversational turns, occurring in the closing stages of their encounters with patients as a 'final check' and typically coming after long turns by the senior doctor in which they explain a procedure or what the patient can expect to happen next (Collins et al. 2022). This is consistent with the senior doctor's role in working towards discharging or referring the patient.

Staples (2015) discusses lexico-grammatical differences between IENs and USNs according to different phases of the consultation (opening, complaint, exam, counsel, and closing). One key observation related to the transition between phases, such as the move from opening to complaint. This transition was marked in the USN data by 'that' clauses, i.e., 'I hear (that) you're having some problems today'. This was seen to be more explicit than alternatives used in the IEN data, such as 'How are you?', which are not clearly distinguishable from the greetings used as part of the opening phase and which can, therefore, lead to confusion, in terms of what is being asked. That clauses also marked a key difference in the exam phase, as USNs more often verbalised their actions, allowing patients to follow their reasoning ('I see that you have a history of diabetes'), which were not as common in the IEN data.

Staples (2015) also shows that differences in the frequency of lexico-grammatical features can highlight a contrasting focus on the communicative functions that those features are used to perform rather than pointing to any issues with linguistic competence. One example is the higher frequency of the past tense by USNs in the counsel phase, which was shown in context to relate to attending to psychosocial factors affecting the patient. In the IEN data, the relatively low occurrence of past tense markers showed that there was little attention given to such factors and nurses appeared to prefer to focus on physical symptoms and treatment. Staples (2015) states that this might reflect cultural differences in relation to, for example, expressions of grief, as well as differences in what is involved in health training. Nevertheless, psychosocial issues can play an important role in the diagnosis and planning of care for patients, and in this study, examining the transitions between phases of a consultation helped to highlight differences in the type of care provided by the respective groups of nurses.

Atkins (2019) similarly identified important formulations that characterised particular phases of the interactions during the examined role-plays between simulated patients and clinicians in training. Specifically, 'tell me * more about' requests were identified as a recurrent feature of the simulated interactions. Atkins (2019) surmises that the higher frequency of this formulation in the simulations, compared with real GP encounters, reflects the challenge of dealing with a shorter, scripted problem presentation from which the candidate must work hard to gain further information. This interpretation is supported by the observation that such formulaic requests were consistently employed at a particular stage in the interactions and was observed across those candidate doctors who performed well in the assessment. Thus, interactions are shaped by not only which linguistic formulations occur but also the moment in the exchange at which they occur.

4.4.2 Interpersonal aspects of spoken health communication

Findings from early corpus studies have demonstrated the significance of healthcare professionals attending to the interpersonal dimension of interactions with patients. Skelton and Hobbs (1999, p. 576), for example, distinguished between 'dominant' and 'supportive' approaches in doctor–patient consultations, which they pursued through three measures: (i) mean number of words per consultation, (ii) relative frequency of question tags (e.g., 'don't you?', 'Isn't it?'), and (iii) mitigated directives. They explain that a high frequency of words is a marker of dominance, whereas facilitative tag questions ('it's sore there, isn't it?') can be seen as a marker of support. Similarly, mitigated directives such as 'maybe you could try these' can be seen as supportive of patients, particularly in contrast with 'aggravated' directives, such as 'try these' (Skelton and Hobbs 1999).

Thomas and Wilson (1996, p. 93) show that individual doctors can favour distinct styles in their interactions with patients. The application of an automatic semantic tagger helped them to distinguish 'a comprehensive psychosocial cancer support service and staff committed to an holistic approach to the treatment of cancer' and one 'without these services' when comparing the approaches taken by two doctors working in neighbouring District Health Authorities in the United Kingdom. Through investigation of key semantic categories, they found that the language of the doctor from the first location was 'interactive […] interpersonally oriented and informal', compared with a more 'informational […], disease-centred and technical' approach evidenced in the language of the doctor from the second location. The 'interactive' approach was reflected in:

- a significantly higher frequency of first- and second-person pronouns;
- the semantic categories 'Cause' and 'Treatment' to explain the course of treatment; and
- the categories 'Groups' and 'Family/kinship' as the doctor referred to the support services available and showed consideration to include the patient's family and friends.

In contrast, the 'informational' approach was evidenced by a higher frequency of modal items and words belonging to semantic categories such as 'Measurement' and 'Learning', which the authors argue reflects a preoccupation with medical explanations using technical details.

It is difficult to imagine a practitioner–patient exchange that does not feature at least some technical vocabulary, and Adolphs et al. (2004) briefly acknowledge a high frequency of 'medical jargon' terms in their keyword list for NHS Direct telephone interactions before focusing on keywords that were more indicative of interactional style than topic. They categorised 43 pertinent keywords according to the categories: negatives, imperatives, pronouns, vague language, affirmations/positive backchannels, and directives (Adolphs et al. 2004). They extended their investigation of keywords to concordance lines and to sequential turns, drawing on concepts from CA to provide a discourse analytic approach. Their observations reveal 'an overarching tendency for nurses and health professionals to use strategies of politeness and the language of convergence in their interaction with the callers' (Adolphs et al. 2004, p. 14), which involves using strategies to minimise the imposition of advice that is given and showing affirmation of the patient's situation and concerns.

One of the additional features observed by Adolphs et al. (2004, p. 18) was the high frequency of the term 'if', which they explain functions to introduce hypotheticality into the discourse, create options for the patient, and mitigate any advice given. Ferguson (2001) similarly investigated the use of if conditionals in doctor–patient consultations, comparing their use with that in research articles and journal editorials. Ferguson (2001, p. 61) characterises if conditionals as a 'useful resource for managing the interaction with politeness and sensitivity'. The use of an if conditional with an absent apodosis, e.g., 'If you ask them to give you the films and just bring them back down' (from Ferguson 2001, p. 76), marks a formulation in which the mitigation of face threats is of particular importance. This demonstrates that the if statement is not being used to explain cause and effect as is its more regular function in the written texts. Ferguson (2001) argues that this is a use of the formulation that is particular to spoken interactions, and this is also the case with the realisation of the protasis and apodosis across different speaker turns. The following example shows that as the doctor stipulates the relevant conditional, it is the patient who is able to provide the resultant information:

Doctor: And if that was to happen now …
Patient: I'd sort of have to look up, like that.

(Ferguson 2001, p. 77)

This co-constructed example is only possible in dialogue and, furthermore, provides a useful demonstration of how different expertise comes together in spoken interactions between health professionals and patients.

Staples (2015) points to cultural differences, particularly in relation to the importance of the interpersonal aspects of interactions with patients to account for observed differences in the frequency of particular linguistic features in the talk of IENs compared with USNs (which we discussed in Section 4.3.1). The preference for prediction modals in USN talk ('I'm going to feel your pulse'), for example, was shown to be important for giving indications about behaviour and was contrasted with a preference for imperative forms in the IEN data ('Let me check your feet'). Second, there was more evidence of hedging in the USN data, particularly in the context of potential disagreement or correction. Staples (2015) suggests that a lack of softeners in the IEN data might correspond with a desire to avoid uncertainty and show authority. However, this commitment to the power asymmetry can inhibit the potential for rapport-building. Understanding these differences and how they might reflect cultural norms is important for identifying areas in which health professionals might require more guidance in terms of understanding the conventions that their patients are more likely to expect.

4.4.3 Interactivity

In addition to linguistic features that show consideration for the interpersonal aspects of spoken exchanges, we also find evidence for the interactivity of spoken health communication, as speakers acknowledge the co-presence of other interlocutors. Paradoxically, research presentations are typically monologic but, nevertheless, show features that attest to the presenter's recognition of the participation of the audience. Qiu and Jiang (2021) identified listener mentions, directives, questions, and appeals to shared knowledge as being indicative of 'engagement' in their corpus of postgraduate research presentations. They also report that these features occur more frequently, to a statistically significant degree, in these oral presentations when compared with written research articles. Webber (2005) similarly studied a corpus of medical conference talks and reports a high frequency of the second-person pronoun 'you', which is used to preface moments when the audience was invited by the presenter to verify the validity of their claims, through directing them to results from the data in visual materials, for instance ('As you can see here …').

Webber (2005) also found that discourse particles (alternatively called 'discourse markers' e.g., 'well', 'now', 'I mean') were frequent in oral medical presentations, functioning as structuring devices in the (spoken) text. Webber (2005, p. 173) argues that 'now' is 'used more in transactional rather than social discourse because it is speaker-focused and indexes a unit in the upcoming text'. Thus, while the high frequency use of discourse particles is consistent with other forms of spoken language (Carter and McCarthy 2017), there is a particular interactive function that relates specifically to oral presentations; because there is no sharing of the conversational floor, there is a greater need for the presenter to guide the listener through the different elements of the text (i.e., the presentation), as they assume an extended conversational turn.

Carter-Thomas and Rowley-Jolivet (2008) likewise report the high occurrence of 'discourse management' strategies in their corpus of medical conference presentations compared with research articles and editorials on comparable topics. Specifically, speakers in medical conference presentations used if conditionals to 'guide their audience through the talk by signposting its structure, chunking it into manageable segments and marking topic boundaries' (Carter-Thomas and Rowley-Jolivet 2008, p. 199). If conditionals are one of the politeness markers deployed when telling the audience what to do, e.g., 'if you take a look at the median palliative index …'.

In addition, Carter-Thomas and Rowley-Jolivet (2008) observe a higher frequency of initial and medial clause positioning for if conditionals in presentations as spoken data compared with written texts, which, they argue, is the result of the real-time processing demands of spoken interactions. In the case of initial positioning, they point to the importance of speakers providing the background for propositions that follow in terms of the conditions under which it holds. Therefore, by positioning this aspect first, they can avoid back-processing by listeners. The high frequency of medial positioning is attributed to the on-line processing of spoken communication in which an if conditional clause is inserted mid-sentence, as if it is an afterthought. Carter-Thomas and Rowley-Jolivet (2008) suggest that this would be 'corrected' during the writing process. These clause positionings emphasise that spoken (healthcare) interactions often involve 'figuring things out' through talk and speakers mentioning things as they occur, which contrasts with the degree of planning typically involved in written texts (see Chapter 5).

4.4.4 Representing different social actors in health and illness

We have seen in this chapter how various social actors can be involved in the experience of health and illness, and the nature of that involvement can be discursively negotiated. Even with respect to the patient, the identification as 'patient' and, subsequently, the manner in which the individual behaves as the patient cannot be taken as given.

Cortes's (2015) investigation of effective and ineffective disease management control in a collection of grammatically tagged texts taken from interviews with English-speaking diabetes patients demonstrates different patient profiles. The 'efficacy' of disease management in this study was determined through patient adherence to taking their prescribed medication. Cortes (2015), subsequently, reports differences in the adherent group's and the non-adherent group's use of a regular feature: personal pronouns. Through examination of the use of first- and second-person pronouns, Cortes (2015, p. 60) explains that the adherent group patients 'consider themselves more experienced and use the inclusive "you" to de-personify their relationship with the illness', whereas the non-adherent group's use of first-person pronouns when referring to the topics diet and exercise shows 'how immersed they are in the struggle to watch their diet and keep their exercise routines'. Cortes's (2015) analysis also demonstrates that the results of a statistical analysis are often not easily interpretable, and it was only through close examination of occurrences in context that Cortes was able to make sense of the quantitative differences in the use of quite 'ordinary' linguistic features, such as personal pronouns and present progressive tense markers.

In related work, Cortes and Connor (2016, p. 249) compiled a corpus of interviews with English-speaking and Spanish-speaking patients to discuss their perspectives on diabetes management as they experienced healthcare in a rural town in the United States. Keyness analysis of grammatical features highlighted linguistic strategies reflecting participants' practices of identification, such as using second-person pronouns, determiners, and inflected verbs 'to distance themselves from their disease'. In Cortes (2015, p. 65), members of the adherent group used specific linguistic features such as postnominal passive constructions ('there's also a pill called metformin') and the *wh* relativiser ('which') to report the medication and the dosage they were taking, whereas the non-adherent group of patients more frequently used the first-person pronoun 'to mark the personal struggle they undergo while attempting to manage their illness'. Members of the non-adherent group also expressed an enduring struggle to succeed and get well, which manifested in the use of the verb 'do' and the present progressive tense (e.g., 'I'm getting there').

Alongside the self-identification of different participants in the health experience, it is also possible to assign characteristics and roles to others. Cheng (2006), for example, investigates the discussion of important stakeholders in a corpus of public speech events collected in 2003 as a record of responses to the severe acute respiratory syndrome (SARS) outbreak in Hong Kong. Cheng (2006, p. 333) reports that 'institutionalised health provision' carries a semantic preference association with 'health', but that the prosody carries a meaning of 'a desired state of existence that has yet to be achieved'. This is shown in references to 'a good opportunity to develop', 'encourage development of', 'to improve' and so on (Cheng 2006, p. 333).

The COVID-19 pandemic offered a comparable situation in which to examine the forward-looking discourses of social actors involved in coordinating a public response. McClaughlin et al. (2021) show in their corpus analysis of UK press briefings during the COVID-19 pandemic that pronouns were used strategically to convey a sense that the government has a plan ('we will continue') and that the then-prime minister is proactive in decision-making

('I can confirm'). However, the vagueness of the practical implementation of such a plan is augmented by forceful instructions that were presented as a collective obligation: 'we must act'/'we must stay' (for a further corpus analysis of the use of pronouns in the UK government's COVID-19 press briefings, see Williams and Wright 2022).

4.5 Chapter summary

In this chapter, we have emphasised the dialogic nature of spoken health communication as an exchange that often involves the coming together of professional and patient expertise. We have, subsequently, seen how interlocutors show a keen awareness for the other participants in the exchange, with features of engagement and interactivity evident even in more one-sided formats, such as research presentations. Furthermore, we can expect that texts such as research presentations, press briefings, and television dramas are likely to have been prepared as written documents. Nevertheless, as Carter-Thomas and Rowley-Jolivet (2008, p. 198) assert, because such texts are designed to be delivered as speech, the process of recontextualisation (i.e., from research article to presentation, from script to performance) deals with the different 'epistemological status, communicative context, and semiotic affordances of each genre', leading to considerable differences 'in the packaging of information [...] and hence in the role and frequency of certain syntactic patterns'. In other words, presenters and script writers alike will show consideration for the 'spoken' element of the texts they are producing and, thereby, incorporate features of spoken language into the content.

Approaching spoken health communication as dialogue places particular importance on the sequence of turns and, in response, researchers have often combined corpus linguistics with interactional approaches to analysis, such as CA. This was the case for Adolphs et al. (2004), who highlighted the mitigation strategies used by telephone operatives when giving health advice; in Collins et al. (2022), concepts drawn from CA contributed to a more comprehensive taxonomy of questioning utterance types used in ED interactions and enabled the authors to demonstrate how doctors elicit information over a series of turns; and Atkins (2019) showed that candidate doctors used particular phrasal constructs to navigate the transitions between phases of simulated consultations. Atkins (2019, p.113) reflects on the combination of corpus linguistics and CA, whereby the corpus linguistics approach enabled her to identify the 'linguistic fingerprint' of simulated consultations in comparison with real GP encounters. Procedures of CA helped Atkins (2019, p. 133) to analyse

> how sequences unfold, turn-by-turn, linking up an understanding of general information about the success or failure of candidates with endogenous

evidence about the success of particular sequences in achieving interactional projects, such as requesting the patient's history, or instances where interactional difficulties and repair ensue.

The delineation of phases over the course of spoken health communication exchanges in the clinic has enabled researchers to make more informed observations of the data in relation to shifting communicative purposes. Register analysis supports linguists in determining which linguistic features are associated with phases of an interaction that orient towards a particular communicative purpose, but in the first instance, the identification of the boundaries of stages in an interaction requires interpretation, and we, as researchers, can benefit from drawing on professional expertise to this end (as shown by Staples 2015). The classification and/or annotation of spoken corpora in this way also reflects a wider trend for supplementing spoken data with rich metadata, pertaining to the social and professional characteristics of the participants involved, along with relevant details about the physical environment, patient case history, paralinguistic elements, etc.

Because opportunities to collect authentic, clinical interactions are somewhat restricted, the pursuit of alternative kinds of spoken health communication data gives us cause to reflect on its authenticity and the corpus compiler's influence on what is captured. Atkins (2019) has commented on the simulated aspects of role-play examinations that cannot be taken as representative of real-word consultations. Nevertheless, interactions such as these, which are a routine part of clinical training, do exist in their 'naturally occurring' state in that, for the participants involved, they are minimally affected by having a researcher as an additional observer, as there is typically someone assuming the role of examiner present in any case. In other contexts, such as focus groups, some degree of guidance on the part of the researchers is required, though this can vary in terms of providing prompts for discussion or asking direct questions. What is important is that we are transparent about how our data are cultivated and that we critically reflect on what is actually represented in that data as a result.

Although the context of the clinic encourages a power asymmetry that will typically place the health professional in a position of authority, we have seen through corpus studies how interactive approaches, whether explicitly patient-centred or otherwise, demonstrate the importance of the interpersonal work done by participants to develop the therapeutic alliance between practitioner and patient. When we turn our attention to other forms of health communication, we can find other power asymmetries, as discussions of health intersect with other domains of society, such as political leadership. We have observed through studies of press briefings how political representatives work to refocus the topic of discussion and have the capacity to discursively represent different stakeholders in public health concerns. In this sense, we can see the value of continuing to conduct corpus studies of health communication across a range of contexts and, following developments in medical consultations, considering how we can make health communication outside of the clinic more dialogic.

Further reading

- Aijmer, K. (2020). Spoken corpora. In S. Adolphs & D. Knight (Eds.), *The Routledge handbook of English language and digital humanities* (pp. 5–25). Routledge. https://doi.org/10.4324/9781003031758

Aijmer offers a comprehensive summary of the development and use of spoken corpora, generally, and while this chapter is not specifically concerned with health(care) communication, readers will benefit from reflections on developments in the design and compilation of spoken corpora, procedures for transcription and annotation, and the analysis of spoken data using established corpus methods in combination with other discourse analytic approaches.

- Collins, L. & Hardie, A. (2022). Making use of transcription data from qualitative research within a corpus-linguistic paradigm: Issues, experiences and recommendations. *Corpora, 17*(1), 123–135. https://doi-org .ezproxy.lancs.ac.uk/10.3366/cor.2022.0237

Collins and Hardie reflect on transcribing practices that can streamline the process of compiling a corpus from transcripts of spoken interactions. Drawing on their experience of working with transcripts generated as part of an ethnographic study of ED interactions, they offer recommendations for how best to capture detailed metadata from spoken (health) encounters to subsequently enrich analysis using corpus software tools.

- Staples, S. (2015). *The discourse of nurse-patient interactions: Contrasting the communicative styles of U.S. and international nurses.* John Benjamins. https://doi.org/10.1075/scl.72

Staples provides a mixed-method analysis of nurse talk, reporting not only quantitative and qualitative discourse analyses of lexical-grammatical and interactional features but also prosodic and non-verbal aspects of spoken interaction. Observations of the language data are supplemented with qualitative interviews with nurses to offer a comprehensive investigation of the situational characteristics that shape nurse–patient talk in US clinical contexts.

References

Adolphs, S., Brown, B., Carter, R., Crawford, P. & Sahota, O. (2004). Applied clinical linguistics: Corpus linguistics in health care settings. *Journal of Applied Linguistics*, *1*(1), 9–28. https://doi.org/10.1558/japl.vl.i1.9

Archer, D.E., Rayson, P., Piao, S. & McEnery, A. (2004). Comparing the UCREL semantic annotation scheme with lexicographical taxonomies. *Proceedings of the 11th EURALEX (European Association for Lexicography) international congress (EURALEX 2004)*, 6–10 July 2004, Université de Bretagne Sud, Lorient, France. Euralex. https://www.euralex.org/elx_proceedings/Euralex2004/089 _2004_V3_Dawn%20ARCHER,%20Paul%20RAYSON,%20Scott%20PIAO %20and%20Tony%20McENERY_Comparing%20the%20UCREL%20semantic %20annotation.pdf.

Aston, G. & Burnard, L. (1998). *The BNC handbook: Exploring the British national corpus with SARA*. Edinburgh University Press.

Atkins, S. (2019). Assessing health professionals' communication through role-play: An interactional analysis of simulated versus actual general practice consultations. *Discourse Studies*, *21*(2), 109–134. https://doi.org/10.1177 /1461445618802659

Barnes, S. & Bloch, S. (2019). Why is measuring communication difficult? A critical review of current speech pathology concepts and measures. *Clinical Linguistics & Phonetics*, *33*(3), 219–236. https://doi.org/10.1080/02699206.2018.1498541

Bednarek, M. (2010). *The language of fictional television: Drama and identity*. Continuum.

Bednarek, M. (2018). *Language and television series: A linguistic approach to TV dialogue*. Cambridge University Press.

Biber, D. & Conrad, S. (2009). *Register, genre & style*. Cambridge University Press.

Biber, D., Johansson, S., Leech, G., Conrad, S. & Finegan, E. (1999). *Longman grammar of spoken and written English*. Longman.

Bigi, S. (2016). *Communicating (with) care: A linguistic approach to the study of doctor-patient interactions*. IOS Press.

Bosse, H.M., Nickel, M., Huwendiek, S., Jünger, J., Schultz, J.H. & Nikendei, C. (2010). Peer role-play and standardised patients in communication training: A comparative study on the student perspective on acceptability, realism, and perceived effect. *BMC Medical Education 10*, 27. https://doi.org/10.1186/1472-6920-10-27

Cameron, D. & Kulick, D. (2005). Identity crisis? *Language & Communication*, *25*(2), 107–25. https://doi.org/10.1016/j.langcom.2005.02.003

Carter, R. & McCarthy, M. (2017). Spoken grammar: Where are we and where are we going? *Applied Linguistics*, *38*(1), 1–20. https://doi.org/10.1093/applin/amu080

Carter-Thomas, S. & Rowley-Jolivet, E. (2008). *If*-conditionals in medical discourse: From theory to disciplinary practice. *Journal of English for Academic Purposes*, *7*(3), 191–205. https://doi.org/10.1016/j.jeap.2008.03.004

Chałupnik, M. & Atkins, S. (2020). 'Everyone happy with what their role is?': A pragmalinguistic evaluation of leadership practices in emergency medicine training. *Journal of Pragmatics*, *160*, 80–96. https://doi.org/10.1016/j.pragma.2020.02.014

Cheng, W. (2006). Describing the extended meanings of lexical cohesion in a corpus of SARS spoken discourse. *International Journal of Corpus Linguistics*, *11*(3), 325–344. https://doi.org/10.1075/bct.17.05che

Cheng, W., Greaves, C. & Warren, M. (2005). The creation of a prosodically transcribed intercultural corpus: The Hong Kong Corpus of Spoken English (prosodic). *International Computer Archive of Modern English (ICAME) Journal, 29*, 5–26. https://icame.info/icame_static/ij29/ij29-page47-68.pdf.

Collins, L.C., Gablasova, D. & Pill, J. (2022). 'Doing questioning' in the Emergency Department (ED). *Health Communication*. Online first. https://doi.org/10.1080/10410236.2022.2111630

Corona Hernández, H., Brederoo, S., de Boer, J. & Sommer, I.E.C. (2022). A data-driven linguistic characterization of hallucinated voices in clinical and non-clinical voice-hearers. *Schizophrenia Research, 241*, 210–217. https://doi.org/10.1016/j.schres.2022.01.055

Cortes, V. (2015). Using corpus-based analytical methods to study patient talk. In M. Antón & E.M. Goering (Eds.), *Understanding patients' voices: A multi-method approach to &e* (pp. 51–70). John Benjamins. https://doi.org/10.1075/pbns.257.04cor

Cortes, V. & Connor, U. (2016). Identifying adherence behaviors through the study of patient talk in English and Spanish. In L. Pickering, E. Friginal & S. Staples (Eds.), *Talking at work: Communicating in professions and organizations* (pp. 235–253). Palgrave Macmillan. https://doi.org/10.1057/978-1-137-49616-4_10

Crawford, P., Brown, B. & Nolan, P. (1998). *Communicating care: The language of nursing*. Stanley Thornes Publishers Limited.

Crystal, D. (1981). *Clinical linguistics*. Springer-Verlag. https://doi.org/10.1007/978-3-7091-4001-7

Cummings, L. (2008). *Clinical linguistics*. Edinburgh University Press. https://doi.org/10.1515/9780748629251

Dahm, M. & Crock, C. (2022). Understanding and communicating uncertainty in achieving diagnostic excellence. *JAMA: The Journal of the American Medical Association, 327*(12), 1127–1128. https://doi.org/10.1001/jama.2022.2141

De Candia, S., Spinzi, C. & Venuti, M. (2013). 'I don't know the answer to that question': A corpus-assisted discourse analysis of White House press briefings. *Critical Approaches to Discourse Analysis across Disciplines, 7*(1), 66–81. https://www.lancaster.ac.uk/fass/journals/cadaad/wp-content/uploads/2015/04/Volume-7_de-Candia_Spinzi-_Venuti.pdf

De la Croix, A. & Skelton, J. (2009). The reality of role-play: Interruptions and amount of talk in simulated consultations. *Medical Education 43*(7), 695–703. https://doi.org/10.1111/j.1365-2923.2009.03392.x

Edwards, D. & Potter, J. (1992). *Discursive psychology*. Sage.

Egan, T. & Jaye, C. (2009). Communities of clinical practice: The social organization of clinical learning. *Health, 13*(1), 107–125. https://doi.org/10.1177/1363459308097363

Fairclough, N. (2015). *Language and power* (third edition). Routledge.

Ferguson, G. (2001). If you pop over there: A corpus-based study of conditionals in medical discourse. *English for Specific Purposes, 20*(1), 61–82. https://doi.org/10.1016/S0889-4906(99)00027-7

Ferguson, G. (2012). English for medical purposes. In B. Paltridge & S. Starfield (Eds.), *The handbook of English for specific purposes* (pp. 243–261). John Wiley & Sons.

Gharaveis A., Hamilton K., Pati D. & Shepley M. (2018). The impact of visibility on teamwork, collaborative communication, and security in emergency departments: An exploratory study. *Health Environments Research & Design Journal, 11*(4), 37–49. https://doi.org/10.1177/1937586717735290

Gut, U. (2021). Spoken corpora. In M. Paquot & S.Th. Gries (Eds.), *A practical handbook of corpus linguistics* (pp. 235–256). Springer.

Hoek, H.W. (2006). Incidence, prevalence and mortality of anorexia nervosa and other eating disorders. *Current Opinion in Psychiatry, 19*(4), 389–394. https://doi.org/10.1097/01.yco.0000228759.95237.78

Hunt, D. (2021). Corpus linguistics: Examining tensions in General Practitioners' views about diagnosing and treating depression. In G. Brookes & D. Hunt (Eds.), *Analysing health communication: Discourse approaches* (pp. 133–160). Springer.

Hunt, D. & Churchill, R. (2013). Diagnosing and managing anorexia nervosa in UK primary care: A focus group study. *Family Practice, 30*(4), 459–465. https://doi.org/10.1093/fampra/cmt013

Hyland, K. (2005). Stance and engagement: A model of interaction in academic discourse. *Discourse Studies, 7*(2), 173–192. https://doi.org/10.1177/1461445605050365

Lave, J. & Wenger, E. (1991). *Situated learning: Legitimate peripheral participation.* Cambridge University Press.

Lofberg, L. & Rayson, P. (2019). Developing multilingual automatic semantic annotation systems. In M. Ji & M. Oakes (Eds.), *Advances in empirical translation studies: Developing translation resources and technologies* (pp. 94–109). Cambridge University Press. https://doi.org/10.1017/9781108525695.006

Magaña, D. (2019). Cultural competence and metaphor in mental health interactions: A linguistic perspective. *Patient Education and Counseling, 102*(12), 2192–2198. https://doi.org/10.1016/j.pec.2019.06.010

Maynard, D.W. & Heritage, J. (2005). Conversation analysis, doctor-patient interaction and medical communication. *Medical Education, 39*(4), 428–435. https://doi.org/10.1111/j.1365-2929.2005.02111.x

McClaughlin, E., Nichele, E., Adolphs, S., Barnard, P., Clos, J., Knight, D., McAuley, D. & Lang, A. (2021). Public health messaging by political leaders: A corpus linguistic analysis of COVID-19 speeches delivered by Boris Johnson. (Report No. SR02). University of Nottingham. https://nottingham-repository.worktribe.com/output/6059760

McEnery, T. & Brookes, G. (2022). Building a written corpus: What are the basics? In A. O'Keeffe & M. McCarthy (Eds.), *The Routledge handbook of corpus linguistics* (second edition, pp. 35–47). Routledge. https://doi.org/10.4324/9780367076399

Mishler, E.G. (1984). *The discourse of medicine: Dialectics of medical interviews.* Ablex.

Miyake, M. & Tremarco, J. (2005). Needs Analysis for Nursing Students Utilizing Questionnaires and Interviews. *Kawasaki Journal of Medical Welfare, 11*(1), 23–34.

Montiel, C.J., Uyheng, J. & Dela Paz, E. (2021). The language of pandemic leaderships: Mapping political rhetoric during the COVID-19 outbreak. *Political Psychology, 42*(5), 747–766. https://doi.org/10.1111/pops.12753

Morgan, S., Pullon, S., McKinlay, E., Garrett, S., Kennedy, J. & Watson, B. (2021). Collaborative care in primary care: The influence of practice interior architecture on informal face-to-face communication-an observational study. *Health Environments Research & Design Journal, 14*(1), 190–209. https://doi.org/10.1177/1937586720939665

Mundt, M.P., Gilchrist, V.J., Fleming, M.F., Zakletskaia, L.I., Tuan, W.J. & Beasley, J.W. (2015). Effects of primary care team social networks on quality of care and costs for patients with cardiovascular disease. *Annals of Family Medicine, 13*(2), 139–148. https://doi.org/10.1370/afm.1754

Parry, R. (2004). Communication during goal-setting in physiotherapy treatment sessions. *Clinical Rehabilitation*, *18*(6), 668–682. https://doi.org/10.1191/0269215504cr745oa

Partington, A. (2002). *The linguistics of political argument: The spin-doctor and the wolf-pack at the white house*. Routledge.

Pilnick, A. (1999). 'Patient counseling' by pharmacists: Advice, information, or instruction? *The Sociological Quarterly*, *40*(4), 613–622. https://doi.org/10.1111/j.1533-8525.1999.tb00570.x

Qiu, X. & Jiang, F. (2021). Stance and engagement in 3MT presentations: How students communicate disciplinary knowledge to a wide audience. *Journal of English for Academic Purposes*, *51*, 100976. https://doi.org/10.1016/j.jeap.2021.100976

Rayson, P. (2008). From key words to key semantic domains. *International Journal of Corpus Linguistics*, *13*(4), 519–549. https://doi.org/10.1075/ijcl.13.4.06ray

Roberts, C., Sarangi, S. & Moss, B. (2004). Presentation of self and symptoms in primary care consultations involving patients from non-English speaking backgrounds. *Communication & Medicine*, *1*(2), 159–169. https://doi.org/10.1515/come.2004.1.2.159

Robinson, J.H., Callister, L.C., Berry, J.A. & Dearing, K.A. (2008). Patient-centered care and adherence: Definitions and applications to improve outcomes. *Journal of the American Academy of Nurse Practitioners*, *20*(12), 600–607. https://doi.org/10.1111/j.1745-7599.2008.00360.x

Roter, D.L. & Hall, J.A. (2006). *Doctors talking with patients/patients talking with doctors: Improving communication in medical visits* (second edition). Praeger Publishers.

Semino, E., Demjén, Z. & Demmen, J. (2018). An integrated approach to metaphor and framing in cognition, discourse, and practice, with an application to metaphors for cancer. *Applied Linguistics*, *39*(5), 625–645. https://doi.org/10.1093/applin/amw028

Skelton, J. & Hobbs, F.D.R. (1999). Descriptive study of cooperative language in primary care consultations by male and female doctors. *BMJ*, *318*(7183), 576–579. https://doi.org/10.1136%2Fbmj.318.7183.576

Skelton, J., Murray, J. & Hobbs, F.D.R. (1999). Imprecision in Medical Communication: Study of a Doctor Talking to Patients with Serious Illness. *Journal of the Royal Society of Medicine*, *92*, 620–625. https://doi.org/10.1177%2F014107689909201204

Slade, D., Manidis, M., McGregor, J., Scheere, H., Chandler, E., Stein-Parbury, J., Dunston, R., Herke, M. & Matthiessen, C.M.I.M. (2015). *Communicating in hospital emergency departments*. Springer.

Staples, S. (2015). Examining the linguistic needs of internationally educated nurses: A corpus-based study of lexico-grammatical features in nurse-patient interactions. *English for Specific Purposes*, *37*, 122–136. https://doi.org/10.1016/j.esp.2014.09.002

Staples, S. (2016). Identifying linguistic features of medical interactions: A register analysis. In L. Pickering, E. Friginal & S. Staples (Eds.), *Talking at work: Corpus-based explorations of workplace discourse* (pp. 179–208). Palgrave Macmillan. https://doi.org/10.1057/978-1-137-49616-4_8

Stern, K. (1997). The Longman Spoken American Corpus: Providing an in-depth analysis of everyday English. *Longman Language Review*, *3*, 14–17. http://www.pearsonlongman.com/dictionaries/pdfs/spoken-american.pdf.

Stewart, M., Brown, J.B., Weston, W., McWhinney, I.R., McWilliam, C.L. & Freeman, T. (2014). *Patient-centred medicine: Transforming the clinical method* (third edition). CRC Press. https://doi.org/10.1201/b20740

Tagliamonte, S. & Roberts, C. (2005). So weird; So cool; So innovative: The use of intensifiers in the television series Friends. *American Speech, 80*(3), 280–300. https://doi.org/10.1215/00031283-80-3-280

Thomas, J. & Wilson, A. (1996). Methodologies for studying a corpus of doctor–patient interaction. In J. Thomas & M. Short (Eds.), *Using corpora for language research* (pp. 92–109). Longman.

Vorbrink, K. (2021). Creating teaching materials for nursing schools using medical TV series. In E. Le Foll (Ed.), *Creating corpus-informed materials for the English as a foreign language classroom. A step-by-step guide for (trainee) teachers using online resources* (third edition). Open Educational Resource. https://elenlefoll. pressbooks.com. CC-BY-NC 4.0. https://dx.doi.org/10.5281/zenodo.4992504

Webber, P. (2005). Interactive features in medical conference monologue. *English for Specific Purposes, 24*(2), 157–181. https://doi.org/10.1016/j.esp.2004.02.003

Weetman, K., Dale, J., Scott, E. & Schnurr, S. (2019). The Discharge Communication Study: Research protocol for a mixed methods study to investigate and triangulate discharge communication experiences of patients, GPs, and hospital professionals, alongside a corresponding discharge letter sample. *BMC Health Services Research, 19*, 825. https://doi.org/10.1186/s12913-019-4612-1

Weetman, K., Dale, J., Scott, E. & Schnurr, S. (2020a). Adult patient perspectives on receiving hospital discharge letters: A corpus analysis of patient interviews. *BMC Health Services Research, 20*, 537. https://doi.org/10.1186/s12913-020-05250-1

Weetman, K., Dale, J., Spencer, R., Scott, E. & Schnurr, S. (2020b). GP perspectives on hospital discharge letters: An interview and focus group study. *BJGP Open, 4*(2), bjgpopen20X10103. https://doi.org/10.3399/bjgpopen20X101031

Weetman, K., Spencer, R., Dale, J., Scott, E. & Schnurr, S. (2021). What makes a 'successful' or 'unsuccessful' discharge letter? Hospital clinician and General Practitioner assessments of the quality of discharge letters. *BMC Health Services Research, 21*, 349. https://doi.org/10.1186/s12913-021-06345-z

West, C. (1984). *Routine complications: Troubles with talk between doctors and patients.* Indiana University Press.

Wiggins, S. (2009). Managing blame in NHS weight management treatment: Psychologizing weight and obesity. *Journal of Community & Applied Social Psychology, 19*(5), 374–387. https://doi.org/10.1002/casp.1017

Williams, J. & Wright, D. (2022). Ambiguity, responsibility, and political action in the UK daily COVID-19 briefings. *Critical Discourse Studies.* https://doi.org /10.1080/17405904.2022.2110132

Zhang, C.X., Crawford, E., Marshall, J., Bernard, A. & Walker-Smith, K. (2021). Developing interprofessional collaboration between clinicians, interpreters, and translators in healthcare settings: Outcomes from face-to-face training. *Journal of Interprofessional Care, 35*(4), 521–531. https://doi.org/10.1080 /13561820.2020.1786360

5

WRITTEN HEALTH COMMUNICATION

5.1 Introduction

There are various ways in which experiences of health and illness can be shaped by written documents or committed to writing. Moilanen et al. (2022, p. 2) reflect on the breadth of written health texts that are available in the form of 'international and national steering documents that aim to regulate and ensure the quality and availability of services'; organisational documents used to plan, record and evaluate care; patient records; annual reports; and patient feedback to name just a few. They conclude that '[h]ealthcare documents increasingly provide rich data that focus on multiple target audiences and perspectives, and this can deepen our understanding of different aspects of health and healthcare' (Moilanen et al. 2022, p. 10).

Having explored various forms of spoken health communication in the previous chapter, here, our focus is on written forms of health communication and how these have been the subject of corpus analyses. First, we reflect on the particular characteristics of written texts that factor into our (corpus) linguistics interpretation of what is documented in those texts prior to outlining the different forms of written health communication that have been of interest to corpus linguists. In addition to discussing written materials that are generated in conventional healthcare contexts such as hospitals and clinics, we also consider the broader experience of health and illness as it is represented in written media texts, as well as how concepts relating to health and illness have been recorded in writing throughout history. Furthermore, in this chapter, we emphasise lived experiences of illness and explore how forms of creative writing can help people to convey what living with certain health conditions is like.

DOI: 10.4324/9781003099659-5

5.2 Investigating language in written health communication

The relative accessibility and 'readiness' of written documents for corpus construction has no doubt contributed to the fact that, in general, corpus studies of written communication far outweigh the number that focus on spoken data (Knight and Adolphs 2021). As discussed in Chapter 2, one of the key considerations for (written) corpora is 'authenticity', referring to the extent to which the researcher is involved in the elicitation and documentation of the language data under study, broadly corresponding with the wider corpus linguistics concern for collecting naturally occurring language. In studies that collect data through an experimental design or questionnaires, the researcher typically has a greater level of involvement compared with the compilation of documents such as patient information leaflets. Examining documents that are produced as a matter-of-course in the delivery of healthcare can minimise the disturbance that research can have on practice yet still provide accurate reflections of health language data as it is encountered by health professionals and patients alike. As such, McEnery and Brookes (2022) point out that the distinctions between different degrees of authenticity are likely to be finer with respect to written documents compared with the wider range that results from the more conspicuous transliteration 'away' from natural language typically involved in studies of spoken data (see Chapter 4). In any case, the procedures involved in converting data into an operational corpus will affect its authenticity, and it is important to consider which aspects of the original communication warrant retention in the form of annotation. We will discuss examples of the documentation of features of written texts, including metadata, throughout this chapter.

boyd (2010) points out that the act of writing an utterance makes it 'persistent', and written communication, unlike much spoken communication, can readily be made available to audiences who were not present at the time and place of production. We have more long-standing archives of written health communication as a result of the continuing development of the technologies used to create and preserve them. By comparison, resources that originated as digital texts are relatively new and spoken interactions are less well-documented. As such, one of the ways in which researchers have approached written texts is diachronically (i.e., looking at how they vary, linguistically, over time), and in this chapter, we will consider how corpus approaches are suited both to studies of health communication over time as well as at particular points in history. It is possible, for instance, for us to study printed or even hand-written health- and illness-related documents in the form in which they were originally created so long as they have been preserved. This preservation will likely involve digitisation and digital archiving, which has improved the storage capacity and accessibility of such repositories. Nevertheless, we can still consider such texts to be shaped by their original means of production and the conventions of their respective written register.

The enduring presence of written documents creates opportunities for new contexts in which the texts can be read and (re)interpreted. Revisiting written health documents can prompt new reflections on social practices that shape healthcare provision and personal health stories can find new audiences, for example. On the one hand, the potential for recontextualisation (Bernstein 1996) means that written texts can have continued and renewed relevance long after their original publication; on the other hand, we have to be careful about attributing meaning to content that was generated in a very different time context. In our own documentation of written forms of health communication, then, we can look to preserve relevant contextual information that can help subsequent readers of the text to appreciate its meaning according to the context in which it was produced. In our analysis of written texts archived at an earlier point in time, we must be careful about potentially misreading particular terms when meanings are closely tied to the sociohistorical context in which they were originally used. In this chapter, we reflect on some of the efforts of corpus linguists to draw on historical data to recover such information and uncover meanings that are situated in a particular historical context.

Most forms of written text can be said to be relatively contrived when compared with more spontaneous forms of spoken communication (and certain types of digital communication) – perhaps because the 'persistence' of written texts generates an elevated sense of permanence and historical record. Certainly, the types of written communication we focus on here – news articles, policy documents, and fictional writing about illness – will have likely gone through drafting and redrafting, planning and revision. There is a high degree of craft in written documents that can be motivated by a range of factors, including careful legal considerations (e.g., in the case of policy documents) or authorial pride (e.g., use of personal pronouns). Many health documents can also be *pro forma*, requiring users to rearticulate their perspective according to a standardised template. While digital resources can be edited and revised with practically no record of previous iterations for the user, the printing and publication of written documents more definitively establishes its enduring form, even if it is later modified, removed, or replaced.

The relative permanence of written texts also has implications for actions that might follow from them, particularly in the context of health and illness. Indeed, if we consider how the details of the medical record at one stage of the patient journey can determine what type of care is offered at the next, then *how* the patient experience is recorded in health documents can have life-changing implications, as we will see in this chapter. To begin our discussion of written health communication, we endeavour to map out the different forms of written health texts that have been investigated using corpus methods before reviewing some of the features that characterise different registers within this mode.

5.3 Forms of written health communication

Our review of corpus studies of written health communication is principally organised around four categories: clinical documents, media texts, historical documents, and literary works. This demonstrates the breadth of genres across which experiences of health and illness have been documented in language as well as the areas in which those undertaking corpus studies of written health texts have directed the majority of their attention. In each case, we will discuss how conventions associated with professional discourses and the wider sociocultural context influence the types of texts that are produced.

5.3.1 Health and illness in the clinic

Clinical encounters that involve health professionals and patients arguably represent the nucleus wherein concepts of health and illness are established and illness identities are ratified through diagnosis and treatment. As Buus and Hamilton (2016, p. 64) assert, clinical documents emphasise that patients 'are constituted by institutional practices and that they have constitutive effects on social identities, social relationships, clinical knowledge and clinical practices'. Buus and Hamilton's (2016) systematic review of language-focused studies of nursing records revealed that such documents are 'dominated by technocratic-medical discourse focused on patients' bodies', are economical in their use of language, and convey little information to the uninitiated reader (p. 64). Despite efforts towards a patient-centred model of care that values 'understanding the whole person' (Brickley et al. 2020), Heckemann et al., (2022, p. 422) found 'little documentation of patient involvement in care-related discussion and decision-making', as evidenced in an analysis of 69 medical records and 57 discharge letters collected from the Swedish healthcare system. Clinical documents privilege a biomedical view that undoubtedly contributes to the clinical processes of diagnosis and treatment but can omit other personal aspects of the patient experience. Ultimately, then, communicative norms of institutional practices may inhibit a more person-centred style of health(care) documentation.

Not only can the clinical record omit pertinent aspects of the 'whole person' but the representation of the patient in these written documents can also have further implications for their involvement in the overall system of care. Aarseth et al. (2016) studied the language of medical certificates written by GPs in Norway, which are used to inform decisions regarding the provision of disability benefits to individuals. They found that the certificates tended to construct patients as passive carriers of symptoms, while the symptoms themselves are represented as active agents affecting those individuals' lives. They caution that this approach over-emphasises work incapacity at the cost of discussing the person's potential and abilities, reducing them to a mere function of their illness and marginalising them in the decision-making related to their own healthcare (Aarseth 2016). This functionalisation, which emphasises the patient as a 'biological object' (Lövestam et al. 2015), reflects a biomedical perspective and is associated with objectivity and information efficiency. Nevertheless, there are limitations with restricting the role of the patient in the decision-making process, beginning with information-gathering and extending to compliance with treatment.

Studies have also shown that prejudices can be imbued in the way in which health information is recorded, for example, in the way that disbelief is expressed in relation to the personal testimonies of Black patients compared with White patients (Beach et al. 2021). When patients are not believed, the consequences can be 'delayed diagnosis, inappropriate treatment, unnecessary pain and suffering, and even death' (Beach et al. 2021, p. 1711). Indeed, we can see how stances recorded at one stage of the patient journey affect the kind of care that the patient then receives at subsequent stages. Goddu et al. (2018) conducted an experimental study that elicited 413 physicians' responses to a patient record that used stigmatising language – compared with a control – and found that doctors more negatively evaluated the patient and prescribed less aggressive pain management. In this instance, stigmatising language involved casting doubt on the patient's pain, portraying the patient negatively, providing irrelevant or unnecessary indicators of lower socioeconomic status, and implying patient responsibility with references to uncooperativeness, e.g., 'he refuses his oxygen mask' vs 'he is not tolerating the oxygen mask' (Goddu et al. 2018, p. 687). Other studies have shown that describing a patient as a 'substance abuser', compared with 'having a substance use disorder' can result in higher levels of agreement with the proposition that the patient was personally culpable and should have punitive measures taken against them (Kelly et al. 2010).

Health service users can also be complicit in creating partial representations that fit with institutional models for what a patient looks like. In a corpus-assisted study of 32 narratives written by patients waiting for initial assessment at a transgender clinic, Zottola et al. (2021) found evidence for a normalised account that they interpret as being designed to maximise the likelihood of 'progressing' to the next stage of care. Having identified pertinent themes through manual reading of the narratives, Zottola et al. (2021) calculated their frequency in the corpus using select terms and found that respondents produced a number of recurring features relating to aspects such as positive and negative coping strategies in order to index an 'acceptable' case. Zottola et al. (2021) suggest that their participants are aware of the need to conform to normative ideals in order to appear 'authentic', embracing stereotypical clothing and activities in their reports and conveying the negative aspects of their current situation in order to match the criteria for being treated. Zottola et al. (2021) highlight the limited empowering potential of this scenario, which appears to allow or encourage one type of story to be told, and individuals seeking treatment subsequently write to this script. Collecting a corpus of such data, thus, allows this regularisation to be studied and highlighted as well as to consider both the shared elements and the individual components that may, indeed, tell us more about each person's experiences.

Even when written health documents are purportedly designed to be read by patients, there are still indications that they are governed by linguistic practices associated with professional medical practice. Patient information leaflets are produced in accordance with guidelines established by regulatory authorities and provide information on the proper and safe use of medicines, including recommended dosage and known side effects. While these leaflets are produced for patients, they are often based on summaries of product characteristics, which are designed for healthcare professionals. There are conventions – and legal requirements – for what is included in patient information leaflets, yet pharmaceutical companies can still determine how the requisite information is presented. Indeed, recognising that patient information leaflets and summaries of product characteristics are written for different communicative purposes (primarily, in terms of readership), Grabowski (2013, 2014) has investigated 'register features' of collections of these documents and, subsequently, reports similarities and differences in functional categories of keywords and clusters, which are discussed in Section 5.4.4.

Richards Golini (2022) highlights a need for increased patient information relating to radiographic examinations, citing reports of limited understanding of which procedures posed radiation risks. Richards Golini (2022) investigated recurrent clusters in a corpus of 221 patient information sheets about radiography (466,949 words), collected from the UK NHS, the British Society of Interventional Radiology, and a US radiology patient information website. The results indicated a preference for a detached style, as demonstrated in the use of the passive voice (e.g., 'you may be given'). This is argued to contribute to a wider pattern of features that Richards Golini (2022) likens to academic prose, which stands in contrast to the 'Plain English Campaign' and related style guides generated by medical institutions to promote readability. Patient understanding is particularly important in contexts such as radiographic examinations in which patients are asked to provide informed consent on the basis of their comprehension of the risks involved in particular forms of treatment.

Patients can also be tasked with making sense of documents designed to capture their experiences into a form – or even terminology – that is amenable to clinical procedures. One example is the widely used McGill Pain Questionnaire, which presents patients with 20 groups of linguistic descriptors that are intended to help them to convey the quality and intensity of their pain experiences (Melzack 1975). Patients are asked to select the appropriate term matching their experience, e.g., 'scalding', 'searing', 'stabbing', etc. However, Semino et al. (2020) highlight potential linguistic problems with the McGill Pain Questionnaire which can affect patients' responses – specifically, their preference for particular terms – and thereby mitigate how effective it is for capturing the breadth of pain-related experiences. Based on their observations of general English corpus data, Semino et al. propose that certain terms may be more closely associated with pain in general English, and, as a result, patients might be more inclined to select a recognised collocate of 'pain'. This suggests that the questionnaire is more suited to capturing patients' linguistic knowledge rather than their pain experience.

TASK 5.1

Based on your intuitions, which of the following words would you expect to be used in relation to 'pain'? Are there some that have a particularly strong association? Would some more commonly be used in English to refer to things other than pain?

- sharp
- burning
- searing
- stabbing
- throbbing
- shooting
- dull
- piercing
- radiating

We can check our intuitions against the evidence of naturally occurring examples collected in a corpus. At https://www.english-corpora.org/ you can carry out searches using a range of corpora (registration may be required). Check the frequencies of the terms listed above in combination with 'pain', i.e., 'searing pain'.

- How do the results compare with your intuitions?
- Does this change depending on what corpus you use?
- You can also check your results against those in the chapter by Semino et al. (2020).

In the same way that patient information leaflets are designed to ensure that patients understand the risks involved with taking certain medications, participants also need to understand the risks associated with taking part in clinical research, which is fundamental to the development of such treatments.

Clinical trials are a key part of the development of healthcare interventions and involve standards for research procedures that are designed to ensure quality outcomes as well as protecting the legal and wellbeing rights of those who participate. Participation is contingent upon consent, and the routine procedure for eliciting consent is to produce patient information documents. Subsequently, participants typically complete an informed consent form based on their comprehension of those information documents. This highlights the importance of ensuring that participant information documents are accessible and accurate, both in relation to medical information and the research procedures involved in clinical trials.

Isaacs et al. (2022) analysed a corpus of participant information and informed consent documents in relation to randomised control trials for cancer treatment. One of the goals of their study was 'to build an open-access corpus of patient information sheets and consent forms and analyze each genre using an interdisciplinary approach to capture multidimensional measures of language quality beyond traditional readability measures' (Isaacs et al. 2022, p. 431). Keyword analysis was conducted using the BE06 as a reference corpus (Baker 2009), alongside established measures for readability, such as word count and the Flesch-Kincaid test (Kincaid et al. 1975). The Flesch-Kincaid test is a commonly used readability test that indicates grades of difficulty, primarily based on word length and sentence length. Isaacs et al. (2022) also investigated 'easability', which was defined in terms of narrativity, syntactic simplicity, word concreteness, referential cohesion, and deep cohesion. Keywords for the patient information sheet data corresponded with higher narrativity scores – compared with consent forms – referring to characters ('patients', 'doctors'), setting ('hospital') and events ('take part', 'surgery'). Isaacs et al. (2022) note a tension between the emphasis on the second person ('you') and mitigation ('if', 'whether', 'may', 'might') observed in patient information sheets compared with the focus on first-person ('I') claims with a greater degree of certainty ('will', 'confirm that', 'give') in consent forms. They, therefore, highlight an issue with asking volunteers to commit, in stronger terms, to a process in which the risks and consequences are not clearly defined.

There are also ethical considerations at the dissemination phase of clinical research in terms of the messages that are conveyed by those who have the credibility and the responsibility to inform wider audiences about health research outcomes. In the early stages of the COVID-19 pandemic, adjustments made to expedite the research publication process – with a view to making important health information more widely available, more rapidly – boosted the popularity of preprint archives such as medRxiv (Redden 2020). However, Redden (2020), among others, expressed concerns as to the quality of this information, as preprint articles have not yet undergone critical peer-review. The impact of this proliferation of COVID-19-related research also impacted the content of health publications that had been through peer-review. In a corpus study of research articles on COVID-19 from top-ranking, Science Citation Indexed journals on the Web of Science, Hyland and Jiang (2021) found evidence of 'hyping' in publications, as authors looked to distinguish themselves within a COVID-19 'infodemic'. This practice was manifest in lexical items conveying themes of certainty ('significant', 'important', 'crucial'), contribution ('necessary', 'essential', 'useful'), novelty ('first', 'timely', 'unique'), and potential ('promising', 'potential', 'apparent') of the research being reported (Hyland and Jiang 2021). In this way, we can see how the discursive representation of health issues relates not only to clinical definitions of what constitutes illness but also to evaluative judgements about certain areas of health research being 'important' and 'necessary'.

Clinical practices are influenced by administrative procedures, which we can also investigate through written documents – relating to government policy, for example. Investigating such documents provides us with a view of how representations established in documentation pertaining to a healthcare domain align (or not) with practice. Diaz (2022), for example, conducted a corpus-assisted discourse analysis of 100 publicly available policy documents relating to opioids and ageing healthcare programs, alongside ethnographic interviews with health service agents, to consider how the implementation of the policy (or at least, how implementation is reported) aligns with the objectives of those who developed it. A collocation analysis of keywords showed that while health professionals focus on the populations that health policies (are designed to) serve, there is a comparable absence in the documents of descriptions of who the target populations are and what their needs are. This, perhaps, reflects the different sites in which these discourses are constructed. The study also highlights that 'frontline' health workers are tasked with interpreting guidelines when it comes to implementing them, introducing a high degree of subjective judgement in how the principles of the policy are enacted.

Brookes (2021, p. 2213) discusses how the UK government policy towards tackling high rates of obesity demonstrates a 'responsibilizing rhetoric' that is consistent with a wider culture of neoliberalism that has characterised political economic practices in the UK since the 1980s. Through this rhetoric, the government minimises its own role in risk management to society, compelling individuals to effectively self-govern.

Koteyko et al. (2008, p. 226) also observe how responsibilities at the governmental level are challenged and defended in response to the problem of the rise of methicillin-resistant staphylococcus aureus (MRSA) in the UK. They combine corpus linguistics techniques with discourse analysis to gain a better understanding of the different interests, values, and normative judgements that were observable in policy documents and news articles (and which, thus, contributed to debates on the matter). Their corpus-assisted analysis of keywords in UK news and policy documents revealed a discursive dichotomy of simple/not simple in relation to identifying the causes of MRSA and initiating a public response. The incumbent UK government foregrounded a common-sense approach to infection control with 'simple' solutions, while challenges to the government highlighted the complexity of the issue and the uncertainty of the related science. Koteyko et al. (2008) argue that contrasting discursive strategies were deployed for the opposing purposes of casting blame and defending oneself against blame. This observation reminds us that ways of representing health challenges can be motivated by political concerns as well as – or even instead of – considerations for wellbeing.

We have seen how various written documents, such as policy documents, research articles, and news articles, interact with and contribute to linguistic conceptualisations of health. In the next section, we turn our attention to the news media, as arguably the most publicly available forms of written texts and thereby an influential contributor to public discourses around health and illness.

5.3.2 Health and illness in the news

The news media remains 'one of the primary means through which people access health information and form their impressions and understandings of health issues' (Brookes 2023, p. 215). News articles, therefore, can serve as an important bridge between the findings of medical research and public understanding of health. News editors and journalists have the capacity to determine not only *what* is covered in the news, but also *how*. As Johnson and Miller (2016, p. 212) argue, '[the] conventions media producers use to organize, make sense of, and give meaning to social phenomena have symbolic power to assert the narratives of certain privileged and dominant perspectives'. News organisations have stakeholders who can influence how topics are covered. News publications must also appeal to their readerships in order to continue to operate; in other words, '[n]ews outlets influence their readers' opinions but must also try to reflect readers' views, otherwise they risk losing those readers' (Brookes and Baker 2022, p. 365).

More generally, those involved in news reporting select information according to the principles of 'newsworthiness', which have been defined in terms of proximity, negativity, eliteness, and superlativeness, for example (Bednarek and Caple 2014). We can, therefore, consider how the same health issue is constructed as 'newsworthy' in how it is discussed across different news publications according to their respective readerships or editorial stances. Furthermore, we can use corpus methods to systematically analyse news content for evidence of ideological patterns. In Section 5.4, we discuss the specific lexical features that corpus approaches have identified as contributing to news representations of health professionals (such as 'foreign doctors') (Baker and McEnery 2014; Brookes and Wright 2020), prospective patients (Jones and Collins 2020), and illnesses and threats to health (Brookes and Baker 2022).

Atanasova et al. (2019) show that the concept of 'recovery', in relation to mental illness, is also discursively negotiated through media representations. They explain that 'recovery' has been conceptualised within the recovery movement as a way of life or attitude involving the growth of new meaning and purpose beyond the effects of mental illness (Deegan 2003). Through their analysis of keywords in national and local newspapers, they show that 'recovery' was more closely aligned with the conventional sense of a return to a normal state of health (Atanasova et al. 2019). Nevertheless, Atanasova et al. (2019) acknowledge that an increase in coverage of 'recovery', which occurs alongside the inclusion of the voices of individuals with mental health issues, offers a more positive alternative to representations of such individuals as violent and unpredictable, which is more widely documented in news coverage (see Bowen 2019). The researchers argue that this finding may be due to their inclusion of regional newspapers, in which there is said to be a greater capacity to report 'good news' stories relating to the local community (Atanasova et al. 2019).

One of the strategies for demonstrating the positive elements of the story was to represent individuals with mental illness according to an 'economy' frame; in this depiction, treatment was presented as a way to facilitate such individuals' return to work, resulting in their contributing to the economy, in contrast to their being represented as an economic burden (Atanasova et al. 2019). Jones and Collins (2020) caution against using the 'economy' frame altogether when discussing recipients of healthcare on the basis that it has been shown to encourage competition between health service users when provisions are limited. In these instances, the commitment of resources to certain treatments is seen as more 'valuable' than others and, consequently, some patients as more 'deserving' than others.

Reali et al. (2016) further demonstrate that the selected framing of a health issue has implications for how that health issue is understood. They combine a corpus analysis of written texts (including news articles, fiction and non-fiction books, emails, and brochures) in different varieties of Spanish with an experimental study, presenting participants with different framings of depression in order to consider the impacts that different metaphorical representations have on perceptions of patient responsibility. Their corpus analysis involved manually coding concordance lines of instances of '*depresión*' and showed that in addition to being represented as a physical disease, depression is typically conceptualised as a place in space (e.g., 'getting out of' depression) or as an opponent (something to 'combat'). Subsequently, they showed that when represented as a place, respondents focused more on social factors and that when depression was presented as an opponent, respondents expressed more blame towards the person with depression and expressed a greater desire to stay away from them (Reali et al. 2016).

Other researchers have similarly investigated metaphorical expressions used in relation to illness in the news media and the use of metaphor is a regular feature of conceptualisations of illness, health interventions, and descriptions of strategies for responding to or coping with illness, generally (see also Semino, 2008). In the first case study for this chapter, we discuss Brookes's (2023) exploration of metaphors used to represent dementia in UK tabloid newspapers.

CASE STUDY:

A longitudinal study of dementia metaphors in UK tabloids (Brookes 2023)

Brookes's (2023) investigation of metaphors used in relation to dementia demonstrates both the opportunities afforded by (digital) archives of written texts and the applicability of corpus methods for investigating language features in large collections of data covering extended timespans.

As Brookes (2023) explains, the term 'dementia' covers a range of discrete diseases including, for example, Alzheimer's disease. Despite the fact that they are reported to affect around 50 million people worldwide (WHO 2017), the effects of these conditions are not well understood. As a progressive syndrome with no pharmacological cure, the individual impacts of dementia are different for each person, will likely worsen over time, and those affected will die with it (though not *of* it). Brookes (2023) reports that representations of dementia typically reduce people to (a decline in) their cognitive faculties and often their literal brain and that these refer to a loss of self that leads to isolation or 'social death'. These representations, thus, draw on metaphorical framings, alongside visual metaphors (see also Brookes et al. 2018), to communicate a sense of decline or loss, which Brookes (2023) states can be dehumanising and, ultimately, stigmatising for those affected.

Brookes (2023) introduces a corpus that captures coverage of dementia over a ten-year period (2010–2019). The compilation of corpora of this size and in relation to news coverage is supported by digital news archives, and Brookes, like many others, uses the online news repository *LexisNexis* to identify and obtain relevant news articles. This repository has a powerful search function that allows us to target specific (combinations of) search terms according to date of publication and within national and regional newspapers, trade magazines, and transcripts of TV/radio broadcasts across 75 different languages. As such, when compiling a corpus from the archive, we need to think carefully about their corpus design, including whether, for example, they want to consider the 'quality' of news publication (i.e., tabloid or broadsheet), what this entails for a presumed readership, and what implications there are for how articles are written. Once the parameters are set, *LexisNexis* allows users to download each result as an individual file. Brookes (2023) opted to focus on UK national tabloids (*Express, Daily Mail, Mirror, Star,* and *The Sun*) and subsequently constructed a corpus of 6,751 articles related to 'dementia', totalling 3,961,272 words.

Based on previous work, Brookes (2023) recognised that metaphorical expressions are common framing devices in discussions of dementia, deployed in their capacity to help to make complex phenomena more accessible through analogy with a more concrete, recognisable concept. One of the challenges with investigating metaphorical expressions is that common source domains, such as WAR (e.g., 'a battle with illness'), can of course also be used in their more conventional semantic sense, and whether a concept is used literally or metaphorically needs to be discerned manually, e.g., by studying concordance lines.

Brookes (2023) is guided by the metaphor identification procedure (MIP) outlined by the Pragglejazz Group (2007), which was developed in order to provide clear guidance on when to mark metaphorical usage, i.e., when 'contextual meaning' contrasts with a more physical and concrete 'basic meaning' (Semino et al. 2018, p. 632). Brookes (2023) generated a list of collocates for the word 'dementia' within a five-word collocation span, with a minimum frequency of ten occurrences, and a mutual information score of 3.0 or above (see Hunston 2022). Having generated a list of collocates, Brookes (2023) studied their concordance lines in order to determine which of the terms indicated the use of metaphor and, following the MIP, retained those that were used metaphorically in at least 50% of cases for further analysis.

Brookes (2023) categorised the use of metaphor (including similes and other figurative expressions) according to the themes of (i) prevalence, (ii) causes, (iii) symptoms and prognosis, (iv) lived experience, and (v) responses. In relation to prevalence, for example, Brookes (2023) found that dementia was described as the 'leading' cause of death in the UK, 'overtaking' other conditions within a metaphorical frame of COMPETITION.

Dementia was written about in terms of VIOLENCE, presented as a 'killer' and resulting in a death 'toll' alongside the numerous people it has 'hit'. It is described as 'robbing' people of their memory and causes are also discussed in violent terms, with certain proteins described as a 'dementia dagger' that 'attacks' parts of the brain. In these examples, we can see how dementia is attributed agency, which is further demonstrated in its reported malevolence as a 'brutal', 'cruel', and 'heartless' disease. This violent experience extends to the 'battle', 'fighting', and 'struggling' that is shown to characterise the lived experience of those with dementia who might also be described in more passive ways, as 'victims' and as being 'stricken' by the condition. Brookes (2023) discusses the use of 'epidemic', used to convey prevalence, as one of the examples that could lead to misunderstandings. He explains that this is a term associated with infectious diseases and, therefore, would not strictly apply – in a literal sense – to dementia.

Brookes (2023) expresses concern over the emphasis on the constructed agency of dementia in contrast with the relatively diminished agency afforded in the coverage to those who experience it. Dementia is reported to move forwards almost inevitably and, in response, all we as individuals and as a society can do is to 'delay' or 'halt' its progression or otherwise 'succumb' to its effects. Considering wider discussions of health, researchers have also articulated concerns about positing the human body as a battlefield on which individuals can 'lose' in the most fatal sense (see also Sontag 1978; Semino et al. 2017). In the context of dementia, Brookes (2023) reiterates that without an effective pharmacological treatment, the WAR framing can be particularly stigmatising, as it is a 'battle' that can only really be considered to be lost. Alternative metaphors can highlight companionship and a 'journey', which individuals can more apparently participate in and which need not be characterised by suffering.

Brookes (2023) acknowledges the potential limitations of his work in that he opted to target tabloid newspapers on the basis of their wide readership and that a collocation analysis will prioritise metaphorical expressions that are lexicalised in close proximity to the search term (dementia). Nevertheless, he concludes that this approach provided a 'productive but practical route into the data' (Brookes 2023, p. 219).

Brookes's (2023) study represents one of a good number of studies of health communication in news media in which corpus linguistics has supported investigations of multiple publications over a relatively long period of time. Price (2022), for example, has investigated stigmatising representations of people with mental illness in a corpus of UK news articles from 1984–2014. Broadly, Price (2022) found that reports over this period of time largely used identity-first forms ('a schizophrenic') to refer to people with mental illness more than person-first forms ('a person with schizophrenia'). Looking to investigate correlations between representations in the media and wider social attitudes towards mental health, Hannaford (2017) similarly combined a corpus analysis of UK press coverage of mental illness between 1995–2014 with findings from the UK National Attitudes to Mental Illness Survey (AMIS) (TNS BMRB 2015). Hannaford (2017) reports an increase in destigmatising coverage of mental illness over the period as well as a decline in coverage of people with mental illness as dangerous, which correlated with a decrease in negative attitudes towards people with mental illness among the public.

Bowen (2019) investigated stigmatising representations of people with personality disorders, as observed in a corpus of UK press coverage from 2008 to 2017, and finds a wide collection of terms demonstrating acts of violence. Subsequently, Bowen (2019, p. 249) warns that readers are likely to be 'drawn into the web of language of violence but less likely to contextualize the biographies of individuals', thereby reducing the people involved to a single attribute that contributes to a stigmatising stereotype of people with personality disorders as violent. Bowen et al. (2019) took a similar approach to investigating representations of schizophrenia, again matching a corpus of representations in UK tabloid newspapers with a corpus of diabetes coverage. In this study, the authors identified an additional category of keywords that they labelled 'Exemplars', which contained references to individuals such as (Peter) Sutcliffe, (Ian) Brady, and (Myra) Hindley. Bowen et al. (2019, p. 149) note that culturally specific references to individuals who have notoriety in the United Kingdom and have committed homicide are 'regarded as a mechanism within the press to heighten the affective response of fear in readers' and thereby contribute to the repeated use of graphic, violent language over the 24-month period that they studied.

Baker et al. (2020, p. 7) studied changes in representations of obesity in the UK press over the period 2008–2017 and found that,

> Consistent over time, is that obesity is viewed increasingly as a problem, both to individuals and to the health service, and what the representations of it as a biomedical problem and matter of personal responsibility have in common is that they locate this problem within the individual, as opposed to the wider social and environmental determinants of health.

They evidence this by showing that words belonging to thematic categories such as education, politics, economics, business and social all became less frequent over time. They contextualise these observations among a wider trend towards neoliberal rationality in the United Kingdom. Bednarek and Carr (2020) likewise investigated coverage of obesity, in 694 newspaper articles from 12 Australian newspapers in the period 2013–2017. Like Price (2022), they observed a tendency to use identity-first forms in the prevalence of the noun 'diabetic' compared with the adjectival 'diabetic' (person), which they state is not consistent with Diabetes Australia's guidelines on using 'people-first' language. They are also critical of the uneven coverage in relation to Australian sub-populations, by state and in relation to Aboriginal and Torres Strait Islander people, that does not align with prevalence rates. The timeframe for this corpus supports Bednarek and Carr (2020) in showing that the number of articles and nature of the coverage is broadly stable, with occasional peaks that correspond with topical events such as National Diabetes Day. These studies further demonstrate that certain aspects of the experience can be foregrounded in the labels used in reference to who experiences them as well as potentially overlooking the experiences of certain communities and contributing to the sense of responsibility placed on individuals for managing their own healthcare.

The media also contribute to determining the lifespan of health problems in that while such issues precede the time of media coverage and exist long after it, their inclusion in media texts as 'newsworthy' can shape not only if but also when they are recognised as a health issue. Diachronic studies, therefore, allow us to assess the apparent newsworthiness of a health topic, based on its coverage in the media. The global COVID-19 pandemic provides an example in which we have the opportunity to track media coverage from the inception of a health event (including its initial outbreak), its definition as a new form of coronavirus, and its status as a global pandemic. Davies (2021) describes the creation of the Coronavirus Corpus as a sub-corpus of the News on the Web (NOW) corpus and offers instructive examples of how such a corpus can be queried to investigate the emergence of key terms over time (e.g., 'flatten the curve') and provide insights into international relations by looking at the collocates of 'China', for instance.

Jaworska (2021) similarly compiled data from United Kingdom, United States, and German news coverage in the early months of 2020 to document the initial outbreak. Jaworska (2021) reports that, in contrast to familiar war metaphors used in the UK and US coverage (manifest in verbs such as 'combat' and 'strike'), there was a relative absence of militaristic language in the German coverage, which focused more on testing (*'testen'*), protecting (*'schützen'*), and informing (*'informieren'*). This approach demonstrates how corpus analysis targeting collocations can help us to understand the impact and perspectives on global health issues, as these are mediated through language and realised at a national level (see also Mahlberg and Brookes 2021).

Since the initial outbreak, the COVID-19 pandemic is unarguably still newsworthy in terms of factors such as negativity and proximity but, perhaps, diminishing in its novelty (Bednarek and Caple 2014). Nevertheless, its relevance can be seen in relation to media coverage of other health issues. Brookes's (2022) keyword analysis of UK news articles referring to both COVID-19 and obesity shows that in a context in which the stakes have been raised, certain publications, particularly the tabloid press, offered a more stigmatising representation of people with obesity as a burden on limited health resources at a time of crisis. Yet on the other hand, Brookes (2022) also observes an increase in coverage referring to race-related health inequalities, thereby encouraging a critical perspective on the social determinants of health, which was not observed in more longstanding UK news coverage of obesity (Brookes and Baker 2021). This occurs alongside greater scrutiny of the government's strategies for addressing the pandemic and associated health risks which, again, was not evident in previous coverage (Brookes and Baker 2022). Brookes's (2022) view is that the pandemic facilitated more exaggerated forms of regular news practice, pushing journalists towards more focused elements of the different areas of concern in the issue of high rates of obesity. Thus, the acute pressures and ubiquity of the COVID-19 pandemic prompted a reconfiguration of the media discussion of obesity that more explicitly contextualised this health concern within a broader national context.

Collins and Koller (2023) use corpus methods to investigate how the COVID-19 pandemic inspired a new vocabulary that reflected the adoption of new social practices ('self-isolate'), the advent of new objects and products ('Covid', 'Comirnaty', or otherwise shifts in semantic meaning that demonstrate changes in behaviour ('zooming'). They demonstrate, using the Coronavirus Corpus of news articles (Davies 2021), how corpus methods are suited to identifying potential neologisms: on the basis of acute and significant rises in frequency, as well as constituting an archival resource in which it is possible to search for the prior and subsequent use of the term. Thus, one of the ways in which we can assess the impact of global events is the extent to which they invoke changes in language.

The full extent of the legacy of COVID-19 remains to be seen, yet we can already see how it has changed the context for understanding other health-related issues. This, again, demonstrates the importance of situating our observations of texts within their sociocultural contexts, and in the next section, we look at how corpus linguists have sought to do just that in relation to written health documents that have come from historical periods for which we have limited contextual information.

5.3.3 Health and illness in history

For many practical reasons, studies of historical language are notably skewed towards written texts. As McEnery et al. (2022, p. 393) tell us, '[l]anguage spoken in the past which had no written form or where written records have been lost in whole or part are, in effect, lost to us', and linguistic approaches that rely on direct access to participants are not possible. McEnery et al. (2022, p. 393) also remind us that 'the survival of texts is linked to cultural value, representations of speech are less commonly found than writing, and literacy levels are likely to greatly influence the types of texts produced'. What we do have access to, in the form of written historical medical texts, are likely to have been generated by high-status medical professionals, social elites, and institutions whose works were deemed worthy of preservation. We can know very little, for example, of the quotidian experiences of health and illness as endured and articulated by 'ordinary' people. Furthermore, the work of converting archived material into a machine-readable format for corpus analysis is another selective process that can also depend upon an understanding of changing meanings and practices.

When there are opportunities to investigate the experiences of 'ordinary' individuals in historical material, there are ethical considerations that can also inhibit the extent to which details of those experiences are widely disseminated. We have argued for the importance of personal narratives in enriching our understanding of experiences of illness, but it is precisely this personal dimension that raises questions about the ethics of making public and scrutinising the often-sensitive details of such accounts. Meyer and Moncrieff (2021) reflect on the open archival practices associated with various national collections of, for example, case files of disability pensions for individuals who served in wars. As Meyer and Moncrieff (2021, p. 63) explain in regard to the British Ministry of Pension Files:

> As well as publicly accessible information such as name, rank, regiment, date of birth and theatres of service, this series contains sensitive details of medical conditions and diagnoses, as well as material concerning stigmatising social circumstances, including domestic violence, prostitution, illegitimacy and even potential criminal activity.

For the researcher, such records provide the rich, contextual information that supports our informed evaluation of the discursive construction of concepts of health and illness, and Meyer and Moncrieff (2021, p. 64) detail some of the work that is already taking place to develop our understanding of British society 'at all levels'.

However, they also emphasise that these are individuals with families, whose lives will be impacted by the revelations that might arise from these archives. Meyer and Moncrieff (2021, p. 69) reflect on the tension between discussing the lives of a vulnerable group as a kind of 'informational colonialism' versus the importance of providing visibility to otherwise marginalised experiences, working to challenge stigma. In their own work, Meyer and Moncrieff (2021) describe their procedures for limiting the amount of metadata available so that researchers can identify cases that might be of interest to them and subsequently apply for full access to the details of the case, after which decisions would be made about what information it is appropriate to disseminate. They thereby stress the importance of holding comprehensive metadata and proper referencing in the management of archive materials, principles that we can also extend to the management of large corpora.

It is not difficult to see how an understanding of the historical context informs our reading of the data. Lehto (2022), for example, considers representations of patients and various health-related professionals in eighteenth-century English using the corpus of Late Modern English Medical Texts. Lehto (2022) highlights two important developments at this time: first, in the wake of the Enlightenment, scientific experiments became more common, for the purposes of collecting objective information on diseases; and second, philanthropy and polite correspondence also prevailed in the era, contributing to the establishment of many voluntary hospitals and dispensaries, subsequently making healthcare more accessible to the middle and lower classes. Lehto (2022, p. 204) remarks that 'the new medical methods and scientific thinking – with statistics, generalisations and experiments – detach the author from the single patient and shift the attention to groups of patients and generalisations'. Meanwhile, compassion is revealed in collocates of terms referring to patients, which include 'poor', 'unhappy', 'unfortunate', and emphasis on the degree to which they 'suffer'. While such broad, sociocultural trends are documented well enough, it remains one of the major challenges of working with historical written data to recover salient information about the contexts in which the texts were produced and consumed by readers in order to facilitate investigations of language variables.

Documenting shifts in the terms used to refer to health concepts can help us to consider how texts are produced in relation to expectations of/from audiences. Schnelle et al. (2022), for example, investigate the morphological, syntactic, and semiotic characteristics of references to menstruation in German herbal texts from the late fifteenth century to the early twentieth century. Changing terminologies used in reference to this particular area of health reflect the wider emergence of a scientific register. Names such as '*Heimlichkeit*' ('secrecy') indicate that menstruation had been considered taboo and metaphorical expressions such as '*Blumenzeit*' ('flower time') were used frequently up until the second half of the seventeenth century. Schnelle et al. (2022) cite the influence of the Enlightenment postulate at this time to account for a shift towards terms that derive from observable properties, such as '*Monatszeit*' ('monthly time') and '*menstruum*' ('menstruation'/'monthly'). However, they also observe that the adoption of the loanword '*menstruum*' involved a juxtaposition of the Latin term with a vernacular expression ('*menstruum gennant*', i.e., 'called menstruum'), which Schnelle et al. (2022, p. 170) explain marks the linguistic manifestation of attempts to combine 'two traditions of knowledge'. Indicative of what they term 'progressive terminologisation', Schnelle et al. (2022, p. 172) observe a decrease in formal variation and in semiotic variation over time as a restricted number of preferred terms become more widely adopted.

Hiltunen and Taavitsainen (2022, p. 1) state that

[t]he register of medical writing is well-suited for historical and diachronic studies, as it has a wide scope with both professional and lay texts and has undergone major alterations resulting from changes in the context of production, reception and use of texts.

They report a growing interest in applying corpus linguistics to the study of medical texts with respect to Language for Specific Purposes (Swales 2000) and to investigate the variation in genres of medicine, reminding us that, historically, the boundaries between medical science, alchemy, religion, and astrology have been 'fuzzy' (Hiltunen and Taavitsainen 2022, p. 6).

Menzel (2022) discusses the issue of what 'counts' as a medical text and demonstrates a computational approach to text classification in an investigation of the Royal Society Corpus. This corpus comprises 48,000 texts (approximately 300 million tokens), covering 330 years over the late modern English period and is enriched with various kinds of contextual metadata as well as being annotated for linguistic and pragmatic features. Menzel (2022) conducts an analysis of morphological, lexical, collocational, and phrasal text elements with a view to determining what are typical linguistic features of scientific journals, compared with other kinds of medical texts. One of the diachronic developments reported by Menzel (2022) relates to text titles which historically had a promotional quality that was expressed in terms such as 'extraordinary' or 'remarkable', but which after 1800 became more concise and content-focused. This provides some context for evaluating the special circumstances that led to research articles on COVID-19 featuring more hyping language, as reported by Hyland and Jiang (2021, see Section 5.3.1), as conventions for less evaluative language have been long-established.

A key feature of McEnery and Baker's (2022) work is the integration of metadata supporting a genre-based analysis of the data. The authors discuss some of the conventions of seventeenth-century genre classification and some of the challenges with making distinctions between genres. Their data come from the one-billion-word Early English Books Online (EEBO) corpus, which includes 44,422 English works of literature, philosophy, politics, religion, geography, history, and a range of other disciplines covering the period 1475 through to 1700, for which we can assume a fairly heterogeneous audience. Focusing on nationality-driven terms for venereal disease and illustrating the value of genre-classification in corpus design, McEnery and Baker (2022) demonstrate how perceptions around venereal disease and its sufferers shifted over the course of the seventeenth century. These terms are discussed in more detail in Section 5.4.3.

In McEnery and Baker's (2022) work, we find that non-medical texts offer a view of how commentators outside of the profession contribute to medical discourses. In the next section, we turn our attention to literary texts to consider how more creative forms of writing provide opportunities for readers to encounter another form of expertise and for those with lived experience to find ways to try and make relatable how illness shapes their everyday experiences.

5.3.4 Health and illness in literature

Creative writing genres can offer distinct opportunities for people to articulate their experiences of health and illness when there is no obvious point of reference for audiences to experience the same physical symptoms or to comprehend the cognitive effects of an illness. Many mental health conditions remain poorly understood, and personal accounts – in whatever creative form of expression they take – are increasingly recognised as important resources for developing our understanding of disorders such as psychosis (Woods 2013). In our second case study of written health communication, corpus methods are applied to help identify patterns in how an autobiographical account encourages readers to appreciate what it is like to experience hallucinations in the context of a schizophrenia diagnosis.

CASE STUDY:

Exploring lived experience through features of mind style (Demjén and Semino 2021)

Demjén and Semino (2021) examine the autobiographical account of Henry Cockburn, who has a diagnosis of schizophrenia, in the co-authored text, *Henry's Demons* (Cockburn and Cockburn 2011), and reflect on the challenges of making relatable the experience of seeing, hearing, and believing things that others cannot perceive. Recognising the high degree of subjectivity of the hallucinatory experiences associated with schizophrenia, Demjén and Semino (2021) identify the concept of 'mind style', drawn from the field of stylistics, as particularly suited to the challenge of discussing how Henry's personal experience can be documented in language.

Mind style is defined as 'any distinctive linguistic representation of an individual mental self' (Fowler 1977, p. 103) and, like the sociolinguistic concept of style, focuses on the particular combinations of language patterns that constitute an individual's way of expressing themselves; however, in the case of mind style, we go beyond what the individual says and also consider patterns in their mental functioning. As such, it is more often applied in the study of fictional texts – in which such mental functioning is made available to us, i.e., by a narrator – and when the individual's mental functioning is in some way distinctive or unusual. Semino and Swindlehurst (1996), for example, apply the concept of mind style to discuss the world view of Bromden, a patient in a mental hospital in Ken Kesey's *One Flew over the Cuckoo's Nest*. They focus on metaphors drawing on the source domain of machinery to demonstrate how the author portrays the narrator's 'idiosyncratic view of the world and his progress towards mental and physical liberation' (Semino and Swindlehurst 1996, p. 143).

The examination of mind style can be based on specific features of language that represent the 'consistent structural options' (Fowler 1977) that contribute to characterisation or, in this instance, provide insights into the author–narrator's mental experiences and thought process in response to those experiences. The focus on patterns, as they manifest in the repeated use of particular features of language, thus, makes it a conceptual model that can be readily combined with the procedures of corpus linguistics analysis. Indeed, McIntyre and Archer (2010) demonstrate how consistency in mind style can be documented, in part, through the quantitative evidence provided by keywords and key semantic domains.

Demjén and Semino (2021) discuss pronoun use, narrative style, visual focus, and the (lack of) representation of others' minds to demonstrate the features that appear to characterise Henry's subjective viewpoint, or individual 'mental world'. Because almost any linguistic feature can be indicative of mind style, Demjén and Semino (2021, p. 339) discuss the need

> to identify in an explicit and rigorous manner any linguistic features that are distinctive and systematic within the relevant text and make a case for their potential contribution to readers' impressions of the mental processes and world view of the relevant character or narrator.

They draw on both previously established aspects of narration that have been found to be relevant to mind style (lexical choices, negation, deictic expressions, interactional behaviour) and a keyword analysis of the chapters written by Henry with a reference corpus of autobiographical material, carried out at the level of semantic domains using Wmatrix (Rayson 2008). Keyness was determined through a measure of effect size (Log Ratio) with a minimum threshold for significance ($p < 0.001$), measured using the Log Likelihood statistic.

In their analysis of extracts from *Henry's Demons*, written by Henry himself, Demjén and Semino (2021) highlight how some features correspond with what is known about more general experiences of psychosis (i.e., not specific to Henry), such as the use of the verb 'feel' preceding speech, indicating that the communications that Henry perceives are not straightforwardly auditory. Henry's narration, specifically, is shown to be characterised by an overuse of singular first-person pronouns ('I', 'me', 'my', 'myself') and underuse of third-person pronouns ('he', 'his', 'him', 'her') and the collective 'we'. That this self-reference is statistically significant is notable, given that the reference corpus (of autobiographies) constitutes a self-reflexive genre in which the use of first-person pronouns is already likely to be frequent.

After investigating the use of these pronouns in context, Demjén and Semino (2021) determine that Henry's self-references reflect a tendency for 'overinterpretation', i.e., to notice small details in his surroundings and interpret them as having some significance to him, personally. This phenomenon has been linked with psychosis. The elevated sense of subjectivity, as an effect of frequent self-reference, can create a sense of uncertainty in that it reminds readers that they are not being presented with objective truths. Uncertainty is further conveyed from Henry's point of view through the regular formulation

'I found myself', which Demjén and Semino (2021) argue demonstrates diminished agency; with a cognitive intermediary between Henry and his physical actions (e.g., 'I found myself walking'), he does not appear to be entirely in control of what he does. Furthermore, these resultant actions do not appear to be anticipated by Henry, conveying disorientation.

Demjén and Semino (2021) also discuss features that are absent from Henry's narration, which is determined by the knowledge of what conventionally appears in such narratives. Specifically, they remark upon a lack of temporal or causal markers that would demonstrate connections between different elements in the narrative. The statistical underuse of third-person references fits within a broader pattern which Demjén and Semino (2021) describe as Henry's 'narrow field of vision' and in-the-moment responses that result in a lack of continuity in relation to events and to the people that Henry comes across.

Demjén and Semino's (2021) study is presented as an example of how a corpus stylistic analysis can provide 'detailed and systematic evidence of how narratives such as [*Henry's Demons*] may enable a deeper appreciation of mental and emotional experiences that are poorly understood and sometimes stigmatized, creating the conditions for greater empathy and acceptance' (p. 352). It is these types of perspectives that are not easy to find in news reports or other kinds of health documentation.

Furthermore, with broader options for what form the text can take, creative writing genres can be effective in helping readers experience events and objects in a comparable way to the author, who can introduce these elements in a manner that reflects how they encountered them. As further studies of mind style are carried out and researchers use approaches from corpus linguistics to document and discern consistent structural elements, creative writers can develop a more informed understanding of how to craft such elements to various effects. This, subsequently, can potentially offer the tools through which to demystify certain health and illness experiences.

Semino (2014) similarly draws on the concept of mind style to examine the narration in the novel, *The Curious Incident of the Dog in the Night-Time* (Haddon 2003). This novel has been lauded by those with lived experience and professionals in clinical psychiatry alike (though not universally) as offering an accurate and compelling representation of the mind and behaviour of a person with autism, although it is never stated in the novel that the narrator, Christopher, has a diagnosis of autism. Semino (2014) applies a corpus stylistic analysis to demonstrate how an interpretation of Christopher as a person with autism is made possible by the stylistic features of the narration. Semino (2014) explains that it is the cumulative effect of implicit cues that facilitates a reading of Christopher as neurodivergent, and, as such, establishing frequency-based patterns through corpus methods allows us to observe and document how those cues are introduced over the course of the novel.

Hunt and Carter (2012, p. 34) discuss thematic categories of keywords identified in the novel *The Bell Jar*, derived from comparison with the Brown corpus as a reference corpus, and assert that a corpus-assisted approach 'helps clarify how the presentation of mental illness is linguistically constructed and illuminates the idiosyncratic characteristics of this fictional narrator's psychological difficulty'. They advocate, therefore, that 'grammatical analysis facilitated using corpus tools could further our understanding of narratives of mental illness and provide replicable evidence to support our existing interpretations' (Hunt and Carter 2012, p. 38). Relatedly, Demjén (2015) has used similar techniques to investigate the journal writing of Plath herself and advocates combining qualitative and quantitative linguistic approaches to help to uncover the implicit features that are present in the narratives of those with lived experience of mental illness.

The exploratory nature of the keyness analysis approach supports the identification of features that are pertinent to the investigation of mind style in the case of specific narrators or characters, as the potential range of features that contributes to mind style is vast and cannot be specified as a framework that will apply across case studies. In the next section, we detail some of the lexical and grammatical features that have been documented through corpus studies and which we can consider to have some relevance to the associated health topic.

5.4 Features of written health communication

Our discussion of clinical documents, news articles, historical texts, and literary works provides us with a range of contexts in which we can explore the written representations of health and illness using corpus methods. As such, in this section, we report some of the linguistic forms and structures that have been identified in reference to depictions of health professionals, ways of characterising the patient, defining illness and threats to health, and conceptualising treatments and solutions. We can, thus, see how these representations compare across registers and how they have developed over time. We begin with examples of how health professionals have been represented throughout history.

5.4.1 Representing health professionals in written health documents

Historical texts provide us with an opportunity to see how modern medicine as a profession emerged as distinct from other related disciplines, such as alchemy, herbology, and astrology. Lehto (2022) explored the corpus of Late Modern English Medical Texts (LMEMT) to look at representations of physicians, surgeons, and apothecaries, as documented in various treatises, public health texts, medical journals, and general periodicals. The professional identifying labels 'physician', 'surgeon', and 'apothecary' were shown to be particularly frequent in the data, and Lehto (2022), subsequently, analysed content (as opposed to grammatical) collocates for these terms. Lehto (2022) found that each of the professional labels was discussed in relation to actions ('take', 'make', 'use'), knowledge ('know', 'known') and other practitioners ('practitioners', 'naturalists', 'chemists'). However, while 'physicians' were associated with their educated peers through the collocate 'college' (of physicians), 'apothecaries' were discussed in relation to other 'quacks', demonstrating a more critical view of their expertise.

Similarly, while descriptive references to 'physicians' and 'surgeons' tended to be more positive, as shown in collocates such as 'eminent', 'great', 'skilful', 'experienced', 'qualified' and 'educated', there were fewer descriptive references to 'apothecaries', and these tended to be negative, e.g., 'dishonest', 'blockheads', and 'ideots'. Lehto (2022) reports that references to money were more prevalent in discussions of apothecaries, which is said to be expected, given that lower fees was one of the reasons for which (poorer) people visited them. Nevertheless, this is another aspect through which negative attitudes towards apothecaries were expressed, characterising them as interested solely in making a profit instead of the wellbeing of patients. Ultimately, physicians were held in the highest esteem of these groups, and this is reflected in the co-occurrence of terms indexing their education and professional expertise.

Menzel (2022) found similarly laudative descriptions of medical professionals in a collection of scientific journals covering the late modern English period, in which positive evaluative adjectives such as 'eminent', 'celebrated', 'judicious', etc. were used to preface mentions of medical professionals. Furthermore, Menzel (2022) reports that there was also a trend for eponymous references to body parts (e.g., 'Eustachian tube', 'Haversian system') in this period. This, to some extent, can be explained by the fact that many such body parts were discovered at this time; nevertheless, we can see this as another form of veneration, and many of these eponymous terms are still used today.

Alongside investigations of how health professionals were written about by others, Ollikainen (2022) refers to self-mentions in medical texts taken from the Early Modern English Medical Texts corpus (which covers the period 1500–1700) to consider how medical writers constructed their own professional identity. Medical writers were shown to refer to both book learning and personal experience in their portrayal of their authority, though in 'discovery narratives' authors were more inclined to demonstrate their skills in deduction more than their prior knowledge. This show of authority and expertise applied in instances of 'failure' as well as success. In this way, they function, to some extent, to provide lessons for the future but also to establish that poor outcomes were not due to a lack of expertise on the part of the author who, nevertheless, made an accurate prognosis. This shows that both from the perspective of commentators and from the authors of medical journals, the expertise and agency of the individual practitioner were foregrounded.

In modern news coverage, we can see how discussion of health professionals intersects with other important political issues, such as immigration, and that rather than focusing on prominent individuals, journalists variously collectivise health professionals according to other characteristics that are made relevant in relation to newsworthy topics. For example, Baker and McEnery (2014) use corpus methods to investigate representations of foreign doctors working in the UK National Health Service over ten years' worth of UK news articles. Categories of collocates of the term 'foreign doctor(s)' demonstrated a focus on their arrival in the United Kingdom ('flown', 'brought', 'coming', etc.), mistakes or incompetence ('killed', 'poor', 'incompetent'), English language ability ('English', 'language', 'speak'), and regulation ('tests', 'training', 'checks'). Baker and McEnery (2014) show that these were all areas through which criticism was directed at foreign doctors, whose supposed limited language skills contribute to a notable number of errors, subsequently, prompting some to call for stricter regulations for accepting and employing doctors from countries outside of the United Kingdom.

Baker and McEnery (2014) highlight a number of contradictions in the press coverage, which they assert are of interest because they indicate that multiple stances can be taken on the same issue. One such contradiction was the proposition that 'foreign doctors' were forcing British doctors into unemployment or to emigrate, reported alongside concerns about staff shortages in the health services. This reiterates the 'argumentative' potential of journalism, through which oppositional stances can be presented based on the available information. Baker and McEnery (2014) extend their analysis to compare how 'doctors' generally were represented, and how the terms 'foreign' and 'foreigner' were used in UK news coverage. Finding similarly negative representations of 'foreign' individuals and groups (e.g., posing a threat) that were not generally observed in discussion of doctors, Baker and McEnery (2014) conclude that foreign doctors are primarily viewed in terms of their non-domestic status ahead of their professional status.

Wright and Brookes (2019) similarly found that health professionals were a key group of social actors in their investigation of English-language ability as a contributing factor to ideologies about national identity in UK tabloid news coverage between 2011 and 2016. Their corpus-assisted study did not begin with a focus on healthcare, but, rather, they were concerned with coverage of debates about language, following the UK Census in 2011 that reported that 99.74% of respondents spoke English as a main or additional language. Their collocation analysis of the phrase 'speak* English' demonstrated that alongside general terms for migrants ('immigrants', 'foreign', 'migrants') and roles in education ('pupils', 'student', 'teachers'), terms for various health professionals ('doctors', 'nurses', 'staff', 'patients') were central to discussions of (English) language ability. Doctors and nurses with reported limited English language ability were presented as a threat to the health and safety of the public, and the extent of this threat was expressed in vague quantification terms ('thousands'). Once again, this is contextualised within concerns about regulatory measures that allow such individuals to practise (for a diachronic study of this corpus, see Brookes and Wright 2020). In summary, health professionals – particularly doctors – have historically been characterised in terms of their professional expertise, and even when they are represented negatively, it is other aspects of the identity (nationality, language ability), separate from their professional identities, that is the subject of criticism.

5.4.2 *Representing patients in written health documents*

In contrast to health professionals, who are shown to be proactive and central to the enactment of health procedures, patients have historically been presented as passive in, or are otherwise absent from, written health documents. Lehto (2022) shows that in texts from the eighteenth century, patients were portrayed as objects of scientific inquiry and of the medical procedures and cures that were administered by skilled and expert health professionals. Price's (2022) investigation of media coverage from 1984–2014 similarly shows how those with mental illness are presented as passive and pitiable. This, in part, is indicated in the subtle distinction between a preference in the press to describe those with mental illness as 'suffering', compared with first-person accounts from people with mental illness, which were more likely to refer to 'experiencing' mental illness.

Jones and Collins (2020, p. 214) highlight issues with the limited representation of who is a potential beneficiary of pre-exposure prophylaxis (PrEP), as a treatment to inhibit the spread of the human immunodeficiency virus (HIV). Their analysis of clusters in UK news coverage between 2014 and 2018 demonstrates that there is very limited discussion of who is at risk of contracting HIV beyond 'men who have sex with men'. They warn that neglecting to inform the public of the fuller range of individuals who are at risk can prevent such individuals from taking appropriate precautionary steps (including accessing PrEP). Furthermore, Jones and Collins (2020) find evidence of the conflation of 'men who have sex with men' with the identity category of 'gay and bisexual men', which they argue contributes to extending a cultural link between HIV and gay men. This is shown to be problematic, as Jones and Collins (2020, p. 222) explain that such an association 'serves to frame sex between men as intrinsically dangerous and thus reinforces the stigmatisation of homosexuality'.

In related work, Collins's (2022) corpus-assisted analysis of news coverage of PrEP from the United States and from the United Kingdom and Ireland in the period 2016–2019 focused on key 'risk' words. Collins (2022) shows that across publications, references to 'at [higher] risk' and 'at-risk individuals' reflect a focus on particular groups, characterising them in terms of their vulnerability. Describing groups as 'at risk' is understood to be informative and arguably, sympathetic and contrasted with more critical, blaming representations frequently found in the *Daily Mail*. These blaming representations foregrounded 'risky' behaviours and lifestyles, comprised descriptors such as 'hedonistic' and 'promiscuous', and warned that the wider provision of PrEP would encourage further 'risky' sexual behaviour. Collins (2022) discusses how such views contribute to the stigmatisation of people who stand to directly benefit from PrEP provision, thereby encouraging maladaptive coping strategies which, in turn, place them at greater risk. This also shows that when the people who are at risk of illness are placed in agentive roles, they are represented as engaging in problematic or damaging behaviours.

The attribution of damaging behaviours to unwell individuals also contributes to the stigmatising representation of those who require health support as threats to others. Bowen (2019) shows that news coverage of people with personality disorders is characterised by violence. A keyword analysis of UK tabloid news articles including a reference to 'personality disorder(s)' between 2008 and 2017, in comparison with a matched corpus representing coverage of diabetes, generated a list of keywords that Bowen (2019) manually categorised according to the following themes:

- Acts of violence (e.g., 'murder', 'killing', 'killed', 'stabbed');
- Descriptions of acts (e.g., 'violence', 'violent', 'deranged', 'disturbing', 'ruthless');
- Implements of violence (e.g., 'knife', 'crossbow', 'knives', 'blade', 'hammer');
- Identity labels (e.g., 'killer', 'evil', 'murderer', 'psycho', 'monster').

Bowen (2019) highlights that the use of these terms is inconsistent with the guidelines provided by the Time to Change (2018) campaign and can lead to social isolation as a result of other people being fearful of engaging with those with a personality disorder.

Balfour (2019) similarly reports associations with violence in news representation of people with schizophrenia. Analysing a corpus of 15 million words of British newspaper articles published between 2000 and 2015, Balfour (2019, p. 59) demonstrates how the lexeme 'schizophrenic' carried a semantic prosody of 'dangerousness'. Collocates such as 'slashed', 'stabbed' and 'beheaded' contributed to representations of people with schizophrenia as perpetrators of violence, alongside the semi-instrumentalisation of such people as 'sword-wielding'. Furthermore, Balfour (2019) reports that the term 'schizophrenic' was associated with other labels of social deviance, such as 'psychopath', 'killer', and 'alcoholic'. Journalists also appeared to offer lay diagnoses on the basis of evidence of violent behaviour, as shown in the collocation of 'schizophrenic' with 'borderline', 'likely', and 'undiagnosed'. These observations demonstrate how entrenched notions of violence are to the identification of schizophrenia as well as exposing a circular logic to the perception of schizophrenia as a result of violent behaviours.

The limited agency of patients can also be seen in the relative lack of textual evidence that actually comes from those with first-hand experience of illness and who receive healthcare. Collins and Jones (2021) report that just 8.4% of instances of direct speech in news coverage of PrEP came from the category of 'lay people' and that newspapers overwhelmingly favoured quoting the perspectives of 'health advocacy groups', 'politicians, government officials and government initiatives', and 'medical and health experts' (66.0% of all quoted sources). Jones and Collins (2020, p. 222) emphasise the value of first-person perspectives, which offer more humanising representations and which '[stand] in contrast to the aggregated representations of infection rates and treatment costs'.

We have discussed, in Section 5.3.4, how literary texts can be effective in offering a view of what it is like to experience particular health issues. Semino's (2014) keyword analysis of the narratorial style of Christopher in *The Curious Incident...* (Haddon 2003) shows how basic grammatical words such as 'and' point to a simple syntactic style. This, in combination with a restricted general vocabulary contrasts with over-lexicalisation in some specialist areas (e.g., maths and science), thereby activating a reading of the narrator as having a developmental disability such as autism.

Additional linguistic features that help to convey Christopher's particular cognitive processes and perspective on the world include the reporting of long passages of verbatim reported speech, which result in the overuse of the term 'said'. Semino (2014) interprets this aspect of Christopher's narration as reflecting his powerful memory but also indicating that he does not have an intuition for selecting pertinent parts of the conversation that will be of benefit to or interest for the reader. This latter proposition is supported by Christopher's more general over-specification of details that have no clear relevance to the development of the narrative and the reported observations of people he encounters, who are prompted to advise him on what to describe and in what level of detail. Semino (2014) situates this characteristic within a wider struggle to relate to the experiences of others, which is reflected in the underuse of references to second persons; in the underuse of 'we', through which Christopher would position himself alongside others; and an absence of mental verbs associated with other characters, showing a lack of instrumental thought. Similar to the observations of Demjén and Semino (2021) in relation to an autobiographical account of someone with psychosis, these literary representations help to show how such mental health issues can inhibit interpersonal relationships.

Hunt and Carter (2012, p. 29) use a corpus stylistic approach in their exploration of Sylvia Plath's (1966) *The Bell Jar* to 'demonstrate the connection between the novel's linguistic features and its depiction of psychological trauma'. Keyword analysis highlights, for example, a characteristic habit on the part of the narrator, Esther, for using similes, through which ordinary objects in Esther's surroundings are likened to forms of death and violence. Similarly, a tendency to refer to 'faces' is reported to reflect Esther's perception of other people as disconnected facades. Key cluster analysis also shows that Esther's experience is characterised by unfulfilled actions, expressed in phrases such as 'I tried' and 'I wanted', as well as negative phrases such as 'I didn't know' and 'I couldn't see', indicating how individuals experiencing mental health issues can perceive themselves in terms of having a restricted sense of agency.

5.4.3 Representing illness and threats to health in written health documents

In this section, we discuss the representations of illness and the depiction of threats to public and individual health. The naming of an illness can reveal important contextual information related to, for example, international relations. In their investigation of the most frequent terms used to refer to venereal disease in the EEBO corpus, McEnery and Baker (2022) found a prevalence of the national terms 'French pox' and 'French disease', alongside 'gonorrhoea' (and its spelling variants), 'running of the reins' and 'lues venerea'. McEnery and Baker (2022) subsequently discuss the historical events over the course of the seventeenth century that could have a bearing on the fluctuating use of terms attributing venereal disease to a locale or national population. The labelling of disease in relation to a place, McEnery and Baker (2022) remind us, has a long-standing history and has continued in the unofficial naming of the SAR-CoV-2 virus as 'The China Virus' – most notably by former US President Donald Trump. The World Health Organization (WHO) (2020) specifically addressed the issue of finding a name 'that did not refer to a geographical location, an animal, an individual or group of people, and which is also pronounceable and related to the disease' in its public media briefing on 11 February 2020, acknowledging that '[h]aving a name matters to prevent the use of other names that can be inaccurate or stigmatizing'.

Semino et al.'s (2020) aforementioned investigation of the McGill Pain Questionnaire was predicated on the concern that already established word associations were influencing patients' selections from the questionnaire and, thereby, confounding the extent to which the written record documented the degree and intensity of actual pain experiences. Semino et al. (2020) searched the Oxford English Corpus, which includes 2.5 billion words of twenty-first century English, for the terms that appear on the questionnaire, noting their general frequency and their use in relation to pain. Terms such as 'shooting', 'sharp', and 'tight' were shown to occur frequently in the context of 'pain', in contrast with low-frequency terms such as 'pulsing', 'rasping', and 'lacerating', which were also reported to occur in more specialised text genres. Collocation analysis further supported Semino et al. (2020) in demonstrating that only nine of the 78 descriptors collocated with 'pain' and that other terms have a stronger association with other semantic fields, for instance, 'drawing' more often collocates with art-related terms such as 'paintings', 'prints', and 'pencil'.

These observations led Semino et al. (2020) to argue for the 'priming effects' that patients' familiarity with general English can have on their recognition of relevant, pain-related terms on the McGill Pain Questionnaire. In support of their argument, they found high correlation between the most frequently selected term and the strongest collocate of 'pain' in a given category on the questionnaire, suggesting that patients simply opt for the term they recognise as most strongly associated with pain. This study reminds us that patients come to the clinic with pre-existing ideas about discourses and language that influence the manner in which they talk about illness, even when the available terminology is presented by representatives of the clinic.

One explanation for the consistent use of particular terms in relation to pain is that they constitute meaningful and accessible metaphors for the physical experience of pain, and we have also seen in the case study reported in Section 5.3.2 that metaphorical expressions are prevalent in the news coverage of dementia (Brookes 2023). Cotter et al. (2021) investigate metaphorical expressions used in news media texts and policy documents related to obesity, focusing on the semantic domains of war ('battle' with obesity), religion (obesity is 'sinful'), addiction (eating is an 'addiction'), and epidemic (obesity is a 'contagious disease'). They found that, proportionally, policy documents contained more metaphorical expressions (1.6 per thousand words) than news articles (1.1) but that war metaphors were the most common in each text type. The prevalence of metaphorical expressions in policy documents suggests that metaphor is not only useful in communicating health issues to the public (i.e., in news articles) but can also be used to strategically mobilise different agents in collective action to 'combat' obesity.

Brookes and Baker's (2022) keyword analysis of news coverage of obesity demonstrates that obesity can be presented as a threat at different levels of society and that the editorial position of the newspapers (politically left-leaning or right-leaning) and the 'quality' format (tabloid or broadsheet) appears to affect which aspects are foregrounded in the coverage. Keywords for left-leaning broadsheets highlighted a focus on risk factors associated with obesity, such as genes ('epigenetics'), diet ('meat', 'vegan'), the food industry ('industry', 'outlets') and government activities ('government', 'authorities', 'department'). Right-leaning broadsheets similarly focused on risk factors for obesity. However, there was more of an emphasis on individual action, as shown in keywords such as 'running' and 'workouts' as well as references to time spent using technology ('mobile'). Tabloid newspapers were shown to focus more on how developing obesity increased the risk of encountering other health issues. This was particularly evident in the coverage of right-leaning tabloids, which included the keywords 'blood [pressure]', 'heart [disease]', 'condition', and 'type 2 diabetes'.

Corpus analyses, therefore, help us to identify the ways in which journalists contextualise health issues such as obesity and variously foreground the role of various social actors. As with the case of PrEP (Collins 2022), conservative views are more closely associated with a discussion of health risks that place responsibility with the individual who is depicted as having a lifestyle that is unhealthy or damaging in some way, which Brookes and Baker (2022) situate within an increasingly neoliberal political climate in the United Kingdom. Once again, we are reminded that readers receive different health messages depending on which publications they read, and journalists can draw on different aspects of the wider sociopolitical context in their representations of illness.

5.4.4 Representing treatments and solutions in written health documents

Health communication is concerned not only with informing people of the potential risks to their health but also offering advice about available treatments. Identifying an appropriate treatment relies not only upon medical expertise but also the expertise of the individual who can evaluate their personal circumstances and assess the impact of the illness. As such, it is crucial that patients are availed of quality information in order to maximise their understanding of the effects of medications, both in terms of what they are designed to treat and any potential side effects.

Grabowski (2014) reports a corpus-driven description of the use and functions of the most frequent clusters found in 100 patient information leaflets extracted from the websites of ten Polish pharmaceutical companies. Grabowski (2014) categorises the most frequent five-word and six-word clusters in terms of having:

- Referential functions: referring to content, circumstances or locations, such as '*zawartość opakowania i inne informacje*' (translation, 'contents of the pack and other information') or '*na stronie internetowej Europejskiej Agencji Leków*' ('on the website of the European Medicines Agency');
- Discoursal functions: contributing to text organisation, indicating cause and effect, for example '*W celu uzyskania bardziej szczegółowych informacji*' ('In order to obtain more detailed information');

- Stance functions: demonstrating the writer's commitment to a proposition (*'lek ten może powodować działania niepożądane'*, 'this medicine may cause undesirable side-effects'), assessment of importance (*'Ważne informacje o niektórych składnikach'*, 'Important information about certain ingredients'), and instructions that can indicate what is considered to be proper, such as *'nie należy wyrzucać do kanalizacji'* ('should not be thrown into sewage system').

It is in these fixed expressions that we see the overlap between information and advice, as in the stance functions, there are value judgements that provide 'a frame for interpretation' (Grabowski 2014, p. 36) and which presumably derive from professional medical evaluation. We can also see evidence of information selection, as further information is available, thereby demonstrating that the composition of these documents involves determining which information should be prioritised. Ultimately, the prevalence of these particular clusters, across the functional categories, highlights the key imperatives of the text type, which are to alert patients to potential side-effects and instruct them on how to properly use medicines as well as what course of action to pursue in the event of any problems arising from the use of medicines.

In related work, Grabowski (2013) reports the differences between patient information leaflets and the related text type, summaries of product characteristics, which highlight how the content is designed for different audiences (patients and health professionals, respectively). Summaries of product characteristics are created to provide information for market authorisation, and, therefore, there is more of an emphasis on precise, technical language regarding composition, dosage, and administering of the medicinal product. This is reflected in keywords referring to names of chemical substances, including 'apriprazole', 'darbepoetin', and 'erythropoietin', as well as terms denoting measurements ('dl', 'mmol', 'mg'). In comparison, patient information leaflets include a higher number of keywords with an advisory function, such as 'carefully', 'remember', 'please', and 'read'.

TASK 5.2

Patient information leaflets have been shown to feature a number of recurring fixed phrases, which serve to provide clear instructions to users about how to take medications. You can access patient information documents for a range of medicines approved for use in the United Kingdom through the Electronic Medicines Compendium at https://www.medicines.org.uk/emc/browse-medicines.

Compile a corpus of patient information leaflets by downloading a selection from the Electronic Medicine Compendium and storing these in a folder as individual text files. You should aim to collect around 20 examples of patient information leaflets which, for the purposes of this task, can be randomly selected. You can then use one the offline corpus analysis software tools introduced in Chapter 3, namely *AntConc*, *#LancsBox* and *WordSmith Tools*, to explore your corpus.

- Begin by generating a word list for your corpus. Are there any lexical items among the most frequent words that reflect the topical focus of the content, or are the most frequent words largely grammatical?

Recurrent clusters can help to identify content that is more specific to the texts in your corpus. Search for clusters (which might be alternatively called 'n-grams' in the tool) of increasing length i.e., two-word, three-word, four-word, five-word, and six-word clusters.

- How easy is it to make sense of these recurrent word strings? Could you reasonably determine what they mean in context?
- At what point (i.e., what length) do the clusters begin to reflect some of the communicative purposes of patient information leaflets, such as how to take the medicine, what the associated risks are, and where to get additional information?
- Do you see examples of the referential, discoursal, and stance functions as described by Grabowski (2013) among the most frequent clusters?

With respect to medications, there is an impetus to provide precise information, and the treatments themselves are developed according to rigorous laboratory procedures. In other circumstances, the solutions presented in response to health threats are more abstract, which can result in greater variation with respect to how those solutions are characterised in the language used to describe them. Koteyko et al.'s (2008) observation of a 'simple/not simple' dichotomy in policy documents and news coverage produced in response to the spread of MRSA in the United Kingdom shows how health challenges can be variously conceptualised to challenge or preserve the reputations of those involved in determining policy.

Keyword analysis showed that the terms 'simple', 'basic', and 'proper' contributed to competing frames for complexities associated with the origins of MRSA and strategies for infection control. Koteyko et al. (2008) demonstrate that 'simple' and 'basic', as they appear in news coverage, often refer to solutions for infection control, such as 'handwashing' and 'cleanliness'. 'Proper' typically appeared within negative judgments, casting blame on those failing to uphold acceptable practices or otherwise highlighting how these were under threat from the spread of MRSA. Other perspectives, typically coming from government representatives, contested the proposition that the solutions to the spread of MRSA are 'simple'. Koteyko et al.'s (2008) study, therefore, shows that different constructions for the causes and solutions associated with MRSA contributed to discourses of blame towards and defence of the government-led response to a national health threat.

5.5 Chapter summary

In our discussion of written health texts, we have emphasised the practical advantages of such texts being largely ready and available for corpus construction. Furthermore, many such documents are generated somewhat organically as part of clinical procedures or otherwise cultivated for more general research purposes in the form of historical archives. The availability of written health texts supports their inclusion in corpus analysis, and the collection of written texts, on a large scale, will increasingly be facilitated by developments in digital archiving procedures. However, those looking to operationalise such collections as corpora must consider the ethical implications of investigating and disseminating personal stories, particularly in relation to medical histories.

The enduring quality of the written word has contributed to the potential to carry out studies that extend over periods of time, throughout history even, and this is a dimension of written health corpora that reiterates the importance of drawing on information about the sociocultural context in our interpretation of the data. Observing how ideologies expressed in the context of illness and healthcare relate to the wider political climate (Koteyko et al. 2008; Jaworska 2021; McEnery and Baker 2022), many corpus studies contribute to a wider collection of critical discourse studies. The combination of critical discourse analysis and corpus linguistics has been effective in areas beyond health communication (Nartey and Mwinlaaru 2019) and has been effectively deployed to expose aspects of health inequalities and stigmatising representations of those with health issues (Brookes 2022) or otherwise in need of treatment (Jones and Collins 2020), both in the media and in the clinic (Zottola et al. 2021). The stigmatisation of people with illness has been a recurring concern in corpus studies of media representations, which has implications for if and how individuals access treatment and how they develop meaningful interpersonal relationships.

Personal narratives are seen to encourage more empathetic views of people with illness, and we have discussed how literary texts have the capacity to replicate, to some degree, the cognitive experiences associated with various (mental) health issues for readers. Written accounts of the patient perspective have particular value when we consider the continued dominance of the biomedical model in clinical documents, which, historically, has minimised the role of the patient in favour of foregrounding the agency of the health professional (Aarseth et al. 2016; Lehto 2022). Despite developments towards a patient-centred model of care, clinical documents still serve to regulate how the patient experience is recorded in a way that does not encourage accurate documentation of the effects of illness (Semino et al. 2020) or attends to the medical agenda in orienting towards diagnosis and triage (Zottola et al. 2021).

As researchers continue to develop the tools that support corpus analysis, we can bridge the gap between the systematic and (semi-)automatic procedures that make large scale analyses of health communication practicable and the manual, qualitative approaches that provide informed and detailed interpretations of such texts on a smaller scale. Future corpus studies will continue to benefit from the integration of rich metadata that supports the contextualised examination of the data, and the growth of digital archives will facilitate more systematic explorations of historical data. Furthermore, the news media continue to be a valuable resource in the documentation of history as it unfolds, and we have shown that corpus approaches are effective in examining how health issues are constructed in this public discourse space, variously impacting people at different levels of society.

Our review of different kinds of written health communication in this chapter has highlighted that representations of patients across texts are characterised in terms of those affected by illness having limited agency and that when people who are the subject of healthcare concerns are recorded in written texts, such accounts are often stigmatising or reconfigure the patient experience according to a biomedical model. As such, corpus linguistics research in this area should endeavour to focus on the inclusion of patients' perspectives in the various written health texts that are collected for analysis, thereby promoting the first-person perspective in written accounts of health(care) and illness.

Further reading

- Brookes, G. & Baker, P. (2021). *Obesity in the news: Language and representation in the press.* Cambridge University Press. https://doi.org/10.1017/9781108864732

This monograph provides a thorough investigation of 36 million words of UK news coverage of obesity, and the authors demonstrate a range of corpus methods to report the prevailing discursive representations in the news, how these differ according to publication types and over time, and how representations of people with obesity differ according to demographic factors such as gender and social class.

- Demjén, Z. (2015). Drowning in negativism, self-hate, doubt, madness: Linguistic insights into Sylvia Plath's experience of depression. *Communication and Medicine, 11*(1), 41–54. https://doi.org/10.1558/cam.v11i1.18478

Demjén shows the effective combination of targeted, qualitative analysis of pronouns and metaphor with a data-driven keyness analysis to investigate the journals of Sylvia Plath and report salient features of a personal narrative in the case of an individual experiencing depression. Demjén discusses how such a combined approach can be applied more widely in investigations of mental illness.

- Taavitsainen, I. (2009). The pragmatics of knowledge and meaning: Corpus linguistic approaches to changing thought-styles in early modern medical discourse. In A. H. Jucker, D. Schreier, & M. Hundt (Eds.), *Corpora: Pragmatics and discourse - Papers from the 29th international conference on English language research on computerized corpora (ICAME 29), Ascona, Switzerland, 14–18 May 2008* (pp. 37–62). Brill. https://doi.org/10.1163/9789042029101_004

This chapter provides a demonstration of how to conduct a corpus-assisted study in historical pragmatics – that is triangulating keyword analysis with qualitative, contextual analysis to delineate genres of medical writing from historical texts. Taavitsainen also discusses some of the methodological challenges of applying corpus methods to historical data, such as spelling variations.

References

Aarseth, G., Natvig, B., Engebretsen, E., Maagerø, E. & Kveim Lie, A.H. (2016). Writing the patient down and out: The construal of the patient in medical certificates of disability. *Sociology of Health & Illness, 38*(8), 1379–1395. https://doi.org/10.1111/1467-9566.12481

Atanasova, D., Koteyko, N., Brown, B. & Crawford, P. (2019). Representations of mental health and arts participation in the national and local press, 2007–2015. *Health, 23*(1), 3–20. https://doi.org/10.1177/1363459317708823

Baker, P. (2009). The BE06 corpus of British English and recent language change. *International Journal of Corpus Linguistics, 14*(3), 312–337. https://doi.org/10.1075/ijcl.14.3.02bak

Baker, P., Brookes, G., Atanasova, D. & Flint, S.W. (2020). Changing frames of obesity in the UK press 2008–2017. *Social Science & Medicine, 264*, 113403. https://doi.org/10.1016/j.socscimed.2020.113403

Baker, P. & McEnery, T. (2014). 'Find the doctors of death': Press representation of foreign doctors working in the NHS, a corpus based approach. In A. Jaworski & N. Coupland (Eds.), *The discourse reader* (third edition, pp. 465–480). Routledge.

Balfour, J. (2019). 'The mythological marauding violent schizophrenic': Using the word sketch tool to examine representations of schizophrenic people as violent in the British press. *Journal of Corpora and Discourse Studies*, 2, 40–64. https://doi.org/10.18573/jcads.10

Beach, M.C., Saha, S., Park, J., Taylor, J., Drew, P., Plank, E., Cooper, L.A. & Chee, B. (2021). Testimonial injustice: Linguistic bias in the medical records of Black patients and women. *Journal of General Internal Medicine*, 36(6), 1708–1714. https://doi.org/10.1007/s11606-021-06682-z

Bednarek, M. & Caple, H. (2014). Why do news values matter? Towards a new methodological framework for analysing news discourse in critical discourse analysis and beyond. *Discourse & Society*, 25(2), 135–158. https://doi.org/10.1177/0957926513516041

Bednarek, M. & Carr, G. (2020). Diabetes coverage in Australian newspapers (2013–2017): A computer-based linguistic analysis. *Health Promotion Journal of Australia: Official Journal of Australian Association of Health Promotion Professionals*, 31(3), 497–503. https://doi.org/10.1002/hpja.295

Bernstein, B. (1996). *Pedagogy, symbolic control and identity*. Taylor and Francis.

Bowen, M. (2019). Stigma: A linguistic analysis of personality disorder in the UK popular press, 2008–2017. *Journal of Psychiatric and Mental Health Nursing*, 26(7–8), 244–253. https://doi.org/10.1111/jpm.12541

Bowen, M., Kinderman, P. & Cooke, A. (2019). Stigma: A linguistic analysis of the UK red-top tabloids press' representation of schizophrenia. *Perspectives in Public Health*, 139(3), 147–152. https://doi.org/10.1177/1757913919835858

boyd, D. (2010). Social network sites as networked public: Affordances, dynamics and implications. In Z. Papacharissi (Ed.), *Networked self: Identity, community and culture on social network sites* (pp. 39–58). Routledge.

Brickley, B., Sladdin, I., Williams, L.T., Morgan, M., Ross, A., Trigger, K. & Ball, L. (2020). A new model of patient-centred care for general practitioners: Results of an integrative review. *Family Practice*, 37(2), 154–172. https://doi.org/10.1093/fampra/cmz063

Brookes, G. (2021). Empowering people to make healthier choices: A critical discourse analysis of the Tackling Obesity policy. *Qualitative Health Research*, 31(12), 2211–2229. https://doi.org/10.1177/10497323211027536

Brookes, G. (2022). 'Lose weight, save the NHS': Discourses of obesity in press coverage of COVID-19. *Critical Discourse Studies*, 19(6), 629–647. https://doi.org/10.1080/17405904.2021.1933116

Brookes, G. (2023). Killer, thief or companion? A corpus-based study of dementia metaphors in UK tabloids. *Metaphor and Symbol*, 38(3), 213–230. https://doi.org/10.1080/10926488.2022.2142472

Brookes, G. & Baker, P. (2021). *Obesity in the news: Language and representation in the press*. Cambridge University Press. https://doi.org/10.1017/9781108864732

Brookes, G. & Baker, P. (2022). Fear and responsibility: Discourses of obesity and risk in the UK press. *Journal of Risk Research*, 25(3), 363–378. https://doi.org/10.1080/13669877.2020.1863849

Brookes, G., Harvey, K., Chadborn, N. & Dening, T. (2018). 'Our biggest killer': Multimodal discourse representations of dementia in the British press. *Social Semiotics*, 28(3), 371–395. https://doi.org/10.1080/10350330.2017.1345111

Brookes, G. & Wright, D. (2020). From burden to threat: A diachronic study of language ideology and migrant representation in the British press. In P. Rautionaho, A. Nurmi & J. Klemola (Eds.), *Corpora and the changing society: Studies in the evolution of English* (pp. 113–140). John Benjamins. https://doi.org /10.1075/scl.96.05bro

Buus, N. & Hamilton, B.E. (2016). Social science and linguistic text analysis of nurses' records: A systematic review and critique. *Nursing Inquiry, 23*(1), 64–77. https://doi.org/10.1111/nin.12106

Cockburn, P. & Cockburn, H. (2011). *Henry's Demons*. Simon & Schuster Ltd.

Collins, L.C. (2022). Pre-exposure prophylaxis (PrEP) and 'risk' in the news. *Journal of Risk Research, 25*(3), 379–394. https://doi.org/10.1080 /13669877.2021.1894470

Collins, L.C. & Jones, L. (2021). External points of view in the PrEPUK News Corpus. *Journal of Corpora and Discourse Studies, 4,* 108–134. https://doi.org /10.18573/jcads.53

Collins, L.C. & Koller, V. (2023). *Viral Language: Analysing the COVID-19 Pandemic in Public Discourse*. Routledge.

Cotter, C., Samos, D. & Swinglehurst, D. (2021). Framing obesity in public discourse: Representation through metaphor across text type. *Journal of Pragmatics, 174,* 14–27. https://doi.org/10.1016/j.pragma.2020.12.015

Davies, M. (2021). The Coronavirus Corpus: Design, construction and use. *International Journal of Corpus Linguistics, 26*(4), 583–598. https://doi.org /10.1075/ijcl.21044.dav

Demjén, Z. (2015). Drowning in negativism, self-hate, doubt, madness: Linguistic insights into Sylvia Plath's experience of depression. *Communication and Medicine, 11*(1), 41–54. https://doi.org/10.1558/cam.v11i1.18478

Demjén, Z. & Semino, E. (2021). Stylistics: Mind style in an autobiographical account of schizophrenia. In G. Brookes & D. Hunt (Eds.), *Analysing health communication: Discourse approaches* (pp. 333–356). Palgrave Macmillan.

Diaz, B.A. (2022). Finding social (mis)alignment in older adult and opioid health policy implementation with corpus-assisted discourse analysis. *Applied Corpus Linguistics, 2*(2), 100020. https://doi.org/10.1016/j.acorp.2022.100020

Fowler, R. (1977). *Linguistics and the Novel*. Methuen.

Galasiński, D. & Ziółkowska, J. (2020). A moment outside time: A critical discourse analytic perspective on dominant constructions of suicide. In Z. Demjén (Ed.), *Applying linguistics in illness and healthcare contexts* (pp. 349–371). Bloomsbury. http://dx.doi.org/10.5040/9781350057685.0023

Goddu, A.P., O'Conor, K.J., Lanzkron, S., Saheed, M.O., Saha, S., Peek, M.E., Haywood Jr, C. & Beach, M.C. (2018). Do words matter? Stigmatizing language and the transmission of bias in the medical record. *Journal of General Internal Medicine, 33*(5), 685–691. https://doi.org/10.1007/s11606-017-4289-2

Golini, R. (2022). Revealing the hidden characteristics of patient information for radiography with a lexical bundles analysis. *Applied Corpus Linguistics, 2*(1), 100014. https://doi.org/10.1016/j.acorp.2021.100014

Grabowski, Ł. (2013). Register variation across English pharmaceutical texts: A corpus-driven study of keywords and lexical bundles and phrase frames in patient information leaflets and summaries of product characteristics. *Procedia - Social and Behavioral Sciences, 95*(25), 391–401. https://doi.org/10.1016/j.sbspro.2013.10.661

Grabowski, Ł. (2014). On lexical bundles in Polish patient information leaflets: A corpus-driven study. *Studies in Polish Linguistics*, *9*(1), 21–43. https://doi.org/10.4467/23005920SPL.14.002.2186

Haddon, M. (2003). *The curious incident of the dog in the night-time.* Jonathan Cape.

Hannaford, E.D. (2017). The press and public on mental health: A corpus linguistic analysis of UK newspaper coverage of mental illness (1995–2014), compared with the UK National Attitudes to Mental Illness. MPhil(R) thesis, University of Glasgow. http://theses.gla.ac.uk/9016/

Heckemann, B., Chaaya, M., Jakobsson Ung, E., Olsson, D.S. & Jakobsson, S. (2022). Finding the person in electronic health records: A mixed-methods analysis of person-centered content and language. *Health Communication*, *37*(4), 418–424. https://doi.org/10.1080/10410236.2020.1846275

Hiltunen, T. & Taavitsainen, I. (2022). Corpora, pragmatics, and historical medical discourse. In T. Hiltunen & J. Taavitsainen (Eds.), *Corpus pragmatic studies on the history of medical discourse* (pp. 1–19). John Benjamins. https://doi.org/10.1075/pbns.330.01hil

Hunston, S. (2022). *Corpora in applied linguistics* (second edition). Cambridge University Press. https://doi.org/10.1017/9781108616218

Hunt, D. & Carter, R. (2012). Seeing through *The Bell Jar*: Investigating linguistic patterns of psychological disorder. *Journal of Medical Humanities*, *33*, 27–39. https://doi.org/10.1007/s10912-011-9163-3

Hyland, K. & Jiang, F. (K.) (2021). The Covid infodemic: Competition and the hyping of virus research. *International Journal of Corpus Linguistics*, *26*(4), 444–468. https://doi.org/10.1075/ijcl.20160.hyl

Isaacs, T., Murdoch, J., Demjén, Z. & Stevenson, F. (2022). Examining the language demands of informed consent documents in patient recruitment to cancer trials using tools from corpus and computational linguistics. *Health*, *26*(4), 431–456. https://doi.org/10.1177/1363459320963431

Jaworska, S. (2021). Investigating media representations of the coronavirus in the UK, USA and Germany: What can a comparative corpus-based discourse analysis contribute to our understanding of the COVID-19 pandemic? In R. Jones (Ed.), *Viral discourse* (pp. 26–37). Cambridge University Press. https://dx.doi.org/10.1017/9781108986465

Jones, L. & Collins, L.C. (2020). PrEP in the press: A corpus-assisted discourse analysis of how users of HIV-prevention treatment are represented in British newspapers. *Journal of Language and Sexuality*, *9*(2), 202–225. https://doi.org/10.1075/jls.20002.jon

Kelly, J.F., Dow, S.J. & Westerhoff, C. (2010). Does our choice of substance-related terms influence perceptions of treatment need? An empirical investigation with two commonly used terms. *Journal of Drug Issues*, *40*(4), 805–818. https://doi.org/10.1177/002204261004000403

Kincaid, J.P., Fishburne, R.P., Rogers, R.L. & Chissom, B.S. (1975). *Derivation of new readability formulas (Automated readability index, fog count, and flesch reading ease formula) for navy enlisted personnel.* Chief of Naval Technical Training: Naval Air Station Memphis. https://eric.ed.gov/?id=ED108134.

Knight, D. & Adolphs, S. (2021). Building a spoken corpus: What are the basics? In A. O'Keeffe & M. McCarthy (Eds.), *The Routledge handbook of corpus linguistics* (pp. 21–34). Routledge. https://doi.org/10.4324/9780367076399-3

Koteyko, N., Nerlich, B., Crawford, P. & Wright, N. (2008). 'Not rocket science' or 'no silver bullet'? Media and government discourses about MRSA and cleanliness. *Applied Linguistics*, *29*(2), 223–243. https://doi.org/10.1093/applin/amn006

Lehto, A. (2022). Unhappy patients and eminent physicians: The representation of patients and practitioners in Late Modern English medical writing. In T. Hiltunen & J. Taavitsainen (Eds.), *Corpus pragmatic studies on the history of medical discourse* (pp. 203–228). John Benjamins. https://doi.org/10.1075/pbns.330.09leh

Lövestam, E., Fjellström, C., Koochek, A. & Andersson, A. (2015). The power of language on patient-centredness: linguistic devices in the dietetic notes of patient records. *International Journal of Applied Linguistics*, *25*(2), 225–245. https://doi.org/10.1111/ijal.12064

Mahlberg, M. & Brookes, G. (2021). Language and COVID-19: Corpus linguistics and the social reality of the pandemic. *International Journal of Corpus Linguistics*, *26*(4), 441–443. https://doi.org/10.1075/ijcl.00043.mah

McEnery, T. & Baker, H. (2022). 'A geography of names': A genre analysis of nationality-driven names for venereal disease in seventeenth-century England. In T. Hiltunen & I. Taavitsainen (Eds.), *Corpus pragmatic studies on the history of medical discourse* (pp. 23–48). John Benjamins. https://doi.org/10.1075/pbns.330.02mce

McEnery, T. & Brookes, G. (2022). Building a written corpus: What are the basics? In A. O'Keeffe & M. McCarthy (Eds.), *The Routledge handbook of corpus linguistics* (pp. 35–47). Routledge. https://doi.org/10.4324/9780367076399-4

McEnery, T., Brookes, G. & Clarke, I. (2022). Corpus studies of language through time: Introduction to the special issue. *International Journal of Corpus Linguistics*, *27*(4), 393–398. https://doi.org/10.1075/ijcl.00050.edi

McIntyre, D. & Archer, D. (2010). A corpus-based approach to mid style. *Journal of Literary Semantics*, *39*(2), 167–182. https://doi.org/10.1515/jlse.2010.009

Menzel, K. (2022). Medical discourse in Late Modern English: Insights from a multidisciplinary corpus of scientific journal articles. In T. Hiltunen & I. Taavitsainen (Eds.), *Corpus pragmatic studies on the history of medical discourse* (pp. 79–104). John Benjamins. https://doi.org/10.1075/pbns.330.04men

Meyer, J. & Moncrieff, A. (2021). Family not to be informed? The ethical use of historical medical documentation. In A.R. Hanley & J. Meyer (Eds.), *Patient voices in Britain, 1840–1948 – Social histories of medicine* (pp. 61–87). Manchester University Press. https://doi.org/10.7765/9781526154897.00011

Moilanen, T., Sivonen, M., Hipp, K., Kallio, H., Papinaho, O., Stolt, M., Turjamaa, R., Häggman-Laitila, A. & Kangasniemi, M. (2022). Developing a feasible and credible method for analyzing healthcare documents as written data. *Global Qualitative Nursing Research*, *7*(9), 23333936221108706. https://doi.org/10.1177/23333936221108706

Nartey, M. & Mwinlaaru, I.N. (2019). Towards a decade of synergising corpus linguistics and critical discourse analysis: A meta-analysis. *Corpora*, *14*(2), 203–235. https://doi.org/10.3366/cor.2019.0169

Ollikainen, K. (2022). Communicating authority: Self-mentions in Early Modern English medical narratives (1500–1700). In T. Hiltunen & I. Taavitsainen (Eds.), *Corpus pragmatic studies on the history of medical discourse* (pp. 251–272). John Benjamins. https://doi.org/10.1075/pbns.330.11oll

Plath, S. (1966). *The bell jar.* Faber & Faber.

Pragglejazz Group. (2007). MIP: A method for identifying metaphorically used words in discourse. *Metaphor and Symbol, 22*(1), 1–39. https://doi.org/10.1080/10926480709336752

Price, H. (2022). *The language of mental illness: Corpus linguistics and the construction of mental illness in the press.* Cambridge University Press.

Rayson, P. (2008). From key words to key semantic domains. *International Journal of Corpus Linguistics, 13*(4), 519–549. https://doi.org/10.1075/ijcl.13.4.06ray

Reali, F., Soriano, T. & Rodríguez, D. (2016). How we think about depression: The role of linguistic framing. *Revista Latinoamericana de Psicología, 48*(2), 127–136. https://doi.org/10.1016/j.rlp.2015.09.004

Redden, E. (2020). Rush to publish risks undermining COVID-19 research. Inside Higher Education. https://www.insidehighered.com/news/2020/06/08/fastpace-scientific-publishing-covid-comes-problems.

Schnelle, G., Odebrecht, C., Lüdeling, A., Perlitz, L. & Fisher, C. (2022). "Die Blumenzeit der Frau": A corpus-based study of the development of medical references to menstruation in historical texts in herbology. In T. Hiltunen & I. Taavitsainen (Eds.), *Corpus pragmatic studies on the history of medical discourse* (pp. 153–176). John Benjamins. https://doi.org/10.1075/pbns.330.07sch

Semino, E. (2008). *Metaphor in discourse.* Cambridge University Press.

Semino, E. (2014). Language, mind and autism in Mark Haddon's *The Curious Incident of the Dog in the Night-Time.* In M. Fludernik & D. Jacob (Eds.), *Linguistics and literary studies: Interfaces, encounters, transfers* (pp. 279–303). De Gruyter.

Semino, E., Demjén, Z., Hardie, A., Payne, S. & Rayson, P. (2017). *Metaphor, cancer and the end of life: A corpus-based study.* Routledge.

Semino, E., Demjén, Z. & Demmen, J. (2018). An integrated approach to metaphor and framing in cognition, discourse, and practice, with an application to metaphors for cancer. *Applied Linguistics, 39*(5), 625–645. https://doi.org/10.1093/applin/amw028

Semino, E., Hardie, A. & Zakrzewska, J. (2020). Applying corpus linguistics to a diagnostic tool for pain. In Z. Demjén (Ed.), *Applying linguistics in illness and healthcare contexts* (pp. 99–127). Bloomsbury. http://dx.doi.org/10.5040/9781350057685.0023

Semino, E. & Swindlehurst, K. (1996). Metaphor and mind style in Ken Kesey's *One Flew over the Cuckoo's Nest. Style, 30*(1), 143–166. http://www.jstor.org/stable/42946325

Sontag, S. (1978). *Illness as metaphor.* Farrar, Straus & Giroux.

Swales, J. (2000). Language for specific purposes. *Annual Review of Applied Linguistics, 20*, 59–76. https://doi.org/10.1017/S0267190500200044

Time to Change. (2018). Responsible reporting – Mind your language. https://www.time-to change.org.uk/sites/default/files/Time%20to%20Change%20Media%20Guidelines.pdf.

TNS BMRB. (2015). Attitudes to Mental Illness: 2014 Research Report. https://www.time-to-change.org.uk/research-reports-publications/campaign.

Woods, A. (2013). The voice-hearer. *Journal of Mental Health, 22*(3), 263–270. https://doi.org/10.3109/09638237.2013.799267

World Health Organisation. (2017). Dementia fact sheet: December 2017. https://www.who.int/mental_health/neurology/dementia/gap_info_sheets/en/.

World Health Organisation. (2020). WHO Director-General's remarks at the media briefing on 2019-nCoV on 11 February 2020. https://www.who.int/director-general/speeches/detail/who-director-general-s-remarks-at-the-media-briefing-on-2019-ncov-on-11-february-2020

Wright, D. & Brookes, G. (2019). 'This is England, speak English!': A corpus-assisted critical study of language ideologies in the right-leaning British press. *Critical Discourse Studies*, *16*(1), 56–83. https://doi.org/10.1080/17405904.2018.1511439

Zottola, A., Jones, L., Pilnick, A., Mullany, L., Bouman, W.P. & Arcelus, J. (2021). Identifying coping strategies used by patients at a transgender health clinic through analysis of free-text autobiographical narratives. *Health Expectations*, *24*(2), 719–727. https://doi.org/10.1111/hex.13222

6
DIGITAL HEALTH COMMUNICATION

6.1 Introduction

Digital technologies are crucial to the current and continuing provision of global healthcare. In its most recent *Global Strategy on Digital Health* document, the World Health Organization (WHO 2021, pp. 7–8) reiterated its position that:

> [S]trategic and innovative use of digital and cutting-edge information and communications technologies will be an essential enabling factor towards ensuring that 1 billion more people benefit from universal health coverage, that 1 billion more people are better protected from health emergencies, and that 1 billion more people enjoy better health and well-being.

The implementation of digital tools in healthcare has already been seen in the form of big data analytics (Khanra et al. 2020), artificial intelligence (Schwalbe and Wahl 2020), smart wearable devices (Chau et al. 2019), and virtual care (Bhavnani and Sitapati 2019) (see Lupton 2017 for a general discussion). Digital tools that enable efficient data capture, storage, and transfer, thereby creating a continuum of care, have the capacity to improve health outcomes, supporting clinical trials, diagnosis, and therapy and facilitating self-management of care 'as well as creating more evidence-based knowledge, skills and competence for professionals to support health care' (WHO 2021, p. 8).

In this chapter, we reflect on the breadth of forms of communication that take place in digital contexts and how this enables the creation of different kinds of interpersonal exchange. We discuss the developing dynamics between

DOI: 10.4324/9781003099659-6

health professionals and 'expert patients', as digital platforms support the sharing of information among various kinds of communities. Corpus studies of digital health communication have shown that the technical properties of different digital spaces can variously encourage personal disclosures around health. We review case studies that have captured how aspects of illness and expert identities are enacted through language as well as demonstrating how people show affiliation with others in these digital spaces to create communities characterised by particular health experiences.

6.2 Investigating language in digital health communication

In their review of assessment and intervention in mental healthcare services, Bucci et al. (2019, p. 282) point to ease of access, low cost, offering choices about healthcare, information sharing, connection with virtual networks, opportunities for peer support, anonymity, and secure, easy, and timely data sharing as the key advantages that digital health technologies offer users. Uneven health service provision means that, for some people, it is not feasible to travel the distance required to reach a clinic and receive care in person; in which case, digital technologies can provide a vital alternative. Digital platforms may also offer a much more acceptable form of healthcare for health anxious individuals when face-to-face consultation might exacerbate their mental distress (Baumgartner and Hartmann 2011). On the basis of facilitating this kind of optionality, and as a result of more comprehensive personal data, Bucci et al. (2019, p. 278) assert that digital healthcare provision takes treatment 'into the context of an individual's everyday life, unconstrained by location and time', thereby encouraging a patient-centred model of care. As a result, corpus studies of language can generate findings relating to otherwise marginalised experiences of illness to better understand the personal contexts of those who are not well-represented in clinical encounters.

The accessibility of digital resources and their capacity for transcending time and place creates increased opportunities for people to find a community of others who can relate to and potentially advise on the health challenges they are facing. Francis (2021) demonstrates how personal disclosures on Twitter by a high-profile user, the rapper Kid Cudi, relating to depression facilitated wider social media conversations about Black men's mental health. Francis (2021, p. 449) explains how:

A Black woman Twitter user created the #YouGoodMan hashtag on October 5, less than 24 hours after Kid Cudi's announcement, and sought to engage Black men on Twitter in conversations about mental health (Nuckolls 2016). According to the creator, the purpose of the hashtag was 'For Black men to confess, ask for help, vent, or get pointed in the direction of mental health professionals' (Nuckolls 2016). Further, the creator noted that '#YouGoodMan is a permission slip for vulnerability in a world that hides depression under toxic expression of masculinity'.

(Nuckolls 2016)

The capacity of digital spaces to support ad hoc communities in this way is indicative of the affordances that distinguish digital formats of healthcare provision from other formats, and from a (corpus) linguistics standpoint, we can consider how such communities are formed and maintained through a shared linguistic repertoire.

Digital spaces often function without the administration of a socially powerful institution, such as a national health service or a media company. As such, they offer researchers the potential to gather a wider range and greater amount of naturally occurring data that is not elicited in the presence of a researcher or a health professional (Hunt and Brookes 2020). Digital platforms have been said to have 'empowered ordinary users by having the option to participate in text production and distribution' (KhosraviNik 2014, p. 287). If we consider the ways in which the patient experience is often reframed according to the institutional biomedical model in paper-based methods of assessment (see Chapter 5), there is greater scope in digital modes for the patient to document their point of view in their preferred terms.

Digital technologies support the creation of participatory, collaborative spaces for open exchange, which stands in contrast to the traditional, unidirectional model of information exchange from healthcare institutions to patients (Chou et al. 2013). The capacity for ordinary people to access health information and participate in discussions without disclosing their identities also contributes to the normalisation and destigmatisation of health challenges. Indeed, participants in online forums are more likely to refer to aspects of their medical record – providing valuable contextual information relating to the health complaint – than to aspects of their personal lives that might compromise their anonymity (Frost et al. 2014). Such information is invaluable for other participants who can make informed assessments about the correspondence of these experiences with their own as well as holding value for corpus linguists looking to discern what is generalisable from what is context-specific.

Despite the promise of openness, egalitarianism, and universality associated with the World Wide Web as a platform for digital (health) communication, there are concerns around the quantity and quality of information that is available, which can be overwhelming for some and varies in terms of its quality as a result of uneven regulation (Bucci et al. 2019, p. 282). Basch et al. (2021, p. 2376) discuss a collection of TikTok posts that parody negative reactions to vaccinations – prior to the treatments being publicly available – which they warn 'reflects a deliberate and dangerous effort to communicate anti-vaccination sentiment'. Such content can subsequently undermine efforts to promote uptake of (COVID-19) vaccines. They go on to explain that while TikTok audiences can be thought of as having high digital literacy, 'they tend to have comparatively low levels of health literacy, limiting their ability to critically evaluate online content, including that found on social media' (Basch et al. 2021, p. 2376). Navigating digital health communication, thus, requires digital literacy skills in the form of being able to identify and manage risks, for instance (Bucci et al. 2019). Systematic studies of the language used to deliver health information, including those using corpus linguistics approaches, can contribute to understanding how to communicate effectively but can also investigate responses to health messages, as these appear in such dialogic digital spaces (Hodson et al. 2022; Cheded et al. 2023), thus offering a view of how such information is received.

Corpus linguists can also benefit from the affordances of digital technologies that contribute to generating more evidence-based knowledge. The growth in corpus studies of digital health(care) communication, as we discuss in this chapter, can, to a large extent, be attributed to a recognition of 'the growing influence of digital (communicative) technologies over the ways that people communicate – and indeed act – in relation to their health' (Brookes et al. 2022a, p. 617). Brookes et al. (2022a) also emphasise the relative ease with which digital texts can be re-operationalised as corpus files, and, once compiled, the increased processing speeds, data storage, and distribution capacity of digital texts (Creeber and Martin 2009) can facilitate collaboration and multidisciplinary analysis. In order to investigate the discourses that are produced such digital contexts – i.e., to be able to discuss features of digital texts compared with non-digital texts – we can direct our attention to what Jones et al. (2015) refer to as 'technologies of entextualisation'; this includes elements such as the semiotic systems available (e.g., language, emoji, images, etc.) as well as the mediating technology (e.g., television, smartphone, etc.). Thus, when considering the relationship between the mode (e.g., written, spoken, visual) and the subsequent communicative interactions – and how these correspond with established social practices – we can ask ourselves: '[h]ow do these new "technologies of entextualisation" and the kinds of texts they result in allow people to different things, or to do old things in different ways?' (Jones et al. 2015, p. 10). As an important aspect of the context in which digital health communication is produced and disseminated, we will see how the fundamental structure of digital platforms has implications for *who* participates in digital health communication and *how* they are able to contribute to such texts.

Despite marking out digital communication in this chapter as distinct from written and spoken forms of communication, it would be misleading to think of digital (health) communication as being entirely separate from those other modes. Bateman (2021) emphasises the continuities that can be found in digital texts that have their origins in spoken and written modes, and we can refer to examples such as online news articles to see this in effect; while the composition and structure of digital news articles exhibit many of the features established in print news, the inclusion of audio-visual media, hyperlinks, and user comments demonstrates how digital tools have been integrated as developments of a recognisable text type. Thus, in thinking about digital texts in terms of their continuities with other text types, we can position 'digital' and 'non-digital' texts on a spectrum. The continuity between these two points also suggests that we can adapt existing techniques for corpus linguistics analysis that have been applied effectively in the study of non-digital texts to continue to investigate digital health communication.

6.3 Forms of digital health communication

We structure our discussion of forms of digital health communication in this chapter according to the distinction between digital health communication with professionals and digital health communication among peers. In terms of the former, we refer to those operating in a professional capacity as healthcare providers or representatives of a (commercial) organisation. With respect to the latter, we are more typically referring to members of the public with some personal experience of a salient health issue.

The boundaries between these two proposed types of interaction are, admittedly, blurred. One of the reported characteristics of digital platforms, and in particular, social media, is the notion of 'context collapse', in which the 'collapsing' of contexts, resulting from the lack of spatial, social, and temporal boundaries online, creates a diverse networked audience for discourse taking place online (boyd 2010, p. 49). In other words, individual users are presented with a potential audience that combines different domains of their social and professional lives, the members of which might not typically be addressed simultaneously (Androutsopoulos 2011). This can influence how textual contributions to online platforms of (health) communication are articulated, as users attend to the various preferences of a diverse, networked audience or demonstrate forms of audience design (Bell 1984) in composing their comments in a way that targets particular members. In digital spaces, this can be quite overt – through @-tagging or hash-tagging, for instance – but it can also be observed in more subtle linguistic choices that index membership to a particular (language) community. These digital features have arguably contributed, in part, to the closing of the gap between 'public' and 'private', as ordinary users can broadcast their messages to a wide, unknown audience, and professional institutions more often engage with individual users specifically. This has coincided with a shift towards personalisation and 'conversationalistion' in public discourses (Fairclough 1993).

Ultimately, individuals might use social media spaces to simultaneously engage in informal, phatic communication, read news headlines, and share information relating to their health needs. Despite the ambiguity of trying to distinguish digital spaces (e.g., social from professional), in adopting these characteristics as a starting point, we can refer to the context-driven patterns of communication that have been reported in corpus studies of health across different digital contexts and observed among different kinds of participants. We, thereby, structure our discussion of digital health communication around those resources that are more explicitly badged as professional communication and those which cultivate peer-to-peer discussions of lived experience.

Zummo (2015, p. 187) similarly differentiates between three types of digital space in which health information is disseminated: (i) sites where health professionals provide the user with generic information about a given medical problem, (ii) sites providing information addressing specific user questions, and (iii) digital discussion groups. As such, we will begin with a discussion of external communication from professional health bodies where the addressee(s) are unknown, such as health websites and blogs. We then turn our attention to forms of digital communication that support interaction between health professionals and non-professional perspectives, in the form of user queries, comments, and feedback. Finally, we will reflect on digital spaces characterised by peer interactions, such as online health forums. Having established the range of types of digital health communication that have figured in corpus studies, we will then consider what linguistic features have been observed in corpus studies in these domains.

6.3.1 Digital health information from professionals

We first consider digital communication produced by health professionals and made publicly available through websites, blogs, or social media platforms. A systematic review of health information seeking behaviours has shown that information seekers overwhelmingly favour search engines as a strategy for identifying relevant health information, but when they do target specific sources, websites dedicated to proving health information were the most commonly sought (Jia et el. 2021). What users cite as the most valued qualities of these websites is their (i) accuracy, (ii) currency of information, and (iii) ease of understanding (Jia et al. 2021).

It is often the case that people visit websites that address specific health conditions when they are deliberating treatment options, and Allen and Saeed (2022) correspondingly consider how the websites of two major dialysis organisations in the United States represent options for people with kidney failure. The websites they examined received an estimated 2.3 million visitors and 598, 900 visitors respectively in the course of one month (January 2021), thereby demonstrating their potential influence but also the unevenness with which sources of information are accessed online. The authors applied corpus procedures to support a thematic analysis of the content of these webpages (totalling 226,968 words) and observed a lack of information relating to conservative kidney management options, despite claims on the websites as to their 'educational' value. Allen and Saeed (2022, p. 4) subsequently determine that such materials 'may be best understood or intended as marketing and not patient education'. Furthermore, the web materials are judged as offering an 'ameliorated view of quality of life on dialysis, that is not aligned with the reported effects of symptom burden, high caregiver burden and high unemployment' (Allen and Saeed 2022, p. 4). As such, the authors caution against the reliability of information provided by organisations that might have a commercial interest in particular treatment options.

Chałupnik and Brookes (2021) also observe a commercial influence in their corpus-assisted critical discourse study of the webpages of the 187 active clinical commissioning groups (CCGs) that make up the NHS in the UK. Focusing on how the CCGs represent themselves and their actions in their web materials, the authors consider how these self-representations reflect and, indeed, enact a wider process of marketisation in UK health services. Chałupnik and Brookes (2021) report that the CCGs present themselves as facilitating patients' self-care and as fulfilling an administrative function that supports a more patient-centred approach. These representations are likened to a wider discourse of 'deliverology' (Mautner 2010), as we see principles of competition, economic performance, and customer service in the external-facing communications with visitors to the site.

Wong et al. (2020) assert that for communities whose lives are more intertwined with digital technologies, which is more common among adolescents and young adults, the affordances of digital tools can help with ease of understanding health information. However, there are other circumstances in which text producers might refrain from utilising digital tools. Mazzi (2016) discusses how the Irish Cancer Society's production of informative healthcare materials was motivated by concerns about limited health literacy as a major public health issue. As such, although the organisation appears to have capitalised on the potential for wider dissemination that is enabled by making such materials available online, the text producers may have refrained from incorporating additional features afforded by the digital context in order to avoid additional demands related to digital literacy. Mazzi (2016, p. 247) emphasises the value of adequate materials that 'tell patients about the bare facts while at the same time successfully addressing key areas of concern' and speculates that these considerations may have underlain the concept of the Irish Cancer Society's booklets. In this interpretation, the affordances of digital technologies do not necessarily entail accessibility, so it is important to consider in what contexts digital tools will help to achieve the primary goal of making health information accessible.

Kinloch (2018) reports a corpus assisted comparative study of the discourses of infertility, according to how they are constructed in different kinds of digital resources, namely clinic websites, blogs, and news articles from organisations based in the UK. Subsequently, Kinloch (2018) is able to consider the different representations afforded by clinical information (websites), lived experience (blogs), and media representations (news articles). Like Chałupnik and Brookes (2021) and Allen and Saeed (2022), Kinloch (2018) reports a marketisation discourse in relation to infertility, which is observed alongside themes representing (i) the transformative effect of infertility, (ii) medicalised (in)fertility, and (iii) parenthood as privilege and imperative. These observations show how discussions of infertility intersect with wider social, medical, and commercial discourses. While each of these themes was observed across the data types analysed, Kinloch (2018) reports that their prevalence was variable across the different digital spaces. For example, the transformative effects of infertility were most prevalently observed in blogs, which more directly reflected lived experience.

Like most forms of digital texts, however, there is a great deal of register variation in the breadth of blogs that contribute to health communication, generally. Furthermore, even when blogs appear to draw on a common professional register – such as the conventions associated with academic writing – other contextual factors can influence the discourses produced. Curry and Pérez-Paredes (2021, p. 469) present a corpus-based contrastive analysis of 'stance nouns + that/*de que*' in a comparable corpus of English and Spanish COVID-19 themed academic blogs from *The Conversation*. They refer to this type of text as 'parascientific' in that the publication is motivated by making the findings of scientific research accessible for a wider audience, as indicated in its tagline, 'Academic rigour, journalistic flair' (https://theconversation.com/uk). In addition to bridging the stylistic domains of academia and journalism, however, Curry and Pérez-Paredes (2021, p. 470) show that texts produced for *The Conversation* can offer insights into 'academic knowledge cultures' and, in their case, specifically in relation to how these cultures 'engage with and disseminate information on COVID-19 to their wider public'.

The wide dissemination of information is a fundamental imperative during public health crises, and in addition to having their own webpages and contributing to blogs, institutions responsible for generating such information have recognised the potential of social media platforms for the dissemination of public health information as well as for fostering meaningful engagement with public users (Guidry et al. 2017). Starbird and Palen (2010) have shown that in emergency situations, Twitter users are more likely to retweet messages that have come from the profiles of official information sources such as news media organisations and emergency management services compared with any other type of social media profile. Social media profiles representing official government and health institutions, therefore, make an important contribution to public discourses.

Ibrahim et al. (2022) reflect on how the Ministry of Health of Saudi Arabia used their official Twitter account to run awareness campaigns during the COVID-19 pandemic, providing updates about the transmission of the virus, the numbers of confirmed cases, and measures taken to overcome the crisis, including advising the public on best protection practices. Ibrahim et al. (2022) discuss the Ministry's use of 'pre-suasion' techniques – that is, measures taken to prepare the addressee(s) to receive an instruction or request (Cialdini 2016). They propose that the principles of pre-suasion can be operationalised through specific language features and present their analysis of frequent lexical forms and manual codes for communicating authority, reciprocity, and unity, for example. The authors do, however, report that pre-suasion and persuasion tactics are often combined and that the boundaries between the two concepts are porous, indicating that these functions are realised discursively, in addition to through specific lexis (Ibrahim et al. 2022).

Producers of digital texts can draw on multiple semiotic resources to compose their messages, and, as a consequence, it is important to consider the coherence between different elements. Jones et al. (2023, p. 3) investigated the tweets of the 13 regional accounts that represent Public Health England on Twitter over the course of what they describe as the 'first major phase' of the COVID-19 pandemic (1 March 2020 to 17 February 2021). They collected the images attached to tweets featuring frequent four-word clusters for subsequent image analysis, informed by Kress and Van Leeuwen's (2020) 'Visual Grammar'. This supported them in coding for image systems such as narrative themes, character, perspective, prominence, compositional vectors, framing etc., and on the basis of these codes, the authors selected a representative sample of tweets to use as materials for facilitating discussions in focus groups. Jones et al. (2023, p. 6) determine that the tweets identified through frequent clusters function to 'either give instructions or present information as a means of giving advice'. However, they state that when analysed in combination with the images, the overall function of the tweet was not always clear. They subsequently confirm, via participant responses in their focus groups, that simple messages with strong alignment between what is represented in text and in image are perceived to be the most effective form of health communication.

Representatives of scientific research also offer important contributions to discussions that take place in social media spaces; Coberley et al. (2023, p. 9) assert that '[r]eal-time science communication about emerging science through social media, such as Twitter, is important during high-risk situations such as the COVID-19 pandemic – not only to save lives but also for the necessary transparency required for credibility'. They report findings from their corpus-based study of modal verbs, as indicators of stance, in different forms of science communication on Twitter. They found consistency between US-based representatives of health science, environmental science, and ocean sciences in their use of modal verbs to convey ability (e.g., 'can'), obligation ('must') and volition ('shall'). These are interpreted as reflecting established conventions for communicating scientific information that are only minimally adapted for social media communication. The authors recommend that researchers continue to monitor expressions of stance in science and health communication for stylistic developments related to the immediacy and brevity associated with social media texts such as tweets.

In this section, we have discussed examples of organisations capitalising on the broadcast functions of social media, disseminating health messaging far and wide for a diverse audience. In the next section, we look at more focused interactions between health professionals and more narrowly defined audiences – the queries of specific individuals, even – as they occur in digital spaces.

6.3.2 Digital interactions with health professionals

Alongside the expansive visibility and engagement afforded by digital tools, users can also create private spaces, inviting select participants to a group chat, for example. It is also possible to make messages visible to specific individuals, e.g., by tagging their unique username or linking a response as a direct reply to a post, which will typically result in a notification, promptly alerting the user to the incoming message. Although such messages can be designed to directly address known individuals, their visibility to a wider, non-ratified audience can also influence how they are composed (Bell 1984). Indeed, Zappavigna (2011, p. 800) has coined the term 'ambient affiliation' to describe the phenomenon whereby social media users participate in co-present, impermanent communities 'by bonding around evolving topics of interest'. A social media user can locate a collective of like-minded peers, with whom they have no prior relationship, simply on the basis of indexing a topic with a hashtag. As such, health information advice can be simultaneously personal and generic, provided in relation to the specific circumstances outlined by an individual contributor but made interpretable for many others who can assess for themselves whether such information pertains to their own health concerns.

A series of studies conducted by researchers at the University of Nottingham draws on data collected from a health information website called Teenage Health Freak (THF), which was designed to respond to adolescents' queries about various health topics and more generally offer visitors to the site basic health information (Brookes and Harvey 2016). As Brookes and Harvey (2016, p. 215) explain:

> The THF is a user-friendly, interactive resource for adolescents, allowing them to email their questions and health-related concerns to the health

professionals who operate the website. The professionals respond to the problem messages in the guise of the persona of Dr Ann, the virtual doctor to whom users of the website directly submit their problems. The responses to the messages that are answered appear on the website and are thus designed to be read not only by the original help seeker but also by a much wider audience. In this sense, the doctors are writing not only for an individual advice seeker but also for a more general adolescent audience. All direct correspondence between Dr Ann and the advice seeker is anonymous.

The anonymity of the service is recognised as a distinct benefit, providing adolescents with a secure platform through which to 'seek advice about sensitive or awkward health-related topics, without fear of being judged or stigmatised by others' (Brookes et al. 2018, p. 101). The resultant candour of the posts to the service has provided an invaluable snapshot of contemporary health concerns among teenagers, including insights into how they articulate those health concerns (Harvey et al. 2008).

The Teenage Health Freak corpus has subsequently been investigated using corpus methods to determine what health issues are of common concern among adolescents (Harvey et al. 2007); to analyse descriptions of experiences of self-harm (Harvey and Brown 2012), mental health issues (Brookes and Harvey 2016) including depression (Harvey 2012), and sexual health concerns (Brookes et al. 2022a) including HIV/AIDS (Harvey et al. 2014); and to critically reflect upon the robustness of the keywords procedure in light of spelling variations in born-digital data (Smith et al. 2014) and the impact of these findings through their dissemination among health professionals, policymakers and other stakeholders (Brooks et al. 2018).

In the first of our case studies in this chapter, we review Hunt and Harvey's (2015) investigation of the Teenage Health Freak data alongside an online forum to consider how experiences of eating disorders are represented in contributions to these digital platforms.

CASE STUDY:

Discursive representations of eating disorders in online health queries (Hunt and Harvey 2015)

Like many investigations of digital health communication spaces, Hunt and Harvey (2015, p. 135) recognise the potential of studying data from the web in enabling researchers to 'investigate discourses around contemporary social issues as well as to understand the unique communicative activities mediated by the Internet'. Specifically, they examine two contexts of online discourse relating to anorexia: the professionally run website Teenage Health Freak that enables users to submit health queries, and a lay-run, pro-recovery anorexia forum.

Hunt and Harvey (2015) remind us of the value of anonymity and the relative accessibility of online communication, particularly in the context of stigmatised health problems such as eating disorders. As such, forms of digital health communication can provide opportunities to investigate discussions of health experiences that otherwise remain marginalised or unspoken. In the case of anorexia, Hunt and Harvey (2015, p. 137) explain that experiences of disordered eating are often characterised by ambivalence, as anorexic patients report experiencing stigma from peers and family members in relation to a condition that they themselves see as an index of personal control (see Rich 2006). As such, those experiencing anorexia may investigate digital spaces in order to find the support and advice that is not available to them in their 'offline worlds'.

Furthermore, the naturally occurring digital communication that takes place in a variety of online contexts is largely free from the influence of the researcher. Interviewees in studies of anorexia have been shown to be resistant to medical treatments and, in particular, the clinical measurements – such as BMI – that are used to conceptualise and monitor health and illness (Rich 2006), which also suggests that individuals might withdraw from professional health services and, instead, engage with like-minded peers. Digital platforms, however, can also be highly influential with respect to how users perceive and articulate their illness as well as the steps they take in managing and treating it. We are told that the forum analysed by Hunt and Harvey (2015) explicitly presents itself as a pro-recovery website, prohibiting users from posting 'pro-anorexia' messages, e.g., presenting anorexia as positive, endorsing anorexia as a lifestyle choice, or encouraging others to remain anorexic.

Hunt and Harvey (2015) carry out a comparative keyword analysis, generating separate keyword lists from their two target corpora by comparing each one with a third reference corpus: the spoken component of the BNC1994. This allowed them to look for similarities and differences between the keyword lists, from which they report a shortlist of those keywords that they determine are related to the topic of eating disorders. They also investigate nomination strategies by looking at the use of the keywords 'anorexic' and 'ED' in each corpus.

One of the notable findings from their keyword analysis was that 'anorexic' appeared among the top 20 keywords for the health query website data, but this was not the case for the forum data, which prompted their particular interest in how users refer to anorexia. They examined the collocates of 'anorexia' in the Teenage Health Freak queries, and these are shown in Table 6.1. The collocates demonstrate how important ways of talking about health concerns can be realised in both grammatical and lexical words. Based on these collocates, Hunt and Harvey (2015) report that users often referred to potential anorexia,

TABLE 6.1 Grammatical and lexical collocates of 'anorexic' (Hunt and Harvey 2015)

Collocate type	Collocate
Grammatical	'I', 'am', 'and', 'to', 'Im', 'my', 'be', 'not', 'but', 'is', 'a', 'me', 'do', 'that', 'I'm', 'because', 'what', 'was', 'or', 'if', 'she'
Lexical	'think', 'want', 'friend', 'friends', 'know', 'really', 'weight', 'say', 'people', 'stone', 'eat', 'help'

submitting queries that sought some kind of diagnostic confirmation, such as 'Am I anorexic?', or 'I think I am anorexic'. This could also take the form of dismissing what a third party, such as their 'friend'/'friends' might 'say' about the user having anorexia, as the individual paradoxically submits a query about a 'problem' that they claim they do not believe they have. Hunt and Harvey (2015) highlight that this is likely a face-saving strategy, with the reported third-party perspective providing justification for the claim to professional help but the denial serving to downplay the severity of the issue.

Hunt and Harvey (2015) show that one of the ways in which anorexia is characterised is through ambivalence in that some users express a desire to be anorexic, referring to the skill of 'successfully' restricting food intake and coping with the discomfort of hunger while acknowledging the damaging effects of living this way. Hunt and Harvey (2015) refer to the harmful cultural ideal of having a slender body as exerting control over these individuals who are struggling to resist the pull of the perceived positive valuations associated with an extreme dietary regimen.

Health queries are shown to feature vocabularies of quantification and measurement as part of a wider 'medicalising' discourse around anorexia. This is manifest in references to weight and height (in numbers and units) as well as the energy value of certain foodstuffs in terms of calories. Hunt and Harvey (2015, p. 43) remark that '[i]n precisely enumerating details of their body size and calorie intake, it thus becomes possible for the narrators to set themselves up against, and compare themselves with, some abstract physical norm', which they interpret as 'a discursive strategy which marks out and clinically sanctions their problematic behaviours'.

Hunt and Harvey's (2015) collocation analysis of the keyword 'ED' showed that in the anxiety forum data, members favoured a view of anorexia that was distinct from the individual, with more frequent references to 'an ED' or 'the ED' and a relative lack of references to 'my/your ED'. Furthermore, the nominal representation of anorexia as 'ED' facilitates a discourse in which the condition is agentive, carrying out verbal ('tells me to do so many things') and material processes ('use anything to try and trick you'). The recurrent use of a definite or indefinite ('the', 'an') article coincides with personification of the disorder.

Hunt and Harvey (2015) also discuss how, in positing anorexia as a separate identity, individuals contributing to their data are able to claim a set of values for themselves that potentially absolves them of responsibility for their deleterious behaviours which are instead attributed to 'the ED'. This, in turn, can be seen as a way of conveying the internal conflict of anorexia as well as a strategy for redirecting disapproving or stigmatising views directed towards them. This strategy can help individuals cope with negative responses they receive in the offline world but also to navigate delicate interactional sequences within the forum itself.

Hunt and Harvey (2015, p. 149) reflect on the 'insights into the relative frequency of linguistic patterns afforded by corpus methods', which allows them to discuss the dominant discourses that are predicated on the aggregation of those lexical and discursive patterns. They contextualise their observations of the data within the wider treatment of anorexia, highlighting a contrast between the coping strategies they observed in the online forum and the types of disempowering experiences that have been reported from interactions with psychiatric professionals (referring to Malson et al. 2004). This highlights that in digital spaces, individuals can potentially express themselves in ways – and to effects – that are distinct from professional psychiatric contexts and that online interactions might offer something beyond, or in addition to, institutional interactions. Hunt and Harvey (2015, p. 151) conclude that their focus on authentic discourse and the data-driven approach to language learning it facilitates make corpus linguistics 'well-suited to pedagogical interventions for healthcare providers' and 'a natural match for the ethos of "evidence-based" care in medicine'.

We can see from studies of the THF data, including Harvey and Hunt (2015), how digital spaces can empower patients to directly address concerns that they have reservations about discussing face-to-face. Zummo (2015, p. 188) similarly argues that the virtual environment in which health professionals address specific user questions offers the possibility of shaping a new form of patient–practitioner relationship 'marked by reversals in the classical form of power relationships', as it is users who set the topic of conversation. Subsequently, Zummo (2015) discusses some of the linguistic patterns that denote (in)formality in patient questions and professionals' responses as part of a corpus of 'Ask the doctor' type exchanges from five health websites. Zummo (2015, p. 196) finds that the computer-mediated context for these interactions did generate some perception of familiarity; however, posts still retained 'a certain stylistic and formal care', which is evidenced in the use of salutations and the low occurrence of informal traits associated with computer-mediated communication (contractions, emoticons, etc.). Zummo (2015, p. 196) concludes that the digital medium leads to 'a different model of doctor-patient relationship' in which patients are unlikely to find diagnoses and treatments but can find a sympathetic, active listener in the health professional who is able to respond.

Advice-giving remains a common function of health professionals' communication within digital interactions, and this involves not only establishing a persona that is credible and trustworthy but also showing sensitivity at the 'relational and interpersonal level' (Locher and Hoffmann 2006, p. 75). Again, this relates not only to the direct addressee who has submitted a health query but also to a wider audience. Thus, Locher (2006) highlights the importance of the 'relational work' and rapport-building that health professionals are likely to participate in to help to foster engagement when they generate public replies to health queries. Advice-givers might more often demonstrate mitigation strategies, for example, as they strive to avoid appearing 'bossy' (Locher 2006).

Baker et al. (2019) reflect on the practice of balancing stock (i.e., preformulated) and unique replies when representatives of the NHS provide responses to online feedback from patients. They assert that personalised, unique replies are not inherently more effective than posting a more generic, formulaic response and that staff are tasked with resolving a tension between, on one hand, engaging with patients to show that they care and, on the other, maintaining a formal, professional style of communication (Baker et al. 2019). There are also concerns regarding what is practical – given pressures on time and resources – as well as for consistency, which might be inadvertently compromised when staff write unique replies and convey implicit attitudes. Baker et al. (2019) state that the 'best practice' in this context will depend on what is understood to be the function of the digital platform, i.e., whether it is to market the practice or whether it is to elicit the honest perspectives of patients. In any case, the exchanges are interpersonal, and there may be an impetus for professionals to use impersonal language in order to mitigate the potential face threats to individual staff members who might be their colleagues or, indeed, themselves.

The significance of the interpersonal aspects of these types of communication encourages us to think of such exchanges as dialogic. Digital health communication more routinely includes the capacity for readers to add comments to blogs, articles, social media posts, etc. Hodson et al. (2022) examine Twitter and YouTube comments directed at the profile of the office of Canada's Chief Public Health Officer (CPHO) during the first wave of the COVID-19 pandemic. Combining a keyword analysis with a grounded theory approach to documenting prevailing themes at the sentence and paragraph level, they report polarised responses to the same public health information and show that close, textual reading is required to identify the subtleties in tone that define the sentiments of user responses. Their observations of these responses are discussed further in Section 6.4.3.

Online news texts that include below-the-line comments also encourage non-professional responses to institutional reporting of events; this feature demonstrates both the wider trend towards the inclusion of user-generated content and the hybridisation of genres in digital spaces, as the fact-based reporting of 'hard news' is juxtaposed with subjective interpretations and experiences (Brookes and Baker 2021, p. 229). Brookes and Baker (2021, p. 255) assert that comments sections 'do appear to grant opportunities for more democratic forms of journalism in which readers can challenge journalists and each other and engage in important debates on topical social issues', thereby extending the representations that are available to the public as a potential counterdiscourse.

Through their corpus analysis of user comments following news articles on obesity from UK publications, Brookes and Baker (2021) find that commenters can offer perspectives on obesity that are more explicitly ideologically charged than those put forward in the articles on which they are commenting. For example, as commenters work to contextualise obesity in relation to broader issues in the United Kingdom, such as the extent of the welfare state and the nation's relationship with the European Union (EU), they take aim at those receiving welfare benefits or the consequences of membership in the EU for immigration. Brookes and Baker (2021) warn that provoking certain kinds of response in the below-the-line comments provides an opportunity for news organisations to introduce, more explicitly, points of view that the news outlet or journalist themselves is reluctant to articulate – in order to adhere to standards of journalistic practices or with a view to avoiding editorialising, for example. Including a trigger for these views in the article can, therefore, be a subtler strategy for drawing out these perspectives; journalists can present themselves as more objective, holding back on their own evaluations of the object of the story, and rely instead on readers to provide the evaluation that accords more generally with the dominant ideological position of the publication and its (perceived) readership.

Collins (2019) similarly observed a contrast in the more informal tone of user comments compared with the cautionary messaging of the articles on sexual health that those comments appeared alongside. Collins (2019) analysed two pairs of UK news articles and user comment threads prompted by the same press release about the rise of antibiotic-resistant gonorrhoea: an article from the *Daily Mail* with 1,883 user comments, and an article from the *Guardian*, with 835 user comments. While the articles reported rates of 'super-gonorrhoea' and discussed safe sex practices, the user comments for both the *Daily Mail* and the *Guardian* were characterised by crude humour about oral sex and about sexless marriages. Commenters appeared to posit two categories of people in opposition: those committed to fidelity – and even inadvertent celibacy – through marriage, and those whom users perceived to be in casual relationships and responsible, through their promiscuity, for the broader development and spread of sexually transmitted infections that are resistant to antibiotics. In this sense, the user comments were more explicit in their castigation of people who did not engage in safe sexual practices compared with the authors of the news articles who focused more on the importance of safe sex practices. More generally, the user comments featured a greater degree of negation than the news articles, pointing to a practice of denial-as-counterclaim and, thereby, suggesting a more deliberative type of exchange (Collins and Nerlich 2015). This reiterates that the user comments space can facilitate debate around different points of view towards (sexual) health concerns and extend the representations provided in news articles.

User-generated content can also be elicited more explicitly as feedback, as users review their experiences with health services, for example. Baker et al. (2019) introduce a corpus constructed from feedback submitted via the NHS Choices online service, comprising 228,113 patient comments (approximately 29 million words of patient feedback) on various aspects and representatives of the health services. Baker et al. (2019) subsequently offer a comprehensive investigation of the key themes in (positive and negative) feedback, the characteristics of comments related to various health professional roles, comparisons between contributors according to different age and sex groups, and the nature of responses provided by representatives of the NHS. We discuss some of the specific features identified through these different types of analysis in Section 6.4.

Baker et al. (2019, pp. 13–14) summarise the motivations for providing feedback as

> concern for other patients; the desire to help the provider; a sense of empowerment; the opportunity to perform the role of 'expert patient'; the hope that the platform operator will act as a means to further and more meaningful interaction; the cathartic value in venting negative feelings and, finally, the positive emotions that are associated with giving praise.

In addition to potentially developing a more patient-centred service, Brookes et al. (2022b, p. 29) assert that the feedback mechanism has the capacity to cultivate a kind of consumer empowerment, 'with the patients cutting providers out of the process and expressing their dismay by taking their "business" elsewhere and encouraging others to do the same'. It is important, then, to analyse digital health discourses such as these as part of the wider commercial practice of hosting customer reviews and the ongoing process of commercialisation in the UK healthcare landscape (Brookes et al. 2022b).

User-generated content, such as user comments and feedback, can provide valuable information and perspectives for other users looking to engage with healthcare services. This demonstrates how non-professionals can provide expertise for the benefit of others, and in the next section, we look more closely at the kinds of peer support that are facilitated by digital forms of health communication.

6.3.3 Digital health communication among peers

Digital communication has facilitated an increasing number of health resources that are separate from health institutions. As Hunt and Harvey (2015, pp. 135–136) report, '[as] well as organisational health websites, much online health communication takes place in condition-specific support groups, in which patients share advice, offer social support and provide narratives of their illness and recovery'. Online support forums are arguably the most prolific form of non-professional digital health communication, cultivating means of self-management and, therefore, patient autonomy whilst also offering social support. The exchanges that take place in online support forums enable contributors to restore a coherent self through the articulation of identity narratives; in other words, participants have the opportunity to define and present themselves in relation to their health concerns according to their own terms, which may be separate from the ways that health professionals operating within a biomedical paradigm may construct them as a patient (Sik 2021). Furthermore, online forums bring together peers who have a shared interest in a given health concern and can exchange experiences and advice.

Online support forums are characterised in terms of the information and emotional support they offer (Yip 2020), and many users of online forums feel more comfortable discussing sensitive and personal issues in online spaces that afford them relative anonymity (Webb et al. 2008). Rudolph Von Rohr et al. (2018, p. 221) stress that people can potentially access the same scientific information online as health professionals do, and forums dedicated to a specific health concern can be effective in collating various sources of information. Furthermore, contributors to forums are often motivated to disseminate important information not only for the purpose of increasing knowledge and awareness but also as part of the discursive practice of establishing expertise, which can also include 'referring to one's professional status, listing numerical facts, displaying empathy, using humour, and mobilizing personal narratives' (Rudolph Von Rohr et al. 2018, p. 219). Linguistic investigations of online forums have demonstrated how users construct their membership identity through diagnosis, advice-seeking, and advice-giving (Stommel and Lamerichs 2014), with disclosure of personal troubles constituting an important component in the enactment of social support (Goldsmith 2004). Members also construct their 'expert' identities through demonstrating a history of interactions with medical professionals or a knowledge of treatments, for example (Galegher et al. 1998).

There are concerns, however, that demonstrating membership to a forum means subscribing to the prevailing ideologies about the topical health concern. Lustig and Brookes (2022), for example, employ a corpus-based discourse analysis approach to examine the discursive practices that contribute to the construction of group norms in a forum for people who self-identify as alcoholics. Although the group reportedly promotes the idea of acceptance of alcoholism, Lustig and Brookes (2022, p. 6) observe that discussions were often driven by accounts of individuals' struggles with achieving and maintaining sobriety, that these struggles were quantified in terms of temporal lengths of sober intervals, and that contributors 'trade in tips on how to drink less, how to drink more safely, and how to mitigate the harmful effects of drinking on their lives'.

McDonald and Woodward-Kron (2016) demonstrate that in a bipolar disorder support forum, senior members modelled what it was appropriate for participants to discuss, and new members adopted these views (as evidenced in their lexico-grammatical and discourse-semantic choices). The processes of socialisation that occur in peer support forums show that there is value in investigating the representations that are offered in these digital spaces, as these are 'consumed, reproduced and challenged by other members of the support groups' (Brookes 2020, p. 46), ultimately contributing to how members understand and experience the health issue. In the bipolar disorder support forum data studied by McDonald and Woodward-Kron (2016), the researchers observed that the advice provided to newcomers by veteran members was often aligned with mainstream biomedical norms, and, more generally, participation in online forums has been shown to lead to users feeling better informed, more confident in their relationship with their physician with better knowledge of the treatment options available, and feeling a greater sense of optimism about their prognosis (Van Uden-Kraan et al. 2008). Thus, we can posit participation in peer-led digital spaces alongside – rather than in conflict with – individuals' interactions with health professionals in institutional spaces.

The multifunctionality of social media means that platforms such as Twitter and Facebook are also spaces where users can access health information and support from other professional and peer users alike. In the second case study of this chapter, we consider discussions of a dietary therapy on Twitter, which function to define what the therapy involves and who it is purportedly for.

CASE STUDY:

Lay representations of the ketogenic diet on Twitter (Maci 2022)

Like others (see Section 6.3.2), Maci (2022, p. 81) sees social media as a kind of digital space where 'the way doctors and patients interact is being reengineered, but also where illnesses and healthcare are communicated outside doctor-patient interaction'. Social media is posited as a resource through which users can check relevant factual health information but above all, Maci (2022, p. 81) argues, 'for receiving and expressing empathy'.

Maci's (2022, p. 82) focus is on Twitter users' discussion of the ketogenic diet (KD): 'a high-fat, low-carbohydrate nutritional treatment used in refractory treatment for epilepsy, migraines and obesity'. Maci (2022, p. 83) explains that this dietary therapy was developed in the 1920s and gained popularity in the United Kingdom and United States in the 1980s, yet there continues to be debates about its efficacy in relation to neurological conditions such as epilepsy and migraines, and information resources online remain 'scarce'. Thus, Maci (2022) considers what information and discursive representations of the KD are offered on Twitter.

Maci (2022) collected tweets from two periods in the spring of 2018 using the query keto* to allow for lexical forms such as 'ketone', 'ketogenic', 'ketodiet', 'ketolife', etc., and adding the hashtags: #keto, #ketodiet, #ketodietapp, #ketofam, #ketofood, #ketogenic, #ketogenicdiet, #ketolife, #ketolifestyle, #ketorecipes, #ketosis, and #ketoweightloss to the query. Maci (2022, p. 85) applies various kinds of corpus analytical procedures to the data to consider the different formulations and themes represented in the data, which amounted to 4,592 tweets (83,189 tokens). Maci (2022) focuses on the discursive representations of, and debates around, the KD and included only the verbal content of the tweets (i.e., and not any images or videos attached to the tweets).

An investigation of clusters in the data directed Maci (2022) to explicit expressions of what the KD is ('keto diet is', 'ketogenic diet is') and who or what it is for ('keto diet for', 'ketogenic diet for'). The KD is described as 'a very low carb diet', as an 'intervention', as a treatment for cancer/diabetes/bipolar disorder, and as a recognised alternative to medication. Based on these results, Maci (2022, p. 91) surmises that references to 'the ketogenic diet' are more commonly associated with discussions of its wider medical use compared with 'the keto diet', which is used to eulogise its effects as a weight-loss treatment.

Maci (2022) also reports findings from a semantic domain analysis, using the USAS provided through the WMatrix tool (see Chapter 2). This approach reiterated a focus on 'medical' (represented in the domains, 'Medicines and medical treatment', 'Disease') and 'dietary' ('Food', 'Drinks and alcohol') aspects, as well as showing frequent references to scientific studies ('Investigate, examine, test, search'), to the initiation and duration of the dietary therapy ('Time: Beginning', 'Time: Period'), food intake or restriction expressed in terms of quantities ('Lack of food', 'Quantities: Little'), and feeling 'healthy' ('Healthy') or 'energetic' ('Interested/excited/energetic') as a result of the KD. In addition, Maci (2022, p. 94) finds discourses around 'Religion and the supernatural', as the KD is described as 'god-sent' and 'magic' or conversely, as a 'myth'. Finally, there is also evidence of the supportive culture of social media interactions, indicated in the semantic domain 'Polite', which captures references to 'thanks' and being 'grateful', as well as the domain 'Evaluation: Good' ('good', 'great', 'super'). The domain 'Evaluation: Bad' also showed that contributors could demonstrate empathy in acknowledging that other users' challenging experiences are the 'worst'.

Maci (2022, p. 93) points to an important consideration for researchers using the predefined semantic categories of the USAS in that references to weight loss could be found in domains referring to 'Money: Debts' ('loss'), as well as 'Failure' ('lose'). Maci (2022) reminds us that the developer of the USAS advises manually checking the results of the automatic tagging and warns that the coarse-grained nature of the system may not match sense distinctions required in specific studies (Rayson 2008, p. 529). Nevertheless, the categorisation supported Maci (2022) in mapping out the key themes associated with discussions of the KD on Twitter, highlighting certain evaluative positions and demonstrating some of the interpersonal aspects of exchanges in this digital health domain.

Maci's (2022) study revealed some of the ways in which social media users brought together by their shared interest in a topic (in this instance, the KD) show support and empathy through their posts. Mpofu (2021) has also shown how peer interactions in digital spaces can cultivate collaborative humour that contributes to the desensitising of challenging health issues, thereby facilitating coping mechanisms among digital communities. Taking an ethnographic approach to analysing data generated by groups of South Africans and Zimbabweans on WhatsApp, Facebook, and Twitter, Mpofu (2021) considers how participants humorously dealt with the COVID-19 pandemic by engaging in meme composing, spreading, and consumption. Mpofu (2021, p. 41) describes humour as a 'weapon of the powerless' and asserts that these digital platforms provide spaces and a language – in the form of memes – through which members critique, question, and rebel against the governing state. Thus, by analysing how these critical perspectives are articulated in such spaces, we can generate insights into how people navigate illness and position themselves in relation to the institutions that determine how healthcare is delivered, including positioning themselves in opposition to those institutions.

There are some potentially negative aspects of peer interactions in social media spaces. Lecompte-Van Poucke (2022), for example, investigates the occurrence of a 'forced positive' discourse being exchanged via posts to two public Facebook pages representing organisations promoting endometriosis awareness: Endometriosis Australia (EA), based in Australia, and MyEndometriosisTeam (MET), based in the United States. Lecompte-Van Poucke (2022) annotated the data according to principles of transitivity analysis as part of a discourse-analytical approach to investigating construals of toxic positivity. The analysis of the EA page showed that individuals with endometriosis are represented as relatively powerless followers, enacting what the authors of the page instruct them to do, such as participate in fundraisers and research, purchase things online, listen to podcasts, and manage their bodies. Representations from the MET page depict followers 'actively battling endometriosis, being strong, staying in control, and pretending to be happy' (Lecompte-Van Poucke 2022, p. 7). Lecompte-Van Poucke (2022, p. 8) is critical of the 'unrealistic or even cruel optimism' that is conveyed through contributions such as 'you are what you choose to become' and 'perseverance, bravery, strength and courage are the markings of an Endo Warrior'. Such sentiments are seen as contributing to a neoliberal ideology which encourages individual entrepreneurship and suggests that people have the capacity to manage or overcome their struggles on their own which may ignore any structural conditions that determine people's circumstances and which may not align with followers' own perspectives on what it means to have endometriosis.

Naslund et al. (2016) conclude that despite the potential risks of digital spaces – which have been cited as concerns surrounding the quality of health information, potential hostility, and socialisation into (harmful) normative ideologies – the benefits of peer-to-peer support outweigh these potential harms, and online forums play an important role in motivating untreated and undiagnosed community members to seek professional help. We have seen how such spaces foster communities, the members of which develop shared discourses and exchange personal stories. In the next section, we focus on the specific lexical and grammatical features that participants in digital spaces deploy to perform these various communicative functions.

6.4 Features of digital health communication

Prior to summarising the types of language features that have been reported through corpus studies of digital health communication, we briefly turn our attention to features of digital communication more generally, as the technological affordances of the mode have enabled particular forms of expression that have, subsequently, become strongly associated with what has variously been termed 'eLanguage', 'computer mediated communication' (CMC) or 'online communication' (see Barton and Lee 2013, for a discussion). Carr (2020, p. 12) recounts how among early studies of CMC, the 'cues filtered out' perspective foregrounded the absence of paralinguistic cues associated with spoken communication, but that as computer technologies have increasingly supported multisensory and immersive communication, 'our assumptions about the types of messages and signals computers can mediate continue to evolve'.

Herring and Dainas (2017) introduced the term 'graphicons' to collectively refer to graphical devices such as emoticons, emoji, stickers, GIFs, images, and videos that regularly feature in digital communication. Among these graphical elements, it is emoji that have arguably received the most attention – often to investigate their propositional and pragmatic meanings in context, as Herring and Dainas (2017) have done in relation to Facebook posts. Escouflaire (2021) provides a typology of the functions of emoji that effectively summarises prior research and specifies three primary functions: expressive, interpretative, and referential. The typology also details, at a secondary level, the relational, politeness, emphatic, structural, and aesthetic functions of emoji. As such, we can document how emoji are used to convey emotions (🫤) to signal implicatures that guide the reader to extract, e.g., non-serious meaning (😌), and to represent objects and ideas (🔑).

The structure of Escouflaire's (2021) typology recognises that emoji can fulfil multiple functions simultaneously, and the most commonly used emoji are understood to have more room for ambiguity and differing interpretations (Godard and Holtzman 2022). Indeed, the syringe emoji (💉), which had previously appeared with blood in the barrel, was modified in order to maximise its versatility, most overtly as indexical of vaccinations following the COVID-19 pandemic (Broni 2021). The continued expansion of emoji characters is often motivated by providing wider representation of, for example, disability experience (🧏, 🦽, 🧑‍🦼, 🦼, 🦯, 🦻, 🦿, 🦾, 🧏), suggesting that they are designed according to relatively unambiguous meanings. Nevertheless, the utility of emoji and other graphicons, such as memes and GIFs, appears to be, in part, due to their versatility and the potential for them to be used to generate customised meanings in the local context of interaction (Wagener 2021). In other words, we can investigate how users continue to repurpose emoji to various effects in their digital (health) communication.

TASK 6.1

In this task we are going to reflect on the various functions of emoji characters in social media exchanges around health. Select a social media platform that enables hashtags and identify a short list of tags that are likely to direct you to content about health, e.g., #health, #mentalhealth, #wellbeing etc. Search for the hashtag and note down your observations of how emoji are used in posts in this thread.

Can you find examples of emoji being used according to the various primary and secondary functions outlined by Escouflaire (2021)?

- **Expressive:** conveying emotion, e.g., 'I don't feel well 😔'.
- **Interpretative:** signalling the presence of implicature and guiding meaning, e.g., 'Being ill is fun 🙄'.
- **Referential:** Referring to a concept inside or outside the message, e.g., 'Been to see the doctor 👨‍⚕️'.
- **Relational:** Maintaining a positive relationship with the recipient, e.g., 'Hope you feel better 😊'.
- **Politeness:** Softening the potential face threat of a message, e.g., 'Try not to worry so much 🖤'.
- **Emphatic:** Strengthening the emotional value of a message, e.g., 'Very frustrating 😣😖😣'.
- **Structural:** Separating, framing and punctuating clauses, e.g., 'I have had enough 😵 How are you?'.
- **Aesthetic:** Adding decorative value, e.g., 'Looking forward to the weekend 🖤, 🖤, 🖤'.

    - Is it often the case that emoji are used to perform multiple functions? Are there any combinations of functions that are particularly common?
    - How would you approach quantifying the occurrence of these functions? Could you devise an annotation system that documents their occurrence and supports a qualitative investigation of how they occur in context?

We have structured the remainder of our discussion about features of digital health communication around themes capturing how contributors to digital texts (i) define illness and discuss specific conditions; (ii) discuss responses to illness, including the role of various social actors; and (iii) express sentiment in relation to health concerns. These themes draw attention to the discursive construction of health and health concerns, directing us to content that provides insights into the damaging effects of illness but also to how people support each other in managing their health concerns. This discussion continues our exploration of how those discourses are collaboratively constructed between health professionals and peer groups and how different digital platforms facilitate particular kinds of interaction.

6.4.1 Defining illness in digital health communication

We have discussed the capacity for digital spaces to facilitate greater input from non-professionals, both in terms of the quantity of health communication and, potentially, the manner in which health concerns are expressed. Indeed, one of the research interests guiding the THF studies was to ascertain how adolescents articulated their extant knowledge and interest in a topic, including the terms they used to refer to it (Harvey et al. 2008). Corpus studies have subsequently generated insights into the vocabulary that people use to discuss illness as well as insights into the discourses surrounding health concerns that tell us something about individuals' associations and relationship with illness.

Brookes et al. (2022a, p. 619) focus on the keywords, 'HIV' and 'AIDS' in the THF corpus, reporting 'a terminological conflation of the two concepts, a misconception that is liable to have profound consequences in terms of how the adolescents conceive of and understand HIV and AIDS'. This misconception is borne out in the prevalence of the lemma 'catch' used in relation to 'HIV', which – as an 'activity verb' (Biber et al. 1999) – implies notions of agency on the part of the subject. This sense of responsibility is further engendered in the formulation of questions asking how to 'prevent catching' HIV. Brookes et al. (2022a, p. 620) assert that compared with less euphemistic constructions such as 'contracted' and 'acquired', the verb 'catch' might imply that HIV is perceived to be as communicable as the common cold, i.e., that it is highly contagious and liable to spread quickly. In related work, Harvey et al. (2014) have shown that health professionals favour the verb 'transmit' and the passive form 'infected with' when referring to HIV (and not 'AIDS'), which more closely aligns with a discourse of viral infections.

There is linguistic evidence to show that simply having an appropriate term is of value to people as they navigate illness; as Brookes (2019, p. 15) argues in the case of 'diabulimia':

> Although this term has yet to gain medical approval, the increasing awareness of it, and the apparent traction that it has gained amongst both non-expert and researcher communities alike (but particularly the former), attest to its suitability for exploring the discourses surrounding this health phenomenon.

Brookes (2019, p. 18) highlights a 'medicalising' discourse around the use of the word in online peer-to-peer interactions, which can be summarised as the process by which ordinary aspects of life become defined in medical terms. This manifests in relation to (i) a discourse of distance and objectivity, (ii) a diagnostic discourse, and (iii) a disorder discourse, which Brookes (2019) shows positions diabulimia in grammatical constructions that have been observed in relation to other – medically recognised – mental conditions.

Referring to the terms used by Conrad (2007), Brookes (2019) considers the 'light' side of medicalisation to be that medical frameworks are useful in equipping members with the concepts and vocabulary to disclose their experiences and that these disclosures are more often treated as urgent and serious. On the other hand, the 'dark' side of medicalisation is that it can entail expectations of and even reliance upon medical intervention, i.e., that a medical problem requires medical solutions.

Harvey (2012, p. 372) similarly observes a 'psychologising' discourse in adolescents' queries to the THF service and acknowledges that the approach can 'give form to, and help to make sense of, a set of inexplicably complex and chaotic symptoms'. However, Harvey (2012) reports that contributors appear to overextend a clinical label of depression to experiences that might otherwise be discussed as more normative feelings of emotional distress. The implications of this discursive strategy are that individuals are absolved of responsibility for their personal problems. Relatedly, Harvey (2012) points to the subtle distinction between the formulations 'I am depressed' and 'I have depression' in terms of encoding different meaning-making, i.e., 'the former describing depressive experiences as a reaction to negative life events, the latter portraying depression as a pathology originating within the individual' (Harvey 2012, p. 349). Recognising these subtle distinctions can help practitioners get a sense of how individuals perceive their illness experience and, potentially, what expectations they might have of the support that health professionals can offer.

In Kinloch's (2018, p. 4) comprehensive corpus-assisted critical discourse analysis of talk around infertility in blogs, clinical health information websites and news articles, four themes captured the ways that contributors discussed infertility:

- the transformative effect of infertility;
- medicalised (in)fertility;
- the marketisation of reproduction; and
- parenthood as privilege and imperative.

Kinloch (2018, p. 95) provides examples of how individual authors of blogs, in particular, are impacted by the effects of infertility, expressed in metaphors such as 'the manacle keeping me chained'. Furthermore, the first-hand experience of blog writers 'transforms' them into voices of authority who have the experiential knowledge to espouse the language of the clinic. For instance, the credibility of a 'diagnosis' of 'unexplained infertility' is questioned (Kinloch 2018, p. 99). Kinloch (2018, p. 307) warns that the medicalisation of the infertility experience posits the (female) body as a site of increased monitoring and intervention as well as feeding into notions of neoliberal self-management in the pursuit of maintaining 'normal' bodily functions, i.e., reproductive capacity.

Relatedly, 'marketisation' discourses contribute to the idea that this capacity to reproduce is recoverable at the right cost, though instances of this type of discourse were more often observed in the data from health information websites and news articles. Parenthood is, thus, represented as a reward for engaging with services and the reproductive marketplace, and there are critical views directed at women who 'leave it too late' or otherwise do not conform to normative ideals of pursuing parenthood. Ultimately, Kinloch (2018, p. 313) finds little evidence of contestation of the dominant discourses of medicalisation, marketisation, and the imperative to parent with only blog authors showing resistance to the idea that they would be entirely defined by their fertility status.

Other kinds of digital spaces directly juxtapose professional and lay perspectives on health issues, and in these spaces, we can get a clearer sense of where there are disparities in those respective positions. In their keyword analysis of news coverage of obesity, Brookes and Baker (2021, p. 239) found that while there was convergence between the articles and the comments in terms of their general discussion of obesity-related health issues ('diabetes', 'disease', 'heart', 'liver'), commenters frequently challenged a proposition in the news articles about links between obesity and certain types of cancer. Brookes and Baker (2021, p. 237) report that there were more references to 'research' and 'study' in news articles than there were in comments, as well as quantificational lexis ('per cent', 'figures', 'increase'). These findings attest to a greater concern among journalists to substantiate their reported claims with data. Discussion between commenters pointed to further areas of debate, such as the links between 'trauma'/'stress' and obesity, with some dismissing a causal link, while others emphasised the interrelations between different aspects of an individual's life. Brookes and Baker (2021) discuss how these differing perspectives among readers are related to contrasting views about personal responsibility and individual responses to challenges, resulting in different attributions of 'blame'. Exploring these discourses gives us a sense of how different ideological positions are reasoned (or not) and address not only the causes of illness but also what might be appropriate solutions.

Further investigation of how health concerns are discursively constructed in health queries has generated insights into how maladaptive behaviours associated with mental health concerns are situated within individuals' lives and how they become habitualised. Harvey and Brown (2012) explored adolescent's accounts of self-harm in the THF corpus; their collocation analysis of the keywords 'cut', and 'self-harm' led to the identification of the following themes of (associated collocates in brackets):

- time, duration, and cycles ('started', 'stop', 'years');
- low mood or depression ('feel', 'depressed');
- support and assistance ('help'); and
- peers ('friends').

Exploring these collocates helped Harvey and Brown (2012, p. 331) to ascertain, through contributors' vivid descriptions, that self-harm practices became habitual and compulsive due to the fact that the relief offered by the act was only temporary, compared with the persistence of the emotional turmoil that triggered the behaviour. Furthermore, we are told that self-harm was discussed as an addiction, which Harvey and Brown (2012, p. 331) interpret as having the effect of minimising personal agency and emphasising contributors' 'inability to control their self-harming activity'.

In addition to providing insights into conceptualisations of specific illnesses, the relative openness of digital spaces can facilitate discussions of illness more generally, as contributors can readily submit queries around concerns that they might not consider to be serious or urgent enough to visit a health professional with. In messages to the THF website, for example, Harvey et al. (2007) remark upon the tendency for contributors to formulate their queries in terms of '(ab)normality', e.g., 'am I normal?'. Indeed, 'normal' was identified as a keyword, which was used in a general sense as well as in relation to physical measurements ('normal size', 'normal weight'). A related keyword, 'worried', demonstrates that users are troubled by this uncertain state of '(ab)normality', and we can infer from this framing that 'normal' is perceived to be equivalent to 'healthy' (and 'abnormal' synonymous with 'unhealthy').

6.4.2 Discussing responses to illness in digital health communication

In the previous section, we focused on articulations of illness and health concerns. We now focus on the features of language used online to discuss responses to health threats. Whether this refers to the social actors who are perceived to have the capacity to enact solutions or the manner in which those solutions are communicated, corpus studies of digital health communication have highlighted patterns in how contributors to exchanges in digital spaces support each other with information, advice, and empathy.

Demmen et al. (2015) investigated an online support group for cancer and end of life care involving patients, family carers, and healthcare professionals. They reported a wide range of violence metaphors ('battling' cancer, for example) used to various effects. Patients' use of violence metaphors appeared to reinforce a sense of agency as the individual is represented as being proactive in response to what is happening to them. However, reference to a 'battle' also foregrounded the difficult nature of the experience and introduced the possibility of 'defeat' as personal failure (Demmen et al. 2015, p. 220). Carers more often referred to the fight that they were engaged in alongside the patient – 'fighting' the system to get particular treatments, for example. Contributions to the online forum also showed that carers engaged in discussions around bereavement that involved the 'devastation' of having lost the person they were caring for. Similarly, while health professionals generally positioned themselves in a protective role over the patient, contributions to the online forum also included disclosures about being regularly 'confronted' by death. The occurrence of violence metaphors was shown to be significantly higher in the online forum compared with interviews and, given the nature of how they were used, Demmen et al. (2015) show that the informality and anonymity of forums can encourage solidarity in bringing people together to discuss shared experiences in a non-institutional context.

While many digital spaces appear to encourage contributors to offer sensitive self-disclosures 'with a level of candour that would be unlikely in more inhibiting offline settings' (Hunt and Brookes 2020, p. 62), when it comes to advice-seeking and advice-giving, we can still expect to see varying degrees of directness as members negotiate their interpersonal relationships. As Stommel and Lamerichs (2014, p. 200) explain: '[a]mong the variations, there are general requests for advice ("What can I do to help myself?" or "Please help"), requests that ask for other members' experience with a certain treatment or medication, or requests asking for a confirmation of one's self-diagnosis'. Yip (2020, p. 1216) found that 70% of thread openers in forums for dealing with anxiety and depression requested support but in indirect ways, such as through self-disclosure. This demonstrates the reciprocity of advice-seeking in that participants offer personal information that can help respondents to identify what information and advice would be pertinent but also that the advice-seeker is complicit in maintaining the social connectedness of the digital space. Furthermore, indirect requests for advice are seen as being 'low contingent' (Curl and Drew 2008), minimising expectations for a response and also accommodating for other kinds of reply that are not explicitly offered as advice.

Locher and Hoffmann (2006) discuss the advice-giving strategies of a constructed professional advisor, 'Lucy', as part of an online query service managed by a team of health professionals. Their keyword analysis of the replies that Lucy provides supports them in arguing that the team of authors show a preference for using 'ordinary' language ('sex', 'herpes', 'penis') and avoiding technical terms, which is interpreted as a deliberate strategy towards minimising the distance between the users who submit queries to the service and the persona offering advice. They discuss, however, the difficulties associated with establishing the appropriate degree of informality and refer to an example of a query questioning the use of what they perceive to be 'vulgar' slang in replies (Locher and Hoffmann 2006). Further submissions to the service celebrate the service's 'accessibility', demonstrating that there are different perspectives on how the professional team balances competency and informality (Locher and Hoffmann 2006, p. 91). Locher and Hoffmann (2006) show that, alongside using accessible vocabulary, there are other strategies for creating informality, such as:

- expressing 'personal' views ('It isn't good to smoke no matter what else you do');
- demonstrating a sense of humour; and
- presenting themselves using a first name only, i.e., 'Lucy'.

Crucially, these stand alongside strategies for:

- establishing competence and credibility – presenting facts and information, describing symptoms and side effects;
- showing empathy – 'Living with an addict in the family is difficult and stressful, regardless of whether or not you live under the same roof with that person'; and
- Presenting options in the giving of advice, which can be delivered as declarative statements ('You might look at other stress outlets'), imperatives ('Give yourself time to wind down before going to bed'), or questions ('Do you have friends/family with whom you feel okay sharing your feelings?').

(Locher and Hoffmann 2006).

Kinloch and Jaworska (2020, p. 75) emphasise the potential of digital spaces, particularly peer-to-peer forums, for providing access to the patients' 'unedited' voices. Of course, disclosures online will likely be constructed with the anticipated audience in mind, nevertheless, Kinloch and Jaworska (2020, p. 75) assert that '[b]ecause of its anonymity, availability and interactivity, the digital seems to offer safe spaces in which there is less pressure on face needs, making it easier to disclose details that might otherwise remain hidden'. They argue this is all the more crucial in the context of illness experiences that are subject to stigmatisation. Their analysis of accounts of postnatal depression (PND) posted to an online forum explores depictions of users' maladaptive responses to illness, which appear to be driven by perceived stigma associated with the condition. Stigma associated with PND is said to derive from the notion that low mood, anxieties, and loss of interest in motherhood, which are characteristic of PND, lie 'outside the model of intensive mothering and hence it is likely to be seen as "abnormal"' (Kinloch and Jaworska 2020, p. 78).

One of the major themes observed through the analysis of the term 'PND' in the online forum data was 'hiding', as contributors described their long suffering but also their reluctance to discuss the matter with health professionals. Contributors explain that they would 'never have admitted' PND, using terms such as 'secret' and referring to themselves as a 'failure' (Kinloch and Jaworska 2020, p. 84). Kinloch and Jaworska (2020) go on to discuss how PND encourages individuals to turn their attention inwardly upon themselves; forum posters looked for explanations that originated with their own bodies or within their personal circumstances. Furthermore, because they were not discussing their experiences with others, prior to engaging with the forum, they relied upon a self-diagnosis of PND. This personalisation can lead to isolation, thereby emphasising the value of the digital forum in encouraging those with PND to engage with others and look to a shared experience, thereby minimising the sense of abnormality associated with PND.

Brookes's (2020) collocation analysis of disclosures of experiences of diabetes uncovers descriptions of practices driven by claims to autonomy. Members of online support groups for diabetes frequently discussed ways of restricting insulin, i.e., 'not taking', 'stopping', 'skipping', etc., as well as making references to weight (Brookes 2020). These findings directed Brookes (2020) to forum exchanges relating to 'diabulimia', in which some contributors recognised insulin restriction as a form of autonomous diabetes management. Brookes (2020) interprets this discourse of autonomy as another manifestation of a broader neoliberal model of public health that emphasises individual responsibility. However, there were also disputes around the association of insulin with weight gain, as members highlighted the associated dangers and risks of insulin restriction, particularly for weight management. Understanding how discourses of autonomy influence self-management practices, particularly with regard to chronic health conditions, is important for navigating issues of compliance with medical advice and avoidance of potentially harmful practices. This case also shows that peer support can manifest in challenging maladaptive behaviours and that expert patients may be better positioned, due to the reduced social distance with the addressee compared with a health professional, to provide guidance towards healthier practices.

The proliferation of peer-led digital health support services means that the role of institutional services may be changing. Studies of the digital communicative practices of such institutions can reveal how these construct their role and contributions to individuals' responses to illness. Chałupnik and Brookes's (2021) corpus-assisted critical discourse study of the websites of CCGs in the UK NHS took as its starting point the terms used by the CCGs to refer to themselves in the website materials – the most frequent of which was shown to be the first-person plural pronoun 'we'. Through a subsequent collocation analysis of 'we', Chałupnik and Brookes (2021) observed that the CCGs focused on accomplished and continuing material actions ('we have published', 'we are working'). Similarly, collocates such as 'provide' pointed to activities located in the 'unrestricted present' (Leech 1966). References to improvements to service and prospective collaborations were shown through the verb collocates 'can' and 'will', while 'want' similarly offered an indication of intent that implies a higher degree of self-determination (Chałupnik and Brookes 2021, p. 652). Chałupnik and Brookes (2021, p. 663) argue that these formulations function as 'forms of prestige advertising, designed with the aim of promoting the brands and activities of the CCGs' in spaces that might otherwise be used for providing important health information. This marketisation is seen as a reflection of the wider commercialisation of health services in the United Kingdom, a context in which CCGs are under pressure to demonstrate their value in competition with other units and one in which responses to illness are increasingly evaluated in commercial terms.

Baker et al.'s (2019) study of patient feedback provided an opportunity to consider how different professional roles (i.e., surgeons, dentists, paramedics, cleaners, midwives, consultants, nurses, managers, opticians, pharmacists, doctors, and receptionists) within health services are discursively constructed by patients. Through a collocation analysis which focused on the evaluative terms that were most strongly associated with references to each professional role, Baker et al. (2019) found that midwives were most likely to be evaluated as 'supportive', pharmacists as 'helpful', and nurses as 'attentive' and 'caring' (2019, p. 104). Receptionists, meanwhile, were evaluated particularly poorly by respondents in the data, through terms such as 'terrible', 'useless', 'rude', 'unhelpful', 'arrogant', and 'aggressive' (Baker et al. 2019, p. 108). However, Baker et al. (2019) assert that negative evaluations often seem to arise from misunderstandings about receptionists' roles and responsibilities and that as the public face of the health services, receptionists are often the target of patients' wider frustrations with the health system (see also Brookes and McEnery 2017). Ultimately, this kind of feedback can provide insights into patients' understanding and expectations about health services, which is likely also informed by wider societal discourses surrounding gender and professional status (see also Baker and Brookes 2021) as well as the respondent's own position in society (in terms of their age, gender, culture, etc.). Indeed, Baker et al. (2019) have also shown how patients index aspects of their age and experience to convey credibility as an 'expert patient' when providing their assessments of health services.

While patient feedback is, by design, evaluative, we have seen from other corpus studies of digital health communication that descriptions of illness and of those involved in responsive action to health concerns are often imbued with evaluations when presented in discourse. The final section in our discussion of features of digital health communication considers evaluation more directly, as we turn our attention to the ways that sentiment is expressed across digital health platforms.

6.4.3 *Expressing sentiment in digital health communication*

Natural language processing (NLP) techniques – the kind that enable corpus linguistics procedures such as tokenisation and POS-tagging – are increasingly being used to process vast amounts of digital data and generate swift summaries of the prevailing sentiments expressed by contributors to, for example, social media texts (Calvo et al. 2017). In many cases, such tools are seen as an alternative to questionnaires and surveys that might previously have been used to elicit patient perspectives on health services. As Dunn (2022, p. 28) explains, many computational linguistics approaches to sentiment analysis adopt a dictionary-based method, i.e., guided by a list of words categorised as 'positive', 'negative', and 'neutral'. What is widely acknowledged, however, is that such an approach 'ignores the finer distinctions' and is not well suited to examining types of pragmatic meaning such as 'metaphor, irony, sarcasm, and humour' (Dunn 2022, p. 28). Referring to some of the corpus studies discussed in this chapter, we can begin to see where some of the challenges lie in relation to capturing sentiment using computational tools.

In their introduction to their comprehensive corpus study of patient feedback, Baker et al. (2019) cite an example of a negative comment that does not contain any explicitly negative language but in which the contributor uses idiomatic language ('took forever'), colloquial forms ('a joke'), adverbs indicating extreme cases ('even'), and punctuation ('!!!') to convey their outrage. Terminology associated with timeframes was shown to contribute to both positive and negative experiences, as patients celebrate the 'years' of good service they have received or decry the 'weeks' they have been waiting for an appointment (Baker et al. 2019, p. 94). As such, many formulations through which a manual reader would likely recognise evaluative positions do not evidently comprise 'positive' or 'negative' words and can even be used to opposite effects.

Opinions can, therefore, be expressed in fairly indirect ways; nevertheless, when searching for the expression of stance in a corpus, we can focus on vocabulary more conventionally associated with evaluation. For instance, drawing on Hunston's (2011) definition of evaluative language, Baker et al. (2019) targeted the most frequent linguistic markers of positive ('good', 'excellent', 'great', etc.) and negative ('bad', 'poor', 'worst', etc.) evaluation from a word list of patient feedback data. A collocation analysis of positive and negative evaluative words revealed a high degree of overlap between terms that could be the subject of either positive or negative feedback, namely people ('staff', 'GP', 'doctors', 'manager', 'dentist') and services ('service', 'care', 'treatment'). Baker et al. (2019) subsequently offer a discussion of the semantic prosody of these terms in the context of their data, showing that the terms 'care' and 'treatment' tended to be used in positive evaluations, while the term 'attitude' was shown to have a generally negative evaluative prosody, even when it was not modified by a negative evaluative word or phrase. The authors reiterate that it is important to examine the use of seemingly neutral words *in situ*, 'in order to apprehend more subtly evaluative meanings' (Baker et al. 2019, p. 52). Similarly, further exploration of the co-text provided insights into the finer aspects of 'care', etc., such as good communication skills, that informed patients' positive evaluations of the service.

Hodson et al. (2022, p. 158) also found that opposing positive and negative views oriented around particular key phrases in their analysis of Twitter and YouTube comments posted in response to content from the profile of the CPHO during the COVID-19 pandemic. The authors highlight the importance of reading key features in context – and the advantages that human qualitative coding provides over algorithmic sentiment analysis – in that while the phrase 'thank you' was key in both the Twitter comments and the YouTube responses, there was a distinct contrast in tone. Hodson et al. (2022, p. 161) explain that on Twitter, 'thank you' was directed at the CPHO and appeared to be sincere, while on YouTube, the phrase was typically used in a sarcastic way, e.g., 'Thank you! Oh yes, please enlighten us with your wisdom Mr Smarty Pants'.

In addition, there are examples of more complex formulations through which commenters rely upon discursive strategies to express evaluations, and these can provide a fuller picture of the context and reasoning behind those perspectives. Brookes et al. (2022b) found that patients were more likely to articulate experiences of health services that they evaluated negatively through narratives, compared with positive accounts. One explanation for this was that patients would provide additional background information as evidence to support their claims about poor service provision, which Brookes et al. (2022b) assert could be in anticipation of their negative evaluations more likely to being challenged. Furthermore, the retelling of the negative experience in detail can be an effective strategy for establishing reliability and legitimacy, providing the content through which others can determine its generalisability. Baker et al. (2019) similarly found that reported speech contributed to evidentiality, allowing readers to judge for themselves the acceptability – or otherwise – of the utterances observed by the author of the post. Brookes et al. (2022b, p. 27) discuss how the inclusion of more detailed narratives contributes to the construction of an experienced patient identity, as well as an imagined community of patients, 'who will share values and priorities'. More elaborate and discursive forms of evaluation can be more persuasive than simple evaluative terms such as 'good' and 'bad' as well as offering more contextual detail upon which readers can base their judgements of not only the subject being discussed but also the credibility of the contributor providing that evaluation.

When studying evaluative discourse, there are advantages to combining quantitative and qualitative forms of evaluation, where possible. In their study of patient feedback, Baker et al. (2019) had the opportunity to investigate typed comments that were attached to a quantitative rating that indicated the likelihood that users would recommend the health service they have encountered to their family and friends (1 - Extremely unlikely; 2 - Unlikely; 3 - Neither likely or unlikely; 4 - Likely; 5 - Extremely likely). This gave the researchers a solid foundation for comparing sub-corpora according to their numerical rating and, subsequently, exploring the more nuanced forms of linguistic evaluation provided with the different quantitative ratings. The analysis demonstrated the complexity of articulations comprising categories of words such as those expressing negation ('not', 'no', 'n't'). Negation words were particularly prominent in comments rated 1–3, and Baker et al. (2019, p. 78) show that these can have complex syntactical relations with other evaluative words, e.g., 'Most of reception staff are barely polite when not rude'. In this example, we can see the limitations of taking the word 'rude', or even the combination 'not rude', as indicative of the sentiment of the whole text.

TASK 6.2

Trustpilot is a review website that hosts user reviews of various businesses and services, including the category 'Health & Medical' services. This category is further sub-divided into clinics, dental services, diagnostics & testing, etc.

Visit the Trustpilot website and select one of the individual services within the Health & Medical category to access reviews for that service.

Note: you are likely to be directed to the version of Trustpilot local to you and, subsequently, services related to your area.

Consider the following questions:

- What do you notice about the number of reviews according to each of the five-star rating options? Are these evenly distributed?
- Filter the reviews according to the highest rating(s), i.e., five and/or four and read through some of the reviews. Do you notice any terms of phraseology that tend to occur in these reviews that directly correspond to the positivity of the rating?
- Repeat the process for reviews with the lowest ratings. Could you characterise these in terms of negative evaluative terms?
- What factors are mentioned in the review, whether positively or negatively, that indicate which aspects are informing contributors' evaluations?
- How do your observations compare with those of Baker et al. (2019)? For example, do references to timeframes and to communication skills appear regularly in the reviews that you have read?
- Are there any examples of a mid-rating (i.e., three stars)? Do these reviews feature good and bad aspects?
- Consider what the implications of your observations are for interpreting the results of a corpus linguistics analysis of the data. Are there any terms that you would be cautious about taking at face value for instance?

6.5 Chapter summary

Compared with other modes, the capacity for more substantial contributions from 'ordinary' people is one of the oft-cited advantages of digital spaces. Tim Berners-Lee (2010), the director of the World Wide Web Consortium (W3C) who devised and implemented the first Web browser and Web server, cites the 'egalitarian principles' on which the World Wide Web was founded and emphasises the need to protect its 'universality', 'decentralization', and 'open standards' that mean that any committed expert can contribute to its ongoing design. We have seen in the studies discussed in this chapter how corpus linguists approach and target digital spaces with the understanding that they are likely to offer perspectives on health issues that might be marginalised in, or altogether absent from, other (particularly institutional) contexts. The accessibility of digital spaces has led to wide participation and also a high degree of user-generated content, which has implications for the health professional-patient dynamic.

We should be cautious, however, in presuming that the capacity for wider access leads to wider representation in the digital data we collect as a corpus. Studies have shown that social media platforms are favoured by users belonging to particular demographic categories; for example, 38.5% of Twitter users are aged between 25–34 (Dixon 2022). Brookes and Baker (2022, p. 14) comment on the demographic (im)balances in their corpus of online patient feedback on cancer care, explaining that,

> 87.09 per cent of the comments in our corpus were provided by patients identifying as White English/Welsh/Scottish/Northern Irish. People from LGBTQ+ backgrounds make up just 1 per cent of respondents, while people who speak English as an additional language make up just 3.5 per cent.

In terms of corpus compilation, we need to consider whether we want to (or can) design our corpora in a way that represents the actual membership of the platform we are investigating (including maintaining any of its imbalances) or whether we attempt to include a more even representation that enables us to look at comparisons between pertinent demographic factors such as age, gender, and so on.

In patients' direct exchanges with health professionals, Zummo (2015) has investigated the language choices through which power is enacted, and in advice-giving situations, we have seen how contributors, both professional (Locher and Hoffmann 2006) and non-professional (Rudolph Von Rohr et al. 2018), balance credibility with appearing approachable. This tension highlights two of the reported priorities in digital health spaces: the sharing of information and the facilitation of supportive communities. Zummo (2015) has discussed how even when doctors cannot show strong commitment to their expert deductions in relation to user health queries, they can demonstrate empathy, highlighting the importance of the interpersonal aspects of digital health exchanges.

Existing corpus studies have revealed how and where professional and lay perspectives are not aligned and how these are debated in digital spaces. Brookes and Baker (2021), for example, have highlighted how user comments offer a more democratic form of journalism. More generally, although there are concerns about the fragmentation of online spaces and the potential for the regularisation of views in online forums, for example (McDonald and Woodward-Kron 2016), we have seen evidence that participants in digital spaces do contest prevailing (biomedical) conceptualisations of health (Brookes and Baker 2021) and do challenge each other on presuppositions (Brookes 2020). This indicates that there is deliberation in digital spaces and that visitors to these spaces will be presented with a range of perspectives beyond institutional perspectives provided by health professionals or the media, for example.

As the dynamic between health professional and patient shifts, we have observed patient perspectives that strive for autonomy and self-management regarding their health (Brookes 2020) but also medicalising discourses that appear to work to diminish the sense of responsibility that individuals have for their own state of ill-health (Harvey 2012; Brookes 2019) or injurious practices (Harvey and Brown 2012). The consideration for individual agency with respect to illness appears to correlate with a corresponding shift towards neoliberal ideologies promulgated by health institutions articulated through marketisation and commercialised discourses (Kinloch 2018; Chałupnik and Brookes 2021). Furthermore, the elevated impetus on individual responsibility can also be encouraged by peers to a point of toxic positivity (Lecompte-Van Poucke 2022). More commonly, though, it appears that while senior members in digital forums can convey the wisdom of their expertise, there is an understanding of how these align with biomedical expertise and that it is important to recognise when engagement with health services is appropriate (McDonald and Woodward-Kron 2016; Brookes 2020).

What appears to be a particular strength of digital spaces is their capacity for social connectedness and the forming of communities around shared health concerns, which can bring together members otherwise separated by time and space. Demmen et al. (2015) showed that carers and health professionals working in cancer support engaged in online forum discussions to talk about the impacts of losing someone to cancer, finding empathetic responses from others with shared experience. McGlashan (2021) similarly demonstrates that one set of perspectives of the COVID-19 pandemic that was recorded in digital form was a collection of online memorials posted to the Church of England's Remember Me website (https://www.rememberme2020.uk/). McGlashan (2021) notes that one of the factors that is likely to have encouraged expressions of online remembrance is that social distancing and lockdown measures introduced in response to COVID-19 meant that it was not possible to conduct many traditional, face-to-face bereavement ceremonies nor to visit friends or relatives in the time that led up to their death. Furthermore, memorials provided an opportunity for authors to construct a representation of the deceased that is absent of illness and, instead, define them in terms of their social bonds, which extend beyond their lifetime ('forever in our hearts'). Thus, digital spaces appear to be valued for the capacity to provide alternative representations, often outside of the biomedical model, affording the contributor the means to formulate identities and experience in their own terms but, nonetheless, finding a receptive audience.

What we have also seen through our review of corpus studies of digital health communication are the discursive strategies through which contributors construct the persona of 'expert', administer advice, and provide readers with the content to extrapolate from their personal experiences. These more elaborate language strategies often warrant an analytical approach that enriches corpus procedures with forms of annotation (Brookes et al. 2022b) or combines these methods with approaches that substantiate the qualitative and interactional dimensions of the data (Locher and Hoffmann 2006; Allen and Saeed 2022). This can be particularly challenging given the amount of data available, and researchers often use corpus methods as a way of focusing on particular features or even a sample of texts prior to carrying out some form of discourse analysis. Coltman-Patel et al. (2022), for example, carried out a keyword analysis of forum threads discussing vaccination, which directed them to focus on the use of insults. The authors subsequently coded the use of these insults to determine how they were being used as rhetorical devices, as contributors navigated their way through conflicts outside the forum orienting around contrasting views about vaccination. Their work further attests to the value of extended and contextualised investigation of keywords that direct us to the discursive aspects of deliberations around health concerns and the interpersonal dynamics of digital forums.

We have also briefly acknowledged the different semiotic systems used in digital (health) interactions. Researchers have reported the potential advantages of wider adoption of emoji in health documents, including capturing experiences of illness symptoms and health information (Lotfinejad et al. 2020). Lotfinejad et al. (2020), for example, recommend the use of the emoji characters ✋ 🧼 in the promotion of handwashing practices. Similarly, Headley et al. (2022, pp. 13–14) discuss the potential value of memes in health promotion materials as part of the efforts of health educators to create 'culturally sensitive, low-literacy, multilingual guides, memes, and decision aids with larger font, inclusive photographs, short sentences, and plain language written in the indigenous language target audience'. We have discussed in

Section 6.3.3 how peer interactions on social media participate in the creation and sharing of memes as a kind of subversive humour and coping mechanism in the face of health challenges, and the interdiscursivity of GIF and meme formats emphasises the significance of acknowledging the mixture of culture references that often feature in its localised meaning. Corpus linguistics approaches to multimodal texts require additional annotation, and because of the additional manual input, integration of modes not readily translatable to a machine-readable format in corpus studies has been somewhat limited. Nevertheless, readers will find some useful demonstrations of how this has been achieved in corpus studies of digital texts, such as social media, generally (Rüdiger and Dayter 2020), and we can anticipate that these will be increasingly adopted in the study of digital health communication.

Further reading

- Collins, L. C. & Baker, P. (2023). *Language, discourse and anxiety.* Cambridge University Press.

Collins and Baker investigate an online forum for anxiety support, exploring more than eight years' worth of contributions from a range of corpus approaches. Referring to keywords, collocations, and clusters, they report prevalent ways of discussing anxiety as well as the strategies of peer support that contribute to creating this online community.

- Locher, M. A. (2006). *Advice online: Advice-giving in an American Internet health column.* John Benjamins. https://doi.org/10.1075/pbns .149

Locher's comprehensive study of the professional support service, 'Lucy Answers' demonstrates a corpus pragmatic approach to investigating advice-giving. Readers are guided through the various strategies through which the team of health professionals foster a persona that has credibility and is encouraging of contributions from people looking for health advice.

- McGlashan, M. (2021). Networked discourses of bereavement in online COVID-19 memorials. *International Journal of Corpus Linguistics, 26*(4), 557–582. https://doi.org/10.1075/ijcl.21135.mcg

McGlashan's corpus-assisted critical discourse study of online bereavement messages shows how digital spaces encourage exchanges between different kinds of audience and observations of frequent words and clusters show how community is enacted among the site's members.

References

Allen, R.J. & Saeed, F. (2022). Dialysis organization online information on kidney failure treatments: A content analysis using corpus linguistics. *Kidney Medicine*, 4(6), 100462. https://doi.org/10.1016/j.xkme.2022.100462

Androutsopoulos, J. (2011). From variation to heteroglossia in the study of computer-mediated discourse. In C. Thurlow & K. Mroczek (Eds.), *Digital discourse: Language in the new media* (pp. 277–298). Oxford University Press. https://doi.org/10.1093/acprof:oso/9780199795437.003.0013

Baker, P. & Brookes, G. (2021). Lovely nurses, rude receptionists, and patronising doctors: Determining the impact of gender stereotyping on patient feedback. In J. Angouri & J. Baxter (Eds.), *The Routledge handbook of language, gender, and sexuality* (pp. 559–571). Routledge. https://doi.org/10.4324/9781315514857

Baker, P., Brookes, G. & Evans, C. (2019). *The language of patient feedback: A corpus linguistic study of online health communication.* Routledge. https://doi.org/10.4324/9780429259265

Barton, D. & Lee, C. (2013). *Language online: Investigating digital texts and practices.* Routledge. https://doi.org/10.4324/9780203552308

Basch, C.H., Meleo-Erwin, Z., Fera, J., Jaime, C. & Basch, C.E. (2021). A global pandemic in the time of viral memes: COVID-19 vaccine misinformation and disinformation on TikTok. *Human Vaccines & Immunotherapeutics*, 17(8), 2373–2377. https://doi.org/10.1080/21645515.2021.1894896

Bateman, J. (2021). What are digital media? *Discourse, Context & Media*, 41, 100502. https://doi.org/10.1016/j.dcm.2021.100502

Baumgartner, S.E. & Hartmann, T. (2011). The role of health anxiety in online health information search. *Cyberpsychology, Behavior and Social Networking*, 14(10), 613–618. https://doi.org/10.1089/cyber.2010.0425

Bell, A. (1984). Language style as audience design. *Language in Society*, 13(2), 145–204. http://www.jstor.org/stable/4167516.

Berners-Lee, T. (2010). Long live the Web. *Scientific American*, 303(6), 80–85. http://www.jstor.org/stable/26002308

Bhavnani, S.P. & Sitapati, A.M. (2019). Virtual care 2.0—A vision for the future of data-driven technology-enabled healthcare. *Current Treatment Options in Cardiovascular Medicine*, 21, 21. https://doi.org/10.1007/s11936-019-0727-2

Biber, D., Johansson, S., Leech, G., Conrad, S. & Finegan, E. (1999). *Longman grammar of spoken and written English*. Longman.

boyd, d. (2010). Social network sites as networked publics: Affordances, dynamics, and implications. In Z. Papacharissi (Ed.), *Networked Self: Identity, community, and culture on social network sites* (pp. 39–58). Routledge. https://doi.org/10.4324/9780203876527

Broni, K. (2021). Vaccine emoji comes to life. *Emojipedia*. https://blog.emojipedia.org/vaccine-emoji-comes-to-life/.

Brookes, G. (2019). Insulin restriction, medicalisation and the Internet: A corpus linguistic study of the discourse of diabulimia in online support groups. *Communication and Medicine*, 15(1), 14–27. https://doi.org/10.1558/cam.33067

Brookes, G. (2020). Corpus linguistics in illness and healthcare contexts: A case study of diabulimia support groups. In Z. Demjén (Ed.), *Applying linguistics in illness and healthcare contexts* (pp. 44–72). Bloomsbury. http://dx.doi.org/10.5040/9781350057685.0023

Brookes, G., Atkins, S. & Harvey, K. (2022a). Corpus linguistics and health communication: Using corpora to examine the representation of health and illness. In A. O'Keeffe & M. McCarthy (Eds.), *The Routledge handbook of corpus linguistics* (second edition, pp. 615–628). Routledge. https://www.routledge.com /The-Routledge-Handbook-of-Corpus-Linguistics/OKeeffe-McCarthy/p/book /9780367076382

Brookes, G. & Baker, P. (2021). *Obesity in the news: Language and representation in the press.* Cambridge University Press. https://doi.org/10.1017/9781108864732

Brookes, G. & Baker, P. (2022). Fear and responsibility: Discourses of obesity and risk in the UK press. *Journal of Risk Research, 25*(3), 363–378. https://doi.org/10 .1080/13669877.2020.1863849

Brookes, G. & Harvey, K. (2016). Examining the discourse of mental illness in a corpus of online advice-seeking messages. In L. Pickering, E. Friginal & S. Staples (Eds.), *Talking at work: Corpus-based explorations of workplace discourse* (pp. 209–234). Palgrave. https://doi.org/10.1057/978-1-137-49616-4_9

Brookes, G., Harvey, K. & Mullany, L. (2018). From corpus to clinic: Health communication research and the impact agenda. In D. McIntyre & H. Price (Eds.), *Applying linguistics: Language and the impact agenda* (pp. 99–111). Routledge.

Brookes, G., McEnery, A., McGlashan, M., Smith, G. & Wilkinson, M. (2022b). Narrative evaluation in patient feedback: A study of online comments about UK healthcare services. *Narrative Inquiry, 32*(1), 9–35. https://doi.org/10.1075/ni.20098.bro

Brookes, G. & McEnery, T. (2017). How to interpret large volumes of patient feedback: Methods from computer-assisted linguistics. *Social Research Practice,* 4(1), 2–13. http://the-sra.org.uk/wp-content/uploads/SRA_Social_Research _Practice_Journal_Issue_04-summer-2017.pdf.

Bucci, S., Schwannauer, M. & Berry, N. (2019). The digital revolution and its impact on mental health care. *Psychology and Psychotherapy, 92*(2), 277–297. https://doi .org/10.1111/papt.12222

Calvo, R., Milne, D., Hussain, M. & Christensen, H. (2017). Natural language processing in mental health applications using non-clinical texts. *Natural Language Engineering, 23*(5), 649–685. https://psycnet.apa.org/doi/10.1017/ S1351324916000383

Carr, C.T. (2020). CMC is dead, long live CMC!: Situating Computer-Mediated Communication scholarship beyond the digital age. *Journal of Computer-Mediated Communication, 25*(1), 9–22. https://doi.org/10.1093/jcmc/zmz018

Chałupnik, M. & Brookes, G. (2021). 'You said, we did': A corpus-based analysis of marketising discourse in healthcare websites. *Text & Talk, 41*(5–6), 643–666. https://doi.org/10.1515/text-2020-0038

Chau, K.Y., Lam, M.H.S., Cheung, M.L., Tso, E.K.H., Flint, S.W., Broom, D.R., Tse, G. & Lee, K.Y. (2019). Smart technology for healthcare: Exploring the antecedents of adoption intention of healthcare wearable technology. *Health Psychology Research, 7*(1), 8099. https://doi.org/10.4081/hpr.2019.8099

Cheded, M., Curry, N., Hopkinson, G. & Gilchrist, A. (2023). Managing precarity at the intersection of individual and collective life: A membership categorisation analysis of conflict and tensions in an online biosocial community. *Organization, 30*(1), 42–64. https://doi.org/10.1177/13505084221131643

Chou, W.Y., Prestin, A., Lyons, C. & Wen, K.Y. (2013). Web 2.0 for health promotion: Reviewing the current evidence. *American Journal of Public Health, 103*(1), e9– e18. https://doi.org/10.2105/AJPH.2012.301071

Cialdini, R. (2016). *Pre-suasion: A revolutionary way to influence and persuade*. Simon & Schuster.

Coberley, D., Speltz, E.D. & Zawadzki, Z. (2023). Using corpus methods to analyze modal verbs in government science communication on Twitter. *Research Methods in Applied Linguistics*, 2(1), 100042. https://doi.org/10.1016/j.rmal.2023.100042

Collins, L.C. (2019). *Corpus linguistics for online communication: A guide for research*. Routledge. https://doi.org/10.4324/9780429057090

Collins, L.C. & Nerlich, B. (2015). Examining user comments for deliberative democracy: A corpus-driven analysis of the climate change debate online. *Environmental Communication*, 9(2), 189–207. https://doi.org/10.1080 /17524032.2014.981560

Coltman-Patel, T., Dance, W., Demjén, Z., Gatherer, D., Hardaker, C. & Semino, E. (2022). 'Am I being unreasonable to vaccinate my kids against my ex's wishes?' – A corpus linguistic exploration of conflict in vaccination discussions on Mumsnet Talk's AIBU forum. *Discourse, Context & Media*, 48, 100624. https://doi.org/10 .1016/j.dcm.2022.100624

Conrad, P. (2007). *The medicalization of society: On the transformation of health conditions into treatable disorders*. Johns Hopkins University Press.

Creeber, G. & Martin, R. (2009). Introduction. In G. Creeber & R. Martin (Eds.), *Digital cultures* (pp. 1–10). Open University Press.

Curl, T. & Drew, P. (2008). Contingency and action: A comparison of two forms of requesting. *Research on Language and Social Interaction*, 41(2), 1–25. https://doi .org/10.1080/08351810802028613

Curry, N. & Pérez-Paredes, P. (2021). Stance nouns in COVID-19 related blog posts: A contrastive analysis of blog posts published in *The Conversation* in Spain and the UK. *International Journal of Corpus Linguistics*, 26(4), 469–497. https://doi.org /10.1075/ijcl.21080.cur

Demmen, J.E., Semino, E., Demjén, Z., Koller, V., Hardie, A., Rayson, P. & Payne, S. (2015). A computer-assisted study of the use of violence metaphors for cancer and end of life by patients, family carers and health professionals. *International Journal of Corpus Linguistics*, 20(2), 205–231. https://doi.org/10.1075/ijcl.20.2.03dem

Dixon, S. (2022). Global Twitter user age distribution as of April 2021, by age group. *Statista*. https://www.statista.com/statistics/283119/age-distribution-of-global -twitter-users/.

Dunn, J. (2022). *Natural language processing for corpus linguistics*. Cambridge University Press. https://doi.org/10.1017/9781009070447

Escouflaire, L. (2021). Signaling irony, displaying politeness, replacing words: The eight linguistic functions of emoji. *Lingvisticæ Investigationes*, 44(2), 204–235. https://doi.org/10.1075/li.00062.esc

Fairclough, N. (1993). Critical discourse analysis and the marketization of public discourse: The universities. *Discourse & Society*, 4(2), 133–168. https://doi.org /10.1177/0957926593004002002

Francis, D.B. (2021). 'Twitter is Really Therapeutic at Times': Examination of Black men's twitter conversations following hip-hop artist Kid Cudi's depression disclosure. *Health Communication*, 36(4), 448–456. https://doi.org/10.1080 /10410236.2019.1700436

Frost, J., Vermeulen, I.E. & Beekers, N. (2014). Anonymity versus privacy: Selective information sharing in online cancer communities. *Journal of Medical Internet Research*, 16(5), e126. https://doi.org/10.2196/jmir.2684

Galegher, J., Sproull, L. & Kiesler, S. (1998). Legitimacy, authority, and community in electronic support groups. *Written Communication, 15*(4), 493–530. https://doi.org/10.1177%2F0741088398015004003

Godard, R. & Holtzman, S. (2022). The multidimensional lexicon of emojis: A new tool to assess the emotional content of emojis. *Frontiers in Psychology, 13*, 921388. https://doi.org/10.3389/fpsyg.2022.921388

Goldsmith, D.J. (2004). *Communicating social support.* Cambridge University Press.

Guidry, J.P.D., Jin, Y., Orr, C.A., Messner, M. & Meganck, S. (2017). Ebola on Instagram and Twitter: How health organizations address the health crisis in their social media engagement. *Public Relations Review, 43*(3), 477–486. https://doi.org/10.1016/j.pubrev.2017.04.009

Harvey, K. (2012). Disclosures of depression: Using corpus linguistic methods to examine young people's online health concerns. *International Journal of Corpus Linguistics, 17*(3), 349–379. https://doi.org/10.1075/ijcl.17.3.03har

Harvey, K. & Brown, B. (2012). Health communication and psychological distress: Exploring the language of self-harm. *The Canadian Modern Language Review, 68*(3), 316–340. https://doi.org/10.3138/cmlr.1103

Harvey, K. Brown, B., Crawford, P., Macfarlane, A. & McPherson, A. (2007). 'Am I normal?' Teenagers, sexual health and the internet. *Social Science & Medicine, 65*, 771–781. https://doi.org/10.1016/j.socscimed.2007.04.005

Harvey, K., Churchill, D., Crawford, P., Brown, B., Mullany, L., Macfarlane, A. & McPherson, A. (2008). Health communication and adolescents: What do their emails tell us? *Family Practice, 25*(4), 304–311. https://doi.org/10.1093/fampra/cmn029

Harvey, K., Locher, M.A. & Mullany, L. (2014). 'Can I be at risk of getting AIDS?' A linguistic analysis of two internet columns on sexual health. *Linguistik Online, 59*(2), 113–134. https://doi.org/10.13092/lo.59.1145

Headley, S.-A., Jones, T., Kanekar, A. & Vogelzang, J. (2022). Using memes to increase health literacy in vulnerable populations. *American Journal of Health Education, 53*(1), 11–15. https://doi.org/10.1080/19325037.2021.2001777

Herring, S.C. & Dainas, A. (2017). 'Nice picture comment!' Graphicons in Facebook comment threads. *Proceedings of the fiftieth Hawai'i international conference on system sciences* (pp. 2185–2194). IEEE Press. https://scholarspace.manoa.hawaii.edu/server/api/core/bitstreams/7543e493-f402-404a-9abc-c6e2a0a726e3/content.

Hodson, J., Veletsianos, G. & Houlden, S. (2022). Public responses to COVID-19 information from the public health office on Twitter and YouTube: Implications for research practice. *Journal of Information Technology & Politics, 19*(2), 156–164. https://doi.org/10.1080/19331681.2021.1945987

Hunston, S. (2011). *Corpus approaches to evaluation: Phraseology and evaluative language.* Routledge.

Hunt, D. & Brookes, G. (2020). *Corpus, discourse and mental health.* Bloomsbury. http://dx.doi.org/10.5040/9781350059207

Hunt, D. & Harvey, K. (2015). Health communication and corpus linguistics: Using corpus tools to analyse eating disorder discourse online. In P. Baker & T. McEnery (Eds.), *Corpora and discourse studies: Integrating discourse and corpora* (pp. 134–154). Palgrave Macmillan.

Ibrahim, W.M.A, Abaalalaa, H.S. & Hardie, A. (2022). Pre-suasive and persuasive strategies in the tweets of the Saudi Ministry of Health during the 2020 coronavirus pandemic: A corpus linguistic exploration. *Frontiers in Communication 7*, 984651. https://doi.org/10.3389/fcomm.2022.984651

Jia, X., Pang, Y. & Liu, L.S. (2021). Online health information seeking behavior: A systematic review. *Healthcare*, *9*(12), 1740. https://doi.org/10.3390/healthcare9121740

Jones, C., Oakey, D. & O'Halloran, K.L. (2023). "I will say the picture of the background is not related to the words": Using corpus linguistics and focus groups to reveal how speakers of English as an additional language perceive the effectiveness of the phraseology and imagery in UK public health tweets during COVID-19. *Applied Corpus Linguistics*, *3*(1), 100053. https://doi.org/10.1016/j.acorp.2023.100053

Jones, R.H., Chik, A. & Hafner, C.A. (2015). Introduction: Discourse analysis and digital practices. In R.H. Jones, A. Chik & C.A. Hafner (Eds.), *Discourse and digital practices: Doing discourse analysis in the digital age* (pp. 1–17). Routledge.

Khanra, S., Dhir, A., Najmul Islam, A.K.M. & Mäntymäki, M. (2020). Big data analytics in healthcare: A systematic literature review. *Enterprise Information Systems*, *14*(7), 878–912. https://doi.org/10.1080/17517575.2020.1812005

KhosraviNik, M. (2014). Critical Discourse Analysis, power, and new media (digital) discourse. In M. Kopytowska & Y. Kalyango (Eds.), *Why discourse matters: Negotiating identity in the mediatized world* (pp. 287–306). Peter Lang.

Kilgarriff, A., Baisa, V., Bušta, J., Jakubíček, M., Kovář, V., Michelfeit, J., Rychlý, P. & Suchomel, V. (2014). The Sketch Engine: Ten years on. *Lexicography ASIALEX 1*, 7–36. https://doi.org/10.1007/s40607-014-0009-9

Kinloch, K. (2018). A corpus-assisted study of the discourses of infertility in UK blogs, news articles and clinic websites. Doctoral thesis, Lancaster University. https://www.proquest.com/dissertations-theses/corpus-assisted-study-discourses-infertility-uk/docview/2150556146/se-2.

Kinloch, K. & Jaworska, S. (2020). Using a comparative corpus-assisted approach to study health and illness discourses across domains: The case of postnatal depression (PND) in lay, medical and media texts. In Z. Demjén (Ed.), *Applying linguistics in illness and healthcare contexts* (pp. 73–98). Bloomsbury. http://dx.doi.org/10.5040/9781350057685.0023

Kress, G. & Van Leeuwen, T. (2020). *Reading images: The grammar of visual design* (third edition). Routledge.

Lecompte-Van Poucke, M. (2022). 'You got this!': A critical discourse analysis of toxic positivity as a discursive construct on Facebook. *Applied Corpus Linguistics*, *2*(1), 1–9. https://doi.org/10.1016/j.acorp.2022.100015

Leech, G. (1966). *English in advertising: A linguistic study of advertising in great Britain*. Longman.

Locher, M.A. (2006). *Advice online. Advice-giving in an American internet health column*. John Benjamins.

Locher, M.A. & Hoffmann, S. (2006). The emergence of the identity of a fictional expert advice-giver in an American Internet advice column. *Text & Talk*, *26*(1), 69–106. https://doi.org/10.1515/text.2006.004

Lotfinejad, N., Assadi, R., Aelami, M.H. & Pittet, D. (2020). Emojis in public health and how they might be used for hand hygiene and infection prevention and control. *Antimicrobial Resistance & Infection Control 9*, 27. https://doi.org/10.1186/s13756-020-0692-2

Lupton, D. (2017). *Digital health: Critical and cross-disciplinary perspectives.* Routledge. https://doi.org/10.4324/9781315648835

Lustig, A. & Brookes, G. (2022). Construction of group norms in a radical acceptance online forum for heavy alcohol users: A corpus-based discourse analysis. *International Journal of Drug Policy, 109,* 103862. https://doi.org/10.1016/j.drugpo.2022.103862

Maci, S.M. (2022). Data triangulation using Sketch Engine and WMatrix: Ketogenic diet on Twitter. In S.M. Maci & M. Sala (Eds.), *Corpus linguistics and translation tools for digital humanities: Research methods and applications* (pp. 81–104). Bloomsbury. http://dx.doi.org/10.5040/9781350275256

Malson, H., Finn, D.M., Treasure, J., Clarke, S. & Anderson, G. (2004). Constructing 'the eating disordered patient': A discourse analysis of accounts of treatment experiences. *Journal of Community & Applied Social Psychology, 14*(6), 471–489. https://doi.org/10.1002/casp.804

Mautner, G. (2010). *Language and the market society: Critical reflections on discourse and dominance.* Routledge.

Mazzi, D. (2016). 'It is natural for you to be afraid…': On the discourse of web-based communication with patients. *Language Learning in Higher Education, 6*(1), 229–251. https://doi.org/10.1515/cercles-2016-0011

McDonald, D. & Woodward-Kron, R. (2016). Member roles and identities in online support groups: Perspectives from corpus and systemic functional linguistics. *Discourse & Communication, 10*(2), 157–175. https://doi.org/10.1177%2F1750481315615985

McGlashan, M. (2021). Networked discourses of bereavement in online COVID-19 memorials. *International Journal of Corpus Linguistics, 26*(4), 557–582. https://doi.org/10.1075/ijcl.21135.mcg

Mpofu, S. (2021). Social media memes as commentary in health disasters in South Africa and Zimbabwe. In S. Mpofu (Ed.), *Digital humour in the COVID-19 pandemic: Perspectives from the global south* (pp. 19–46). Palgrave Macmillan.

Naslund, J.A., Aschbrenner, K.A., Marsch, L.A. & Bartles, S.J. (2016). The future of mental health care: Peer-to-peer support and social media. *Epidemiology and Psychiatric Sciences, 25,* 113–122. https://doi.org/10.1017/S2045796015001067

Nuckolls, D.L. [@DaynaLNuckolls]. (2016). #YouGoodMan is for Black men to confess, ask for help, vent, or get pointed in the direction of mental health professionals @ TheCosby. http://twitter.com/DaynaLNuckolls/status/783654446521720833

Rayson, P. (2008). From key-words to key semantic domains. *International Journal of Corpus Linguistics, 13*(4), 519–549. https://doi.org/10.1075/ijcl.13.4.06ray

Rich, E. (2006). Anorexic dis(connection): Managing anorexia as an illness and an identity. *Sociology of Health and Illness, 28*(3), 284–305. https://doi.org/10.1111/j.1467-9566.2006.00493.x

Rüdiger, S. & Dayter, D. (Eds.). (2020). *Corpus approaches to social media.* John Benjamins. https://doi.org/10.1075/scl.98

Rudolph von Rohr, M.-T., Thurnherr, F. & Locher, M.A. (2018). Linguistic expert creation in online health practices. In P. Bou-Franch & P. Garcés-Conejos Blitvich (Eds.), *Analyzing digital discourse* (pp. 219–250). Springer. https://doi.org/10.1007/978-3-319-92663-6_8

Schwalbe, N. & Wahl, B. (2020). Artificial intelligence and the future of global health. *The Lancet, 395*(10236), 1579–1586. https://doi.org/10.1016/S0140-6736(20)30226-9

Sik, D. (2021). From lay depression narratives to secular ritual healing: An online ethnography of mental health forums. *Culture, Medicine, and Psychiatry, 45*, 751–774. https://doi.org/10.1007/s11013-020-09702-5

Smith, C., Adolphs, S., Harvey, K. & Mullany, L. (2014). Spelling errors and keywords in born-digital data: A case study using the Teenage Health Freak Corpus. *Corpora, 9*(2), 137–154. https://doi.org/10.3366/cor.2014.0055

Starbird, K. & Palen, L. (2010). Pass it on?: Retweeting in mass emergency. *Proceedings of the 7th international ISCRAM conference – Seattle, USA, May 2010*. International Conference on Information Systems for Crisis Response and Management. https://cmci.colorado.edu/~palen/starbirdpaleniscramretweet.pdf.

Stommel, W. & Lamerichs, J. (2014). Interaction in online support groups. In H.E. Hamilton & W.Y.S. Chou (Eds.), *The Routledge handbook of language and health communication* (pp. 198–211). Routledge.

Van Uden-Kraan, C.F., Drossaert, C.H., Taal, E., Seydel, E.R. & van de Laar, M.A. (2008). Self-reported differences in empowerment between lurkers and posters in online patient support groups. *Journal of Medical Internet Research, 10*(2), e18. https://doi.org/10.2196/jmir.992

Vanheule, S., Desmet, M. & Meganck, R. (2009). What the heart thinks, the tongue speaks: A study on depression and lexical choice. *Psychological Reports, 104*(2), 473–481. https://doi.org/10.2466/pr0.104.2.473-481

Wagener, A. (2021). The postdigital emergence of memes and GIFs: Meaning, discourse, and hypernarrative creativity. *Postdigital Science and Education, 3*, 831–850. https://doi.org/10.1007/s42438-020-00160-1

WHO. (2021). *Global strategy on digital health 2020–2025*. World Health Organization. Licence: CC BY-NC-SA 3.0 IGO.

Wong, C.A., Madanay, F., Ozer, E.M., Harris, S.K., Moore, M., Master, S.O., Moreno, M. & Weitzman, E.R. (2020). Digital health technology to enhance adolescent and young adult clinical preventive services: Affordances and challenges. *The Journal of Adolescent Health: Official Publication of the Society for Adolescent Medicine, 67*(2S), S24–S33. https://doi.org/10.1016/j.jadohealth.2019.10.018

Yip, J.W.C. (2020). Evaluating the communication of online social support: A mixed-methods analysis of structure and content. *Health Communication, 35*(10), 1210–1218. https://doi.org/10.1080/10410236.2019.1623643

Zappavigna, M. (2011). Ambient affiliation: A linguistic perspective on Twitter. *New Media & Society, 13*(5), 788–806. https://doi.org/10.1177/1461444810385097

Zummo, M.L. (2015). Exploring web-mediated communication: A genre-based linguistic study for new patterns of doctor–patient interaction in online environment. *Communication & Medicine, 12*(2–3), 187–198. https://doi.org/10.1558/cam.31897

7

CONCLUSION

In this closing chapter, we reflect on the continued application of corpus linguistics methods to the study of health communication, taking stock of the insights that we have collected in our review of the extant research and looking ahead to consider how corpus linguistics can develop, alongside advancements in healthcare, to ensure that those using corpus linguistics methods can continue to make a meaningful contribution to the study of health communication as well as to practice in the design and delivery of healthcare. We begin by summarising the evidence attesting to the value of approaching health communication from a corpus linguistics perspective.

7.1 Giving corpus linguistics and health communication a health-check

In Chapters 1–3, we established the fundamental principles of corpus linguistics and demonstrated how the well-established techniques of frequency analysis, keyword analysis, collocation analysis, cluster analysis, and concordance analysis have contributed to our understanding of the lexis and grammar of 'health talk' as well as of discursive representations of various health concepts, identities, processes, and experiences. In structuring our subsequent chapters according to the modes of spoken, written, and digital health communication, we aimed to capture the breadth of forms of communication in which health is made salient and, equally, in which researchers have used corpus linguistics methods to document and analyse the language that characterises those contexts. This attests to the pervasiveness of health in the human experience, and our coverage has by no means been exhaustive of the contexts in which there are opportunities to capture health communication. The fact

DOI: 10.4324/9781003099659-7

that researchers have utilised corpus linguistics methods across these domains attests to the flexibility of corpus approaches as well as to their capacity to feature in mixed methods approaches alongside other language-oriented methods. This includes being combined with the broad set of approaches that can be collectively referred to as discourse analytic techniques (see Brookes and Hunt 2021), but also methods beyond linguistics, which we have only been able to minimally discuss in this book.

The continued application of corpus linguistics alongside other, complementary methods will only enrich and enhance what we can possibly know about experiences of health. Such mixed methods approaches are also likely to become increasingly necessary, as the contexts in which health is discussed continue to emerge and diversify. This is true of the application of corpus methods across other areas of study, though in relation to its deployment in health communication specifically, there are some fundamental principles that seem to be of mutual interest to researchers with a foundation in language-based research, or the social sciences more broadly, and those approaching health communication from the perspective of what might be termed the 'natural sciences'.

We discussed in Chapter 1 that the principles of evidence-based medicine have been argued to align well with the empirical basis of corpus linguistics methods. The diagnostic process is, arguably, analogous to the procedures of corpus linguistics: health professionals collect empirical data through physical examination or the testimony of the patient during a consultation, supplement this with contextual information relating to the patient's personal circumstances, and make evaluations based on patterns they have observed across comparable cases. Furthermore, much like the process of understanding the population-level effects of illness is formalised through large-scale clinical trials, corpus studies can similarly ensure the quality and generalisability of their observations through a commitment to a rigorous process of participant recruitment and corpus design, striving for data that is balanced and representative, and of sufficient quality to be able to provide statistically meaningful results.

In our discussions of different modes of health communication, we have reflected on questions of representation, and in studies of spoken, written, and digital health communication, there appears to be developments towards better representation of non-professional perspectives on health. This, in turn, has led to the proliferation of discursive representations of health and illness which, in many cases, take us beyond the traditional biomedical model. Corpus studies have revealed a high degree of interpersonal and interactive features that attest to the dialogic nature of many spoken health interactions (e.g., Webber 2005). In written texts, we observed a growing interest in the creative forms of expression that can engage readers in, for example, the 'mind style' of someone experiencing illness (Demjén and Semino 2021), thereby encouraging empathy with the illness-related perspectives being articulated. In the digital domain, we reported on the growing significance of peer-support spaces in which the prevailing type of expertise was shown to be lived experience of managing illness over time and finding alternative solutions alongside engaging with institutional health services (e.g. Kinloch and Jaworska 2020).

Healthcare interactions, then, appear to be increasingly characterised by the coming together of perspectives in dialogue; 'expert patients' resolve their knowledge with that of their health professional, meanwhile new members to a forum engage with the views of those with more longstanding participation. What we also observed, at the macro level of discourse, was the influence of neoliberal discourses (e.g., Brookes and Baker 2021), marketisation (Chałupnik and Brookes 2021), as well as the 'psychologising' of emotional experiences among adolescents (Harvey 2012). These observations remind us that our experiences of health, as articulated in micro contexts of interaction, inevitably intersect with macro level social and political discourses. In Chapter 5, we discussed the efforts of those who have drawn upon archive materials as well as various contemporary sources to inform their interpretation of corpora of historical medical texts, and, in more recent studies, researchers have augmented their observations of more contemporaneous texts with findings from survey data (e.g., Hannaford 2017). The need for judicious selection and interpretation of these materials alongside the results of corpus linguistics analysis, reiterates that it is the human analyst, and not the computer, who must contextualise the outputs of computational procedures of analysis and develop explanations.

7.2 Looking ahead

When looking to the future of corpus linguistics and health communication, it is worthwhile reflecting on some of the themes that have emerged from our previous chapters, as many of these gesture towards challenges for the field to confront. Some of these have to do with the challenges associated with representing certain types of language use as well as language produced within particular contexts.

As part of our exploration of spoken health communication in Chapter 4, we noted how qualitative studies in this area have tended to focus (particularly in the early days of the field of health communication) on spoken interactions between healthcare professionals and their patients, particularly those taking place within clinical contexts. While this focus has diversified over time, there remains a strong focus on this kind of data in qualitative studies of health communication to this day. Yet we might also note that the same cannot be said for corpus studies of health communication, of which studies of such spoken interactions make up a very small minority.

There are likely to be a number of reasons for this; foremost among them, perhaps, being the challenge of obtaining ethical consent for collecting such language use, which often entails the disclosure of personal and sensitive information in busy clinical environments that involve lots of other professionals and patients engaged in similar kinds of interactions. The ethical considerations and obligations that attend to researching such contexts represent an area of continuous debate for qualitative health communication research. For those adopting more quantitatively inclined approaches, such as corpus linguistics methods, the larger scale of the data is likely to inflate the scale of such ethical challenges with larger numbers of participants being involved. We are currently witnessing a revival of debates surrounding the ethical compilation, storage, analysis, and distribution of corpora (Brookes and McEnery, forthcoming). Those employing corpus linguistics methods to study health communication data should engage with such debates, not only to inform their own practices but also to share their perspectives in order to support wider development in this area.

Even if we are able to obtain informed consent for collecting such data, we are also likely to encounter challenges with capturing and doing analytical justice to the richness of such encounters. Corpus data and methods are still lagging some way behind qualitative approaches in their capacity to represent and facilitate the analysis of dialogic interactions. The multiparty structure of such interactions is, at present, not easily represented in corpus data, meanwhile the turn-by-turn perspective on such encounters that is afforded by qualitative approaches is currently not so easily achieved through standard corpus analytical techniques. Collins and Baker (2023) offer an example of how the codes applied to functional discourse units in online forum posts can be studied as the unit of analysis and subject to measures of frequency and distribution as a corpus. Referring to the coding framework developed by Egbert et al. (2021), they coded for functions such as 'giving advice and instructions' or 'describing or explaining the past' in a forum for anxiety support and, subsequently, were able to report rates of occurrence of each code as well as the combinations and sequences in which the codes occurred over the course of replies within discussion threads. In other words, they captured some aspects of the relationship between what is posted at the beginning of a thread and the linguistic content of the responses it elicited. Developments such as these point to the ways in which corpus linguistics approaches can contribute to the study of sequences of texts, which have otherwise relied upon qualitative approaches.

It has also been long recognised that effective therapist–client interaction requires both verbal and non-verbal communication (Westland 2015). Qualitative approaches applied to the study of health(care) interactions have begun to document more systematically the multimodal dynamics of health-care interactions, for example, through the use of wearable cameras and eye-tracking technology. Such devices, when worn by the interactants under study, can help analysts to consider how features such as gesture and eye gaze contribute towards the communicative force of what is being said. For example, Tsuchiya et al. (2022) examined how team leaders in emergency care teams articulate requests multimodally through both language use and eye-movement patterns. The researchers recorded the participants in simulated scenarios in which the team leaders wore eye-tracking glasses before undertaking interactional linguistic and multimodal analyses of video, audio, and eye-movement data. By attending to the multimodal dynamics of the interactions, Tsuchiya et al. were able to demonstrate how, while the senior team leader issues requests with multimodal emphasis (by gazing at the recipients of the requests while also addressing them verbally), the junior doctor leading a team often communicated only monomodally when making similar requests (see also the study by Atkins and Chałupnik 2023).

While these studies are qualitative in nature, corpus linguistics techniques have been used to study similar aspects of interaction (Adolphs et al. 2015). However, such multimodal corpus analytical procedures remain far from standard in corpus linguistics methodology and are difficult to implement at scale. Developments in this area, along with our understanding and processes relating to ethical approval, could see increased take up of, and exciting developments in, corpus linguistics approaches to studying medical interactions.[1]

Of course, the concept of multimodality refers not only to features in spoken interactions but also applies to all forms of communication. Written health texts, for example, are often richly multimodal in their composition, often incorporating imagery and the use of carefully designed fonts, colours, layouts, and so on (Brookes et al. 2021). As part of our exploration of written health communication in Chapter 5, we observed how most corpus research in this area focuses on newspaper texts. The authors of several of these studies have lamented their corpora do not represent the imagery originally used in the articles they analysed (e.g., Brookes and Baker 2021), as this limitation obscures from the analytical view the way in which visual depictions of health-related topics might combine with linguistic representations. This limitation results from a combination of the limitations of the databases from which corpus texts are drawn and the complexities of rendering images in a machine-readable format conducive to corpus analysis.

Baker and Collins (2023) report a study of obesity representations in the press that incorporates image representations and subsequently investigates text–image relations using conventional corpus techniques such as keyness and collocation analysis. They use the automatic image annotation tool, *Google Cloud Vision*, to generate a series of tags that capture elements of the images and which can be integrated into the text files that form their corpus. While there are some caveats with using a proprietary tool for which there is limited information regarding the development of the coding labels and which appears to document components of the image with varying levels of specificity, Baker and Collins (2023) demonstrate the potential of a practical tool that enabled them to report how images can variously support or mitigate more explicit representations of people with obesity reported in the text. It remains to be seen what, if any, approaches to multimodal corpus analysis will become established within the field, but this is an exciting area of development in which corpus studies of health communication could be at the forefront.

The theme of multimodality also emerged in our exploration of digital health communication in Chapter 6. Relevant here is the need for corpus resources to represent emerging communicative technologies and developments in existing formats, which continue to shape the landscape of health communication. Researchers (e.g., Lin et al. 2021) have highlighted the adjustments and compensations that have been made in response to the global COVID-19 pandemic, such as the use of teleconsultation to facilitate the delivery of healthcare at distance. Through an online survey that examined mental health providers' perceptions of different delivery modes for therapy, Lin et al. (2021) found that therapists had concerns about implementing common therapeutic skills, namely facilitative interpersonal skills (Anderson et al. 2009) such as warmth, hopefulness and empathy, as well as helping skills (Hill 2019) such as 'restatement' and 'intentional silence'. They emphasise that 'nonverbal behaviors, such as gestures, facial expressions, body movements, and voice pitch can sometimes reflect the client's real mental status, facilitate diagnoses of certain symptoms, and shed light on therapist-client interactions' (Lin et al. 2021, p. 456).

It is, we hope, clear by this point in the book that linguistic research can help us to understand and potentially improve the effectiveness of these kinds of interactions. Indeed, Shaw et al. (2020) undertook just such a study. Using a conversation analysis approach, the researchers examined the communication strategies through which video-mediated medical consultations were accomplished. Their broader objective was to produce recommendations for both patients and clinicians in order to improve the communicative quality of such consultations. They identified the need for evidence-based guidance, in combination with training and support, to help the participants in such interactions to work through technical problems more efficiently, thereby reducing the potential for misunderstandings to occur.

Corpus linguistics methods could similarly be applied to such data, potentially achieving more generalisability in the trends observed. There is already an emerging body of corpus linguistics research which explores the (multimodal) features of virtual professional interactions (e.g., Knight et al., forthcoming). Such work is likely to open up new methodological approaches and propose new principles which could be applied in corpus analyses of virtual healthcare encounters. Ethically, the videos of these encounters might also be more straightforward to gather, in terms of obtaining informed consent for data that patients essentially 'own', and if recorded, such video material could potentially be gathered through crowd-sourcing methods. Of course, all of this requires careful ethical consideration, but such possibilities could make scalable, multimodal corpus analysis of healthcare encounters a more realistic prospect. Advancements in the tools for carrying out multimodal corpus linguistics research, thus, have the potential to enrich studies of spoken, written, and digital health communication alike.

Beyond virtual interactions, digital technologies continue to influence the delivery of healthcare. One area of direct relevance to communication concerns the use of automated conversational agents, which are increasingly being employed to provide information and customer service in healthcare as well as many other industries (Chang et al. 2022), ranging from chatbots to smart conversational interfaces such as Apple Siri or Amazon Alexa (Laranjo et al. 2018, p. 1249). The development of these natural language processing systems that provide and/or elicit information, create patient records and discuss the results of clinical tests, has often been with the intent of creating systems that are more 'person-like' (Chang et al. 2022). Conversational agents that offer 'social presence' have been evaluated positively, and this is understood to promote higher levels of engagement, improving users' perceptions of credibility (Dippold et al. 2020). A perceived lack of empathy, on the other hand, is often cited as a criticism of conversational agents in qualitative studies, though the proposed correlation between perceived (lack of) empathy and individuals' attitudes towards medical chatbots has not been evidenced to a statistically significant degree (Chang et al. 2022).

When conversational agents appear 'human-like', this can raise expectations about interactive capabilities, which, in turn, can negatively impact the interaction when the service's limitations are exposed (Gnewuch et al. 2017). Ultimately, chatbots appear to be most effective when the user's goals and the service are in alignment. While users value a personable and empathetic conversational agent, often what they care most about is that the service can precisely and accurately address their queries and provide critical health information (Chang et al. 2022). It might be possible to refer to corpus studies of digital health interactions, like those described in Chapter 6, to establish the strategies that have been developed in human-to-human digital interactions to optimise information exchange and/or automated conversation and, indeed, to even use corpus techniques to evaluate the queries and responses exchanged when a health chatbot is employed.

7.3 The impact of corpus studies of health communication

Corpus linguistics research has the potential to positively impact policies and practices in the real-world. In 2006, Brown et al. considered the potential for corpus linguistics methods – being grounded in empiricism, based on typically large datasets, and supported by statistical analyses – to help linguists to navigate the positivist paradigm in which medicine is situated in order to support the development of so-called 'evidence-based' practice in healthcare. The vision put forward was one that essentially involved researchers and health(care) professionals alike drawing on the authentic linguistic routines of patient groups, as represented in vast and well-designed corpora in order to better understand patients' experiences and concerns as well as the particular linguistic apparatus they use to articulate these.

There is some evidence to suggest that Brown et al.'s enthusiasm was not misplaced. For example, Brookes et al. (2018) discuss how findings from the THF project were disseminated to health(care) practitioners, including those working in adolescent health, and presented in ways that helped the professionals to use the research to improve their understanding of adolescents' health issues, ultimately, to inform their practices. Meanwhile, Baker et al. (2019) describe how their corpus research on online patient feedback helped their stakeholder partners in the UK NHS to not only reach a deeper understanding of areas of patient priority and concern but also to develop a more critical appreciation of the feedback mechanism itself. Baker et al. (2019) demonstrated that the feedback tool was likely to garner certain kinds of feedback, skewed towards more extreme ratings (both positive and negative) as well as illustrating some of the ways in which patients use language for persuasive purposes in their feedback. These examples, and there are plenty more besides, should provide cause for optimism about the positive contributions that corpus linguistics research can make towards health(care) practice and, in turn, public health.

Yet, at the same time, we should also remain reflective and critical about how we, as users of corpora, can improve our analytical approaches and the ways we engage with those outside the field. Baker et al. (2019) describe how, before turning to corpus linguistics, their contacts in the NHS had originally tried out other digital approaches to text analysis, such as sentiment analysis. The name 'corpus linguistics' is not particularly transparent, so it might be the case that those in the field have to work that bit harder to increase the visibility of the approach and to making the distinction between corpus linguistics and other approaches clearer. For this, it is important that we go beyond our traditional disciplinary silos to demonstrate to others, within and beyond the academy, what corpus linguistics has to offer. For those working in the field of health communication, this includes working to reach those working in health(care) with our research.

To help others to better understand how corpus linguistics differs from other digital approaches to text analysis, there is value in 'showing' what these differences are through systematic and critical comparisons of the kinds of insights that different approaches can (and cannot) provide. We have carried out this kind of work ourselves, for example, Brookes and McEnery's (2019) critical evaluation of topic modelling, Hunt and Brookes's (2020) interrogation of linguistic inquiry and word count, Brookes and McEnery's (2020) comparison of corpus linguistics and culturomics, and Collins's (forthcoming) discussion of the distinctions between corpus linguistics and other approaches based on natural language processing. In the future, research such as this should continue to investigate what emerging approaches have to offer. This will help us and those new to corpus linguistics to understand how it differs to other digital approaches to text analysis and even how approaches might be combined.

Awareness of the approach is likely not to be the only barrier to corpus linguistics making a real-world impact on health(care) practice in the future. Another potential stumbling block concerns differences between (corpus) linguistics and medicine regarding standards of 'proof' and what counts as 'evidence'. As the studies described over the course of the preceding chapters demonstrate, corpus studies of health communication tend to base their findings on (often) small, specialised corpora which represent language use in a particular (clinical) context or otherwise around some health-related topic. Some have raised doubts as to whether such datasets, which often represent convenience samples, are likely to meet the kinds of thresholds for evidence represented by the medical 'gold standard' of randomised controlled trials (Hunt and Brookes 2020; Hunt 2021). For example, Hunt argues that

> Smaller, opportunistic corpora are less likely to be representative of the complexity and diversity of language practices in the domain of interest and their analyses more likely to be skewed by, say, longer texts or individual participants who speak more. Although larger corpora can easily be compiled from online interactions, such datasets typically lack reliable information about participants, their diagnoses and their demographic characteristics that are the mainstay of clinical research.
>
> *(Hunt 2021, p. 156)*

Such arguments do not devalue the contribution that corpus linguistics can make to disciplines within and beyond linguistics, and Hunt (2021, p. 157) also rightly points out that 'adhering to the standards of evidence characteristic of other academic disciplines is obviously not a necessary condition for conducting high-quality discourse analysis'.

Moreover, while the option of statistical analysis might make our findings more immediately appealing to health(care) professionals and medical researchers from a positivist paradigm, we should think carefully before inflating our datasets and making our analyses all the more quantitative in service of such cross-disciplinary approval. Corpus studies of health communication often provide their most interesting and – and in our view, most valuable

– findings through more contextualised analysis of discourse afforded by close reading of the data and the use of techniques at the more qualitative end of the cline, such as concordance analysis. We should proceed cautiously, then. As our datasets grow larger and our methods more quantitative, we risk removing our analytical gaze ever further from the very contexts that shape and give meaning to the lived experiences of health and illness being told through the language we study.

Note

1 Readers interested in the practical aspects of carrying out multimodal corpus linguistics research should consult the IVO project website: ivohub.com.

References

Adolphs, S., Knight, D. & Carter, R. (2015). Beyond modal spoken corpora: A dynamic approach to tracking language in context. In P. Baker & T. McEnery (Eds.), *Corpora and discourse studies: Integrating discourse and corpora* (pp. 41–62). Palgrave Macmillan. https://doi.org/10.1057/9781137431738_3

Anderson, T., Ogles, B.M., Patterson, C.L., Lambert, M.J. & Vermeersch, D.A. (2009). Therapist effects: Facilitative interpersonal skills as a predictor of therapist success. *Journal of Clinical Psychology, 65*(7), 755–768. https://doi.org/10.1002/jclp.20583

Atkins, S. & Chałupnik, M. (2023). A multimodal linguistic analysis of gaze and active listenership in emergency department team interactions. In K. Tsuchiya, F. Coffey & K. Nakamura (Eds.), *Multimodal approaches to healthcare communication research: Visualizing interactions for resilient healthcare in the UK and Japan* (pp. 47–64). Bloomsbury.

Baker, P. & Brookes, G. (2022). *Analysing language, sex and age in a corpus of patient feedback: A comparison of approaches.* Cambridge University Press.

Baker, P., Brookes, G. & Evans, C. (2019). *The language of patient feedback: A corpus linguistic study of online health communication.* Routledge. https://doi.org/10.4324/9780429259265

Baker, P. & Collins, L.C. (2023). Creating and analysing a multimodal corpus of news texts with Google Cloud Vision's automatic image tagger. *Applied Corpus Linguistics, 3*(1), 100043. https://doi.org/10.1016/j.acorp.2023.100043

Brookes, G. & Baker, P. (2021). *Obesity in the news: Language and representation in the press.* Cambridge University Press. https://doi.org/10.1017/9781108864732

Brookes, G., Harvey, K. & Mullany, L. (2018). From corpus to clinic: Health communication research and the impact agenda. In D. McIntyre & H. Price (Eds.), *Applying linguistics: Language and the impact agenda* (pp. 99–111). Routledge.

Brookes, G. & Hunt, D. (Eds.). (2021). *Analysing health communication: Discourse Approaches.* Palgrave Macmillan.

Brookes, G. & McEnery, T. (2019). The utility of topic modelling for discourse studies: A critical evaluation. *Discourse Studies, 21*(1), 3–21.

Brookes, G. & McEnery, T. (2020). Corpus linguistics. In S. Adolphs & D. Knight (Eds.), *The Routledge handbook of English language and digital humanities* (pp. 378–404). Routledge.

Brookes, G. & McEnery, T. (Forthcoming). Corpus linguistics and ethics. In P. De Costa, A. Ahmed & C. Cinaglia (Eds.), *Ethical issues in applied linguistics scholarship*. John Benjamins.

Brookes, G., Putland, E. & Harvey, K. (2021). Multimodality: Examining visual representations of dementia in public health discourse. In G. Brookes & D. Hunt (Eds.), *Analysing health communication: Discourse approaches* (pp. 241–269). Palgrave Macmillan.

Brown, B., Crawford, P. & Carter, R. (2006). *Evidence based health communication*. Open University Press.

Chałupnik, M. & Brookes, G. (2021). 'You said, we did': A corpus-based analysis of marketising discourse in healthcare websites. *Text & Talk, 41*(5–6), 643–666. https://doi.org/10.1515/text-2020-0038

Chang, I.-C., Shih, Y.-S. & Kuo, K.-M. (2022). Why would you use medical chatbots? Interview and survey. *International Journal of Medical Informatics, 165*, 104827. https://doi.org/10.1016/j.ijmedinf.2022.104827

Collins, L. (Forthcoming). Healthcare. In M. Mahlberg & G. Brookes (Eds.), *The Bloomsbury handbook of corpus linguistics: Interdisciplinary perspectives*. Bloomsbury.

Collins, L.C. & Baker, P. (2023). *Language, discourse and anxiety*. Cambridge University Press.

Demjén, Z. & Semino, E. (2021). Stylistics: Mind style in an autobiographical account of schizophrenia. In G. Brookes & D. Hunt (Eds.), *Analysing health communication: Discourse approaches* (pp. 333–356). Palgrave Macmillan.

Dippold, D., Lynden, J., Shrubsall, R. & Ingram, R. (2020). A turn to language: How interactional sociolinguistics informs the redesign of prompt: Response chatbot turns. *Discourse, Context & Media, 37*, 100432. https://doi.org/10.1016/j.dcm.2020.100432

Egbert, J., Wizner, S., Keller, D., Biber, D., McEnery, T. & Baker, P. (2021). Identifying and describing functional discourse units in the BNC Spoken 2014. *Text & Talk, 41*(5–6), 715–737. https://doi.org/10.1515/text-2020-0053

Gnewuch, U., Morana, S. & Maedche, A. (2017). Towards designing cooperative and social conversational agents for customer service. In Y.J. Kim, R. Agarwal & J.K. Lee (Eds.), *Proceedings of the thirty-eighth International Conference on Information Systems (ICIS) - Transforming society with digital innovation, ICIS 2017*. Association for Information Systems. https://aisel.aisnet.org/icis2017/HCI/Presentations/1/

Hannaford, E.D. (2017). The press and public on mental health: A corpus linguistic analysis of UK newspaper coverage of mental illness (1995–2014), compared with the UK national attitudes to mental illness. MPhil(R) thesis, University of Glasgow. http://theses.gla.ac.uk/9016/

Harvey, K. (2012). Disclosures of depression: Using corpus linguistic methods to examine young people's online health concerns. *International Journal of Corpus Linguistics, 17*(3), 349–379. https://doi.org/10.1075/ijcl.17.3.03har

Heritage, J. & Maynard, D.W. (2006). Problems and prospects in the study of physician-patient interaction: 30 years of research. *Annual Review of Sociology, 32*, 351–374. https://doi.org/10.1146/annurev.soc.32.082905.093959

Hill, C.E. (2019). *Helping skills: Facilitating exploration, insight, and action* (Fifth edition). American Psychological Association. https://psycnet.apa.org/doi/10.1037/0000147-000

Hunt, D. (2021). Corpus linguistics: Examining tensions in general practitioners' views about diagnosing and treating depression. In G. Brookes & D. Hunt (Eds.), *Analysing health communication: Discourse approaches* (pp. 133–160). Palgrave Macmillan.

Hunt, D. & Brookes, G. (2020). *Corpus, discourse and mental health.* Bloomsbury.

Kinloch, K. & Jaworska, S. (2020). Using a comparative corpus-assisted approach to study health and illness discourses across domains: The case of postnatal depression (PND) in lay, medical and media texts. In Z. Demjén (Ed.), *Applying linguistics in illness and healthcare contexts* (pp. 73–98). Bloomsbury. http://dx.doi.org /10.5040/9781350057685.0023

Knight, D., O'Keeffe, A., Fitzgerald, C., Mark, G. & McNamara, J. (Forthcoming). Indicating engagement in online workplace meetings: The role of backchannelling head nods. *International Journal of Corpus Linguistics.*

Laranjo, L., Dunn, A.G., Tong, H.L., Kocaballi, A.B., Chen, J., Bashir, R., Surian, D., Gallego, B., Magrabi, F., Lau, A.Y.S. & Coiera, E. (2018). Conversational agents in healthcare: A systematic review. *Journal of the American Medical Informatics Association, 25*(9), 1248–1258. https://doi.org/10.1093/jamia/ocy072

Lin, T., Stone, S.J., Heckman, T.G. & Anderson, T. (2021). Zoom-in to zone-out: Therapists report less therapeutic skill in telepsychology versus face-to-face therapy during the COVID-19 pandemic. *Psychotherapy (Chicago, Ill.), 58*(4), 449–459. https://doi.org/10.1037/pst0000398

Shaw, S.E., Seuren, L.M., Wherton, J., Cameron, D., A'Court, C., Vijayaraghavan, S., Morris, J., Bhattacharya, S. & Greenhalgh, T. (2020). Video consultations between patients and clinicians in diabetes, cancer, and heart failure services: Linguistic ethnographic study of video-mediated interaction. *Journal of Medical Internet Research, 22*(5), e18378. https://doi.org/10.2196/18378

Webber, P. (2005). Interactive features in medical conference monologue. *English for Specific Purposes, 24*(2), 157–181. https://doi.org/10.1016/j.esp.2004.02.003

Westland, G. (2015). *Verbal and non-verbal communication in psychotherapy.* W.W. Norton.

INDEX